Complications of Diabetes Mellitus

Complications of Diabetes Mellitus

A Global Perspective

Jahangir Moini, MD, MPH
Professor of Science and Health (Retired)
Eastern Florida State College
Palm Bay, Florida

Matthew Adams, MD, MBA
VitreoRetinal and Cataract Surgeon
Florida Eye Associates
Melbourne, Florida

Anthony LoGalbo, PhD
Associate Professor
Florida Institute of Technology
School of Psychology
Melbourne, Florida

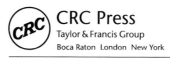

CRC Press
Taylor & Francis Group
Boca Raton London New York

CRC Press is an imprint of the
Taylor & Francis Group, an **informa** business

First edition published 2022
by CRC Press
6000 Broken Sound Parkway NW, Suite 300, Boca Raton, FL 33487-2742

and by CRC Press
4 Park Square, Milton Park, Abingdon, Oxon, OX14 4RN

CRC Press is an imprint of Taylor & Francis Group, LLC

Library of Congress Cataloging-in-Publication Data
Names: Moini, Jahangir, 1942– author. | Adams, Matthew, 1985 November 14- author. | LoGalbo, Anthony, author.
Title: Complications of diabetes mellitus: a global perspective / by Jahangir Moini, Matthew Adams, Anthony LoGalbo.
Description: First edition. | Boca Raton, FL: CRC Press, 2022. |
Includes bibliographical references and index. |
Summary: "Diabetes mellitus is a global epidemic with severe complications that can be of great cost. This book focuses on the complications of hypertension, heart attack or heart failure, stroke, blindness, nephropathy, neuropathy, amputations, and death, along with the prevalence and prevention of disease development"— Provided by the publisher.
Identifiers: LCCN 2021062189 (print) | LCCN 2021062190 (ebook) | ISBN 9781032128344 (paperback) |
ISBN 9781032128948 (hardback) | ISBN 9781003226727 (ebook)
Subjects: MESH: Diabetes Complications—physiopathology |
Global Health Classification: LCC RC660.4 (print) | LCC RC660.4 (ebook) |
NLM WK 835 | DDC 616.4/62—dc23/eng/20220113
LC record available at https://lccn.loc.gov/2021062189
LC ebook record available at https://lccn.loc.gov/2021062190

ISBN: 9781032128948 (hbk)
ISBN: 9781032128344 (pbk)
ISBN: 9781003226727 (ebk)

DOI: 10.1201/9781003226727

Typeset in Palatino
by codeMantra

*To the memory of my parents, who taught me the value of
perseverance and hard work.
To my wife Hengameh, my daughters Mahkameh and Morvarid
and also my precious granddaughters, Laila and Anabelle,
thanks for your understanding and tremendous support.*

J. Moini

*I dedicate this book to Francis Kretzer, PhD, whose favorite poem was "Flower
in the Crannied Wall" by Alfred Lord Tennyson, which reads as follows:*

*Flower in the crannied wall,
I pluck you out of the crannies,
I hold you here, root and all, in my hand,
Little flower – but if I could understand what you are,
root and all, and all in all,
I should know what God and man is.*

M. Adams

*To my family for their unwavering love and support,
and to my professors, supervisors, colleagues, and patients –
I have learned a great deal from you all.*

A. LoGalbo

Contents

Part I: Introduction

Part II: Microvascular Complications of Diabetes

Part II: Macrovascular Complications of Diabetes

Preface

Today, diabetes mellitus is one of the most common chronic diseases, with more than 462 million people affected by type 2 diabetes alone. In the United States, over 34.2 million people are affected. The disease has been globally prevalent since the early 1980s. Modern lifestyles such as increased caloric intake and decreased physical activity are huge contributors to diabetes. Obesity has increased globally, especially in the United States, with approximately 72% of people being overweight or obese. The pandemic of diabetes is linked to a large variety of factors. These include genetics, nutrition, automation, urbanization, food costs, foods that are higher in calories and fat, and a more sedentary lifestyle. There are a variety of complications created by diabetes, which include hypertension, stroke, heart attack, blindness, neuropathy, nephropathy, amputations, and death. The total estimated financial cost of diabetes mellitus in the United States, in 2017 alone, was $327 billion. This cost is expected to increase to $2.2 trillion globally by 2030, and when the complications of diabetes are figured in, this cost will be much higher. The cost of treatment, disability, and premature death are all included. Improvements in the outcomes of diabetes require better testing, earlier diagnosis, patient education, more access to care, and improved quality of care. This book includes information about the history of diabetes, pathophysiology of diabetes, metabolic syndrome, the role of insulin in metabolism, hypoglycemia, hyperglycemia, various types of diabetes, and the prevalence, mortality, risk factors, and various complications of diabetes.

Acknowledgments

The authors appreciate the contributions of everyone who assisted in the creation of this book, Karthikeyan Subramaniam and his team from CodeMantra, and, and Greg Vadimsky and the CRC Press/Taylor & Francis team, Shivangi Pramanik, Himani Dwivedi, and Linda Leggio. The authors also wish to acknowledge Dr. Morvarid Moini for contributing artwork.

Authors

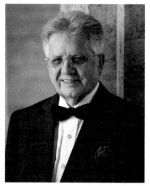

Jahangir Moini, MD, MPH, was Assistant Professor at Department of Epidemiology and Preventive Medicine, School of Medicine, Tehran University of Medical Sciences, for 9 years. For 18 years, he was the Director of Epidemiology for the Brevard County Health Department. For 15 years, he was the Director of Science and Health for Everest University in Melbourne, Florida. He was also a Professor of Science and Health at Everest University for a total of 24 years. For 6 years, he was a Professor of Science and Health at Eastern Florida State College, but is now retired. Dr. Moini has been actively teaching for 39 years, and for 22 years, he has been an international author of 47 books. His book *Anatomy & Physiology for Health Professionals* has been translated into Japanese and Korean languages.

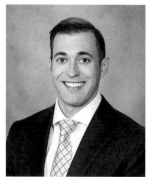

Matthew Adams, MD, MBA, received his medical degree from Baylor College of Medicine. During medical school, he also received an MBA from the Jones Graduate School of Business at Rice University. During his residency at Baylor College of Medicine, Dr. Adams received training in ophthalmology and completed a fellowship in vitreoretinal surgery at the Mayo Clinic. He now serves the community of Brevard County, Florida, as a board-certified ophthalmologist for Florida Eye Associates, where he performs vitreoretinal and cataract surgery.

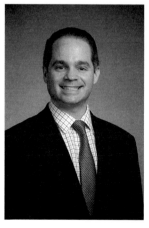

Anthony LoGalbo, PhD, is a board-certified Clinical Neuropsychologist and Associate Professor in the School of Psychology at Florida Tech in Melbourne, Florida, where he teaches graduate coursework and conducts Applied Research in the Clinical Psychology (PsyD) program. He is also the Clinical Director and primary supervisor of Florida Tech's Sports Concussion Management Program, and the Clinical Neuropsychology Director at the Health First Florida Memory Disorder Clinic. Previously, he was in clinical practice at Florida Hospital (AdventHealth) in Orlando, serving both inpatients and outpatients through the Neuroscience Institute and Department of Sports Medicine and Rehabilitation. He earned a PhD in medical/clinical psychology with a focus on neuropsychology at the University of Alabama at Birmingham. He completed a Clinical Psychology internship in the Department of Rehabilitation Medicine at the University of Washington Medical School and Harborview Medical Center in Seattle, Washington, followed by an advanced fellowship in Neuropsychology and Gerontology at the Geriatric Research, Education, and Clinical Center (GRECC) at the VA Puget Sound Health Care System in Seattle and American Lake, Washington. He is board certified by the American Board of Professional Psychology (ABPP) with specialization in clinical neuropsychology, and maintains a part-time private clinical practice focusing on clinical and forensic neuropsychological assessment.

PART I
INTRODUCTION

CHAPTER 1 Pathophysiology of Diabetes

Diabetes mellitus is a disease state that is related to the availability and effectiveness of insulin in the body. *Type 1 diabetes* involves a total lack of insulin, resulting from autoimmune destruction of pancreatic beta cells. Autoimmune destruction occurs in genetically susceptible people, triggered by environmental factors and progressing over months to years. This eventually results in symptomatic hyperglycemia and the classic signs and symptoms of the disease. *Type 2 diabetes* is characterized by the body's peripheral tissues being resistant to the effects of insulin. Both classifications of diabetes lack the signaling effect of insulin, while glucagon and other metabolic signals are of normal or high levels. Diabetes mellitus is due to an imbalance in carbohydrate metabolism and resultant effects upon other metabolic pathways. Insulin resistance causes the body to react, even though it is present at extreme levels. This form differs from type 1 diabetes in that the liver can still manufacture glycogen. Lipolysis is controlled due to the presence of insulin. Plasma **lipoproteins** are usually elevated, often due to poor nutrition and obesity. Pancreatic failure leads to decreased insulin production and secretion. The brain continually requires glucose in order to function normally. Hypoglycemia is often caused by drugs used to treat diabetes mellitus, which include insulin and the oral antihyperglycemic medications.

THE FUNCTION OF INSULIN IN METABOLISM

Insulin is an anabolic hormone, normally present in individuals that consume healthy diets. It is a signaling factor that stimulates storage of excess nutrients, including glycogen and triglycerides, in the form of adipose fat. Insulin mostly affects the liver, adipose tissue, and striated muscles. Its synthesis and release is stimulated by glucose, but potentiated by amino acids. In the liver, insulin stimulates **glycogenesis**, fatty acid synthesis, glycolysis, and the **pentose phosphate pathway**. In adipose tissue, insulin stimulates uptake of glucose and fatty acids, and triglyceride synthesis. This is also known as *energy storage*. In skeletal muscles, insulin stimulates glucose uptake, glycogenesis, and synthesis of proteins. Insulin does not influence metabolism of glucose in the brain or red blood cells.

The liver can manufacture glucose, but glycogen synthesis is reduced. Without insulin, **gluconeogenesis** is uncontrolled. Therefore, blood glucose levels increase, and blood glucose remains in the body. The muscle and fat tissues are simultaneously starved for glucose. Glucagon secretion is not linked to blood glucose levels, yet insulin is important in the regulation of glucagon secretion. Gluconeogenesis, **glycogenolysis**, and lipolysis are processes in the body that become stimulated. Increased lipolysis causes elevation of **free fatty acids** in the blood. Fatty acid molecules are partly taken up by the liver, and incorporated into *lipoproteins*. This increases levels of very-low-density lipoprotein (VLDL) and low-density lipoprotein (LDL), risk factors for heart disease. **Ketone bodies** are produced by excessive lipolysis, unable to be inhibited without insulin. Dangerous *ketoacidosis* can develop if ketone levels are extremely elevated. Administration of insulin is required.

Glucose Metabolism

Glucose is a molecule made up of six carbons. It is a very efficient form of fuel for the body. When metabolized in the presence of oxygen, it is broken down to form carbon dioxide and water. The brain and nervous tissues use glucose as the source of most of their required energy. Other tissues and organ systems use fatty acids and ketones as fuel. The brain is unable to synthesize or store sufficient glucose to last for more than several minutes. A continual glucose supply from the systemic circulation is required for the cerebrum to function normally. Brain death can be due to severe and prolonged hypoglycemia. Significant brain dysfunction occurs because of only moderate hypoglycemia. Glucose is obtained from the circulation by tissues. Hypoglycemia is extremely dangerous in comparison to hyperglycemia. There is rigid control of blood glucose levels while fasting, and they remain between 70 and 99 mg/dL, which is equivalent to between 4.0 and 5.5 mmol/L. After eating, blood glucose levels rise. Insulin is released from the beta cells of the pancreas, allowing glucose to be transported into the body cells. Approximately 66% of the glucose contained in each meal is removed from the blood, and stored in the liver or skeletal muscles as glycogen. When the liver and skeletal muscles become saturated with glycogen, remaining glucose is converted into fatty acids by the liver. These are stored as triglycerides in the adipose tissue's fat cells.

Blood glucose levels decrease to below normal between meals. The liver then converts the stored glycogen back into glucose via glycogenolysis. The glucose is released as part of a homeostatic mechanism regulating blood glucose within normal ranges. Skeletal muscles contain stored glycogen, but do not contain the enzyme glucose-6-phosphatase. This enzyme allows glucose to be broken down, enabling it to pass through cell membranes and enter the bloodstream.

DOI: 10.1201/9781003226727-2

The enzyme only has limited usefulness in muscle cells. The liver synthesizes more glucose from amino acids, glycerol, and lactic acid via gluconeogenesis. Glucose is either directly released into the circulation, or stored as glycogen.

The **glycemic index** is a value that is assigned to foods, based on the speed in which they cause increases in blood glucose levels. Foods that are low on the glycemic index (GI) scale usually release glucose slowly and steadily, while foods high on the glycemic index release glucose quickly. The lower GI foods aid in weight loss, but those high on the scale aid in energy recovery after exercise, or to prevent hypoglycemia. Therefore, people with diabetes or prediabetes should consume more of the lower GI foods. This is because faster release of glucose from the higher GI foods results in spikes in blood sugar levels. Good glucose control is maintained by the slow and steady release of glucose from the lower GI foods. Table 1.1 summarizes examples of the lower and higher GI foods.

Carbohydrates in food are well known with regard to increasing blood glucose. The total amount of carbohydrates consumed, as well as the actual food choice itself, plays roles in this. For example, one serving of white rice quickly spikes blood glucose – just like eating pure sugar. Therefore, it is very important to choose good sources of carbohydrates in order to prevent diabetes mellitus and many other conditions. Good carbohydrate choices can also reduce risks for heart disease and cancer. The GI rates the effect of each type of food upon blood glucose, compared with the same amount of pure glucose. A food with a GI of 25 boosts the blood glucose only 25% as pure glucose. A food with a GI of 95 or higher has the same effect as pure glucose. To summarize further, low GI foods include most but not all fruits and vegetables, beans, grains that have not been heavily processed, low-dairy

foods, and nuts. Moderate GI foods include corn, couscous, and a few of the healthier breakfast cereals that are wheat-based. The high GI foods include white bread, most crackers, bagels, cakes, croissants, doughnuts, and most of the packaged breakfast cereals. Suggestions by dietitians regarding replacing higher GI foods with lower ones include the following:

- Instead of a baked potato – Bulgur (which is a cereal made from whole wheat that is partially boiled and then dried)

- Instead of white bread – Whole-grain bread

- Instead of cornflakes – Bran flakes

- Instead of instant oatmeal – Steel-cut oats

- Instead of white rice – Brown rice

Foods that contain no carbohydrates and are not assigned a GI include fish, meat, most nuts, poultry, herbs, oils, and spices. The GI is also affected by the ripeness of foods, the type of cooking method, the type of sugar contained, and the amount of processing that has been done before being sold. The GI is not the same as the **glycemic load** (GL), which is not based on the amount of food eaten, but is based on the number of carbohydrates in the food source, and how these affect blood glucose. Therefore, it is important to consider both the GI and the GL when selecting foods to help support healthy levels of blood glucose.

The benefits of a low glycemic diet include improved blood glucose regulation, increased weight loss, and reduced cholesterol levels. A low GI diet can reduce blood glucose and improve sugar management in individuals with type 2 diabetes. This diet can increase short-term weight loss, but additional study is needed to determine how long-term weight management is affected. The diet can lower total cholesterol

Table 1.1: Lower and Higher Glycemic Index (GI) Foods

Lower GI Foods (20–49)	Higher GI Foods (70–100)
Oat bran	Grits
Apples	Pineapple
Green beans	Soda
Asparagus	Potatoes
Barley	Most breads
Almonds	Rice
Skim milk	Candy
Blueberries	Most Chinese foods
Chickpeas	Sweet tea
Avocado	Pretzels
Peanuts	Most breakfast cereals
Low-fat or Greek yogurt	Pastries

and LDL cholesterol. The diet should mostly contain fruits, non-starchy vegetables, whole grains, legumes, meat, seafood, oils, nuts, seeds, herbs, and spices. It should limit breads, rice, cereals, pasta, starchy vegetables, baked foods, snacks, and beverages that have been sweetened with sugar. The lowest GI fruits include apples, strawberries, and dates, while the highest GI fruits include watermelon and pineapple. The lowest GI vegetables include boiled carrots and boiled sweet potatoes, while the highest GI vegetables include boiled potatoes and boiled pumpkin. The lowest GI grains include barley and quinoa, while the highest GI grains include white bread and white rice. Legumes such as soybeans, kidney beans, chickpeas, and lentils are all low GI foods. Lower GI dairy products or dairy alternatives include soymilk, skim milk, and whole milk, while higher choices in this classification include ice cream and rice milk. The highest GI sweetener is pure table sugar, while the lowest is fructose.

Carbohydrate tolerance is a term that refers to the body's individualized ability to tolerate carbohydrates. Not everyone tolerates them the same, and there are three different subtypes of carbohydrate tolerance: Low, medium, and high. These can be determined via glucose challenge tests or glucose tolerance tests. The dietary requirements for each type of carbohydrate tolerance are listed below:

- *Low* – 25% carbohydrates, 40% fats, 35% proteins
- *Moderate* – 35% carbohydrates, 35% fats, 30% proteins
- *High* – 50% carbohydrates, 30% fats, 20% proteins

Fat Metabolism

The most efficiently utilized form of fuel is fat, providing 9 kcal/g of stored energy. Carbohydrates and proteins each provide 4 kcal/g. About 40% of calories in the average diet of many countries are obtained from fats. This is equivalent to the percentage obtained from carbohydrates. Fats are a primary source of energy during resting or exercise. The use of fats for energy is just as vital as the use of carbohydrates. When carbohydrates and proteins are consumed in excess of what is needed by the body, they are converted into triglycerides, which are stored in adipose tissue. Each triglyceride contains three fatty acids, linked by a molecule of glycerol. Fatty acids are processed to be used as energy sources by lipases. These are enzymes that break triglycerides down into their component molecules.

The glycerol molecule enters the **glycolytic pathway**. It is used with glucose to produce energy, or to produce more glucose. Fatty acids are moved to tissues, where they are metabolized for energy. Most body cells can use fatty acids interchangeably with glucose for energy. This occurs everywhere except in the brain, nervous tissue, and red blood cells. Many cells utilize fatty acids for fuel, but fatty acids cannot be converted into glucose needed by the brain for energy. Much of the initial breakdown of fatty acids occurs in the liver, mostly when excess fatty acids are being utilized for energy. The liver uses just a small amount of fatty acids for its energy needs. The remainder are converted into ketones, which enter the bloodstream. As fat is broken down, such as when fasting, many ketones are released into the bloodstream. Ketones are organic acids, so the release of excessive ketones, such as in diabetes, can cause ketoacidosis. This is an acute complication of diabetes mellitus.

Protein Metabolism

Proteins are needed in order for body structures to be formed. These structures include genes, enzymes, contractile muscle components, hemoglobin, some hormones, and the bone matrix. Proteins are made from *amino acids.* Unlike the fatty acids or glucose, the body has a limited ability to store excess amounts of amino acids. Most of the stored amino acids are inside body proteins. Amino acids that are excessive in comparison to what is needed for protein synthesis are converted into fatty acids, glucose, or ketones. Then they are stored, or used as fuel for metabolism. Fatty acids cannot be converted into glucose. Therefore, proteins are broken down, with the amino acids used as a primary substrate for gluconeogenesis. This occurs when metabolic needs exceed food intake.

HYPERGLYCEMIA

Hyperglycemia is the primary manifestation of diabetes mellitus. It develops from impaired insulin secretion plus varied amounts of peripheral insulin resistance. Hyperglycemia may also occur in newborns after glucocorticoid hormones are administered, or because of excessive infusion of IV solutions containing glucose. This is common in poorly monitored hyperalimentation over a long period of time. Hyperglycemia causes osmotic diuresis. This is due to glycosuria, which leads to urinary frequency, plus polyuria and polydipsia. Orthostatic hypotension and dehydration can result. Hyperglycemia also causes weight loss, nausea, vomiting, blurred vision, and a predisposition to bacterial or fungal infections. Poorly controlled hyperglycemia that continues for years leads to vascular complications that affect the microvascular or macrovascular vessels, or both. There is **glycosylation** of the glomerular proteins in the kidneys. This may result in **mesangial cell** proliferation, expansion of the matrix, and vascular endothelial damage. There is usually a thickening of the glomerular basement membrane.

CLASSIFICATIONS OF DIABETES MELLITUS

Diabetes mellitus, diabetic ketoacidosis, and nonketotic hyperosmolar syndrome are the most common conditions linked to carbohydrate metabolism. Type 1 and type 2 diabetes are distinguished by various features. Impaired glucose regulation is related to impaired glucose tolerance or impaired fasting glucose. These strong risk factors for diabetes mellitus may be present for many years before the disease actually manifests. Diabetes is linked to higher risks for cardiovascular disease, but in most cases, common microvascular complications do not develop. In type 1 diabetes mellitus, there is insufficient insulin produced, due to autoimmune pancreatic beta cell destruction. This situation may be initiated by environmental factors, if an individual is genetically susceptible. The beta cells are continually destroyed over months or years, until their mass has decreased to a point at which insulin concentration can no longer control plasma levels of glucose. Type 1 diabetes most often develops in childhood or adolescence. In the past decades, it was the most common form of diabetes diagnosed in people younger than age 30. However, type 1 diabetes can also develop in adults, often seeming to be type 2 diabetes at first, and described as *latent autoimmune diabetes of adulthood*. In non-Caucasians, some cases of type 1 diabetes are idiopathic and do not apparently related to autoimmunity. It is not fully understood how beta cells are destroyed, but there are interactions between environmental factors, **autoantigens**, and **susceptibility genes**.

Proteins within the beta cells classified as autoantigens include glutamic acid decarboxylase, insulin, and insulinoma-associated protein. These proteins are likely exposed or released as beta cells experience normal turnover, or when they are injured by an infection or other condition. A cell-mediated immune response is then activated. *Insulitis*, the destruction of the beta cells, then occurs. The glucagon-secreting alpha cells, however, are not damaged. Antibodies to autoantigens can then be found in the serum. These antibodies appear to be a response to beta cell destruction, but not a cause of this destruction. Type 1 diabetes usually manifests with symptomatic hyperglycemia, and sometimes diabetic ketoacidosis (DKA). Some patients endure a long but transient phase of nearly-normal glucose levels following acute onset of the disease. This is called the *honeymoon phase*, because insulin secretion is partly recovered. Those at high risk for type 1 diabetes include brothers, sisters, or children of people with the disease. These relatives can be tested for the presence of islet cell or antiglutamic acid decarboxylase antibodies. These antibodies precede the onset of clinical type 1 diabetes. There are no proven methods of prevention against the disease for high-risk people. Therefore, screening usually occurs only in research studies. All patients with type 1 diabetes must receive insulin. Most patients can be taught how to adjust their insulin doses, and continuing patient education is encouraged because it is very helpful.

With type 2 diabetes mellitus, there is inadequate secretion of insulin. Early in the disease, insulin levels are commonly very high. This situation may continue later on in disease development. Peripheral insulin resistance and the increased production of glucose by the liver cause levels of insulin to be insufficient to normalize levels of plasma glucose. Insulin production becomes reduced, and the hyperglycemia worsens. Type 2 diabetes usually develops in adults and is more common with continued aging. Plasma glucose levels spike higher following meals in older adults compared to younger adults. This is most common following high carbohydrate loads. The levels require a longer period of time to return to normal. This is partly due to increased accumulation of visceral and abdominal fat, plus decreased muscle mass. Type 2 diabetes has become more common than ever in children. Childhood obesity has now reached epidemic levels of prevalence. About 40%–50% of new pediatric cases are type 2 diabetes, and more than 90% of adults with diabetes have this form. Genetic factors are clear, influencing the prevalence of type 2 diabetes ethnic groups such as Hispanics, American Indians, and Asians. Several genetic polymorphisms have been discovered, but no individual causative gene has been identified.

The pathogenesis of type 2 diabetes is not fully understood due to its complexity. Once insulin secretion cannot compensate for insulin resistance, hyperglycemia develops. Though insulin resistance is characteristic, beta cell dysfunction and impaired insulin secretion are common. There is impaired initial-phase insulin secretion as a response to IV glucose infusion, low pulsatile insulin secretion, and increased proinsulin secretion signaling impaired processing of insulin. There is also an accumulation of islet amyloid polypeptide, which is a protein usually secreted with insulin. Hyperglycemia

Table 1.2: Differences between Type 1 and Type 2 Diabetes

Characteristics	Type 1 Diabetes	Type 2 Diabetes
Age of disease onset	Usually before age 30	Usually after age 30
Relationship to obesity	No	Yes, in most cases
Ketoacidosis requiring insulin	Yes	No
Endogenous insulin in the plasma	Very low to undetectable	Can be low, normal, or elevated based on the degree of insulin resistance, defects in insulin secretion
Occurrence in twins	Up to 50%	More than 90%
Relationship to certain HLA-D antigens	Yes	No
Islet cell antibodies present	Yes	No
Islet pathology	Insulitis; selective loss of most beta cells	Smaller, normal-looking islets; there are often amyloid (amylin) deposits
Complications such as retinopathy, nephropathy, neuropathy, and atherosclerotic cardiovascular disease	Yes	Yes
Hyperglycemia response to oral antihyperglycemics	No	Initially yes in most cases

may reduce insulin secretion because high glucose levels desensitize the beta cells. This causes glucose toxicity with beta cell dysfunction, or both. Usually, years pass as these changes to occur along with insulin resistance.

In type 2 diabetes, obesity and weight gain influence insulin resistance. Though genetic determinants are present, diet, exercise, and lifestyle are extensively involved. Adipose tissues increase the plasma levels of free fatty acids, which can impair insulin-stimulated glucose transport and the activity of muscle glycogen synthase. The adipose tissues are believed to have endocrine functions. They release *adipocytokines* that may be metabolically favorable or unfavorable. Adiponectin is an example of a metabolically favorable adipocytokine. Unfavorable adipocytokines include IL-6, leptin, resistin, and tumor necrosis factor-alpha. Insulin resistance occurring later in life is also related to intrauterine growth restriction and low birth weight. This may be in conjunction with prenatal environmental influences upon metabolism of glucose.

Type 2 diabetes may present with symptomatic hyperglycemia, but this condition is often asymptomatic. The disease is commonly detected because of routine tests. Initial symptoms may be complications of diabetes, indicating that the disease may have been developing for a long time. A hyperosmotic coma can occur first. This is often related to stressors or impaired glucose metabolism from corticosteroids and other drugs. Type 2 diabetics with slight elevations of plasma glucose are started on a proper diet and exercise regimen. This is followed by a single oral antihyperglycemic drug if indicated. Additional oral drugs (as combination therapies) may be added. When 2 or more drugs are ineffective, insulin is administered. With greater glucose elevations upon diagnosis, lifestyle changes and oral antihyperglycemics are usually started simultaneously. Differences between type 1 and type 2 diabetes are summarized in Table 1.2.

Gestational diabetes mellitus (GDM) develops during pregnancy, characterized by a reduced ability to metabolize carbohydrates. This is usually due to a deficiency of insulin or insulin resistance. The condition disappears after the infant is delivered. However, in a large number of cases, it returns years afterward, as type 2 diabetes mellitus. Placental lactogen and extensive destruction of insulin by the placenta appear to play roles in precipitating GDM. Usually, pregnant women are screened for GDM between 24 and 28 weeks of gestation, via the 50 g, 1-hour glucose tolerance test. If the patient has risk factors for GDM, she will be screened in the first trimester. Risk factors include any previous pregnancy that involved GDM or a neonate heavier than 4,500 g at birth, unexplained fetal death, family history of diabetes in close relatives, previous persistent glycosuria, and a body mass index (BMI) over 30 kg/square meter (m²). With gestational diabetes, results are most accurately obtained via a glucose tolerance test. If the result is 140–199 mg/dL, a full glucose tolerance test is done. If the glucose is 200 mg/dL or higher, insulin is given. When 2 or more results are abnormal, the patient is placed on a controlled diet for the remainder of the pregnancy. If needed, insulin or oral hypoglycemics are administered. Rigid control of plasma glucose during pregnancy eliminates risks of adverse outcomes almost completely.

Pregnancy can worsen preexisting type 1 and type 2 diabetes, but is not believed to worsen diabeticnephropathy,neuropathy,orretinopathy. Gestational diabetes starts in most cases during pregnancy in those that are overweight, hyper-insulinemic, and insulin-resistant. However, GDM can develop in thin women that are rela-tively insulin-deficient. The disease occurs in 1%–3% of all pregnancies, but has been docu-mented as being significantly higher in Mexican Americans, American Indians, Asians, Indians, and Pacific Islanders. During pregnancy, dia-betes causes more fetal and maternal morbid-ity, as well as mortality. The baby is at risk for hypoglycemia, respiratory distress, hyperbili-rubinemia, hypocalcemia, and **hyperviscosity**. If preexisting or gestational diabetes is not well controlled during organogenesis, up to about 10 weeks of gestation, there is an increased risk of serious congenital malformations, as well as spontaneous abortion. Further on in pregnancy, poor diabetic control increases risks for fetal **macrosomia**, **preeclampsia**, and spontaneous abortion. Fetal macrosomia is usually described as a weight above 4,000 g at birth, but often over 4,500 g. Gestational diabetes may cause fetal macrosomia even if the blood glucose is nearly normal. To reduce risks to the fetus and mother, a diabetes team comprised of physicians, nurses, nutritionists, pediatricians, and social work-ers should be involved in treatment. Any com-plications, regardless of seriousness, must be quickly diagnosed and treated. A delivery plan is created, with an experienced pediatrician present. Neonatal intensive care must be avail-able. Insulin is sometimes used, with human insulin preferred because it reduces antibody formation. Treatment should involve self-mon-itoring of blood glucose, insulin administration, more physical activity, a carbohydrate-regu-lated meal plan, and sufficient intake of calcium and iron.

Neonatal diabetes affects infants and their ability to produce or use insulin. It is a mono-genic condition that is controlled by a single gene. Neonatal diabetes develops within the first 6 months of life. Since there is not enough insulin produced, the glucose levels increase. This rare disease only occurs in 1 of every 100,000–500,000 live births. It can be mistaken for type 1 diabetes. There are two types of neo-natal diabetes. The *permanent* form is lifelong, while the *transient* form disappears during infancy. However, the transient form can recur later in life. Onset of neonatal diabetes can be linked to abnormal pancreatic development and the speeds of beta cell dysfunction. The condi-tion can be genetically linked between patients and offspring. Symptoms include polydipsia, polyuria, dehydration, dry mouth, tiredness, and dark-colored urine. When dehydration is severe, signs include hypotension, sunken eyes, weak pulse, tachycardia, and fatigue. Ketoacidosis develops if the disease is severe. Related to neonatal diabetes is intrauterine growth restriction, with the fetus not grow-ing to reach a normal weight within the womb. After birth, the infant may have hyperglycemia or hypoglycemia. Permanent and transient neo-natal diabetes are both genetically inherited from the mother or father.

The disease may be of autosomal dominant, autosomal recessive, spontaneous, or X-linked causes. Transient neonatal diabetes occurs within a few days to weeks after birth. Insulin dose requirements are usually lower than with permanent neonatal diabetes. The transient form usually resolves within 12 weeks. Affected infants relapse in 50% of cases, usually during childhood or young adulthood. The pancreas, central nervous system, and various body tis-sues are predominantly affected. About 70% of cases are from defects initiating over-expression of the father's genes. This may occur by paternal DNA being defected by uniparental **isodisomy** on chromosome 6. Another cause is when the mother's genes, in the chromosome 6q24 region, are affected by DNA methylation.

Diagnoses of neonatal diabetes are based on fasting plasma glucose, random plasma glucose, oral glucose tolerance, ketoacidosis, and analy-ses of chromosomes and genes.

There are also other specific forms of diabetes mellitus, which are heterogeneous. They differ widely in their etiology and pathophysiology, primarily in relation to insulin secretion and the mechanism of its action. There may also be an abnormality of signal transduction inside the beta cells. These specific forms are as follows:

- Diseases of the exocrine pancreas
- Drug- or chemical-induced diabetes
- Genetic defects of beta cell function
- Genetic defects in insulin action
- Infection-induced diabetes
- Other endocrinopathies
- Other genetic syndromes linked to diabetes
- Rare forms of immune-mediated diabetes

HYPOGLYCEMIA

Hypoglycemia that is not related to exogenous insulin therapy is uncommon. It is character-ized by low plasma glucose levels, symptomatic stimulation of the sympathetic nervous system, and dysfunction of the central nervous system (CNS). Hypoglycemia can be caused by many drugs and disorders. Most often, symptomatic hypoglycemia is due to drugs used in the treatment of diabetes mellitus, including oral antihyperglycemics or insulin. When hypoglycemia occurs for other reasons, the body is often highly able to compensate. Acute hypoglycemia initially causes levels of glucagon and epinephrine to surge. Cortisol and growth hormone levels also sharply increase, which are important for recovery from extended hypoglycemia. The threshold for these hormones' release is usually higher than that for hypoglycemic symptoms.

Insulin-controlled causes of hypoglycemic include exogenous administration of insulin, and anything that encourages insulin secretion, such as **insulinoma**, which is a tumor that secretes insulin. Clinically, if hypoglycemia occurs, the patient is identified as having a healthy appearance, or manifestations of illness. Causes of hypoglycemia can then be divided into those either related to medications or not. *Pseudohypoglycemia* occurs because of delayed processing of blood specimens, using untreated test tubes. Erythrocytes and leukocytes, especially if they are increased such as in polycythemia or leukemia, then consume glucose. *Factitious hypoglycemia* is a real condition induced by nontherapeutic administration of insulin or sulfonylureas.

According to the American Diabetes Association, the complete classifications or subtypes of hypoglycemia include the following:

- *Severe hypoglycemia* – There is dizziness or a complete loss of consciousness; the patient usually requires assistance in administering carbohydrates or glucagon; neuroglycopenic symptoms resolve after administration.

- *Symptomatic hypoglycemia* – Symptoms occur as the plasma glucose concentration reaches 70 mg/ dL or lower.

- *Asymptomatic hypoglycemia* – Even with a plasma glucose concentration of 70 mg / dL or lower, there are no typical symptoms.

- *Probable symptomatic hypoglycemia* – Symptoms occur but do not match low plasma glucose levels.

- *Pseudohypoglycemia* – With poor glycemic control, the patient has symptoms of hypoglycemia even with plasma glucose levels higher than 70 mg/dL.

- *Moderate hypoglycemia* – Neurological symptoms are present, which may prevent the patient from taking oral glucose and often require assistance to do so.

- *Mild hypoglycemia* – There are adrenergic, mild neurological symptoms, preventable by oral intake of glucose.

Responses to Hypoglycemia

In normal individuals, hypoglycemia is a rare occurrence. However, in patients with diabetes mellitus that are treated with insulin, glucose counterregulatory responses are altered. This is especially true after repeated occurrences of hypoglycemia or after exercising. Severe hypoglycemia causes cognitive dysfunction. The patient may become obtunded or experience seizures. If the condition is prolonged, it can result in coma or death. Thresholds of the body's responses to hypoglycemia are varied, based on the individual's glycemic control. Therefore, severe outcomes of hypoglycemia, plus the reduction of counterregulatory and symptom responses, mean that hypoglycemia is a primary limiting factor regarding glycemic management of diabetes mellitus.

In diabetic patients, a plasma glucose level less than 3.9 mmol/L (70 mg/dL) is recommended as an alerting intervention value for hypoglycemia. If repeated, hypoglycemia episodes result in the patient becoming unaware of the condition. There is impaired glucose counter-regulation, and the individual is predisposed to severe hypoglycemia. The pathogenesis of hypoglycemia in insulin-treated diabetic patients usually involves no decrease in circulating insulin that has been exogenously administered, a lack of glucagon secretion, and a regulated increase in sympathoadrenal activity. This combines adrenomedullary with sympathetic neural activity. Previous hypoglycemia, exercise, and sleep cause defective glucose counter-regulation and hypoglycemia unawareness. These make up hypoglycemia-related autonomic failure. Abnormal glucose counter-regulation is related to a 25 times higher risk for severe **iatrogenic** hypoglycemia. When severe, hypoglycemia results in altered mental status. The patient is unable to provide self-care. There may be loss of consciousness or seizures. Glucagon or parenteral glucose therapy is required. Severe hypoglycemia is more common in infants, adolescents, those with longer disease duration, and those with lower glycosylated hemoglobin (HbA1c).

Patients receiving insulin experience many episodes of asymptomatic hypoglycemia, averaging two per week, and one episode of severe hypoglycemia per year, often accompanied by a seizure or coma. Hypoglycemia becomes progressively more frequent with type 2 diabetes, with this frequency becoming nearly as common as with type 1 diabetes. Endogenous insulin deficiency develops over time. Today, because of better treatments becoming available, rates of severe hypoglycemia have decreased and become relatively plateaued. The dangers of hypoglycemia include changes in the white and gray matter of a developing brain. Up to 6%–10% of people with type 1 diabetes die from hypoglycemia and its complications. Deaths have occurred as patients are asleep, possibly linked to prolonged QT and other cardiac arrhythmias. The mortality rates with type 2 diabetes are not documented sufficiently, but have likely occurred.

Treatment goals are to restore blood glucose levels to between 4.4 and 5.6 mmol/L (80 and 100 mg/dL) and to prevent recurrent episodes. When not severe, the patient needs immediate oral intake of simple carbohydrates that can be quickly absorbed. If severe, IV dextrose or IM glucagon is required. It is of the most importance to determine the causative factors. Causative comorbidities include **Addison's disease** and **celiac disease**. Continuous glucose monitoring is sometimes needed.

Late Hypoglycemia of Occult Diabetes

Late hypoglycemia of occult diabetes is a form of *reactive hypoglycemia*, which refers to hypoglycemia that results from abnormal responses to rapid increases in blood glucose levels, due to diet or stress. Reactive hypoglycemia is common and often improperly diagnosed and treated, but can be resolved by diet and lifestyle changes. Reactive hypoglycemia occurs 2–5 hours after food intake. Its three main subtypes are *alimentary* (within 2 hours), *idiopathic* (at 3 hours), and *late* (at 4–5 hours). With late hypoglycemia of occult diabetes, there is a delay in early insulin release from the pancreatic beta cells. This results in an initial exaggeration of *hyperglycemia* during a glucose tolerance test. In response to this hyperglycemia, exaggerated insulin release causes the late hypoglycemia in 4–5 hours. Affected patients are usually very different from those with early hypoglycemia that occurs in 2–3 hours after food intake. They are usually obese and often have a family history of diabetes mellitus. Treatment is directed at weight reduction. Patients often respond to reduced carbohydrate intake when small meals that are well-spaced occur at multiple times during the day. Therefore, they are all considered to be potential diabetics. Periodic medical evaluations must occur.

KEY TERMS

- Addison's disease
- Autoantigens
- Carbohydrate tolerance
- Celiac disease
- Free fatty acids
- Gestational diabetes mellitus
- Gluconeogenesis
- Glycemic index
- Glycemic load
- Glycogenesis
- Glycogenolysis
- Glycolytic pathway
- Glycosylation
- Hyperglycemia
- Hyperviscosity
- Hypoglycemia
- Iatrogenic
- Insulinoma
- Isodisomy
- Ketone bodies
- Lipoproteins
- Macrosomia
- Mesangial cell
- Neonatal diabetes
- Pentose phosphate pathway
- Preeclampsia
- Susceptibility genes

REFERENCES

American Diabetes Association. (2021). *Blood Sugar Testing and Control – Hypoglycemia (Low Blood Sugar)*. American Diabetes Association. https://www.diabetes.org/healthy-living/medication-treatments/blood-glucose-testing-and-control/hypoglycemia

Becker, G., and Goldfine, A.B. (2015). *The First Year: Type 2 Diabetes: An Essential Guide for the Newly Diagnosed (The Complete First Year)*. Da Capo Lifelong Books.

DeFronzo, R.A., Ferrannini, E., Zimmet, P., and Alberti, G. (2015). *International Textbook of Diabetes Mellitus*, 2 Volume Set, 4th Edition. Wiley-Blackwell.

Draznin, B. (2018). *Atypical Diabetes: Pathophysiology, Clinical Presentations, and Treatment Options*. American Diabetes Association.

Draznin, B. (2016). *Managing Diabetes and Hyperglycemia in the Hospital Setting – A Clinician's Guide*. American Diabetes Association.

Dwyer, D. (2012). *Glucose Metabolism in the Brain*. Academic Press.

Eljamil, A.S. (2015). *Lipid Biochemistry: For Medical Sciences*. iUniverse.

Europe PMC. (2011). *Glucose Counterregulatory Responses to Hypoglycemia*. Europe PMC. https://europepmc.org/article/PMC/3755377

Felner, E.I., and Umpierrez, G.E. (2013). *Endocrine Pathophysiology*. Lippincott, Williams, and Wilkins.

Freeman, J. (2018). *The Type 1 Life: A Road Map for Parents of Children with Newly Diagnosed Type 1 Diabetes*. Freeman.

Gardner, D.G., and Shoback, D.M. (2017). *Greenspan's Basic and Clinical Endocrinology*, 10th Edition. McGraw-Hill Education / Medical / Lange.

Garg, R., and Hudson, M. (2014). *Hyperglycemia in the Hospital Setting*. Jaypee Brothers Medical Publishing.

Grant, P. (2016). *Gestational Diabetes: Your Survival Guide to Diabetes in Pregnancy*. Sheldon Press.

Gurr, M.I., Harwood, J.L., Frayn, K.N., Murphy, D.J., and Michell, R.H. (2016). *Lipids: Biochemistry, Biotechnology and Health*, 6th Edition. Wiley-Blackwell.

Harvard Health Publishing / Harvard Medical School. (2020a). *Glycemic Index for 60+ Foods*. The President and Fellows of Harvard College. https://www.health.harvard.edu/diseases-and-conditions/glycemic-index-and-glycemic-load-for-100-foods

Harvard Health Publishing / Harvard Medical School. (2020b). *A Good Guide to Good Carbs: The Glycemic Index*. The President and Fellows of Harvard College. https://www.health.harvard.edu/healthbeat/a-good-guide-to-good-carbs-the-glycemic-index

Health.am. (2007). *Hypoglycemia – The Hypoglycemic States / Postprandial Hypoglycemia (Reactive Hypoglycemia)*. Health.am Inc. http://www.health.am/db/more/postprandial-hypoglycemia-reactive-hypoglycemia/

Healthline. (2021). *What Is the Glycemic Index?* Healthline Media. https://www.healthline.com/nutrition/glycemic-index#what-it-is

Holt, R.I.G., Cockram, C., Flyvbjerg, A., and Goldstein, B.J. (2017). *Textbook of Diabetes*, 5th Edition. Wiley-Blackwell.

Hussain, J., El-Banna, M., et al. (2017). *Hyperglycemia and Its Complications*. Lap Lambert Academic Publishing.

Hussain, S.S., Oliver, N., and Klonoff, D.C. (2016). *Insulin Pumps and Continuous Glucose Monitoring Made Easy*. Churchill Livingstone.

Hypoglycemia Support Foundation. (2021). *Frequently Asked Questions about Hypoglycemia*. Hypoglycemia Support Foundation, Inc. https://hypoglycemia.org/questions/

Janson, L.W., and Tischler, M. (2012). *Medical Biochemistry: The Big Picture*. McGraw-Hill/Medical/Lange.

Martin, C.G., and Waters, M.J. (2018). *Low Blood Sugar, The Hidden Menace of Hypoglycemia*. CreateSpace Independent Publishing Platform.

NIH – National Institute of Diabetes and Digestive and Kidney Diseases. (2021). *Monogenic Diabetes (Neonatal Diabetes & MODY)*. U.S. Department of Health and Human Services/National Institutes of Health/USA.gov. https://www.niddk.nih.gov/health-information/diabetes/overview/what-is-diabetes/monogenic-neonatal-mellitus-mody

Nikolic, B., and Jovanovic, A. (2012). *Hyperglycemia: Causes, Symptoms and Treatment Options (Endocrinology Research and Clinical Developments)*. Nova Science Publications Inc.

Porth, C.M. (2015). *Essentials of Pathophysiology*, 4th Edition. Wolters Kluwer.

Scharfmann, R., Shield, J.P.H., and Mullis, P.E. (2007). *Development of the Pancreas and Neonatal Diabetes: 1st Seminar in Developmental Endocrinology*, Volume 12. S. Karger.

Stone, M. (2014). *Hypoglycemia: What It Is, What It Isn't, and How to Fix the Root Problem*. CreateSpace Independent Publishing Platform.

Szablewski, L. (2018). *Glucose Homeostasis and Insulin Resistance*. Bentham Science Publishers.

Umpierrez, G.E. (2014). *Therapy for Diabetes Mellitus and Related Disorders*, 6th Edition. American Diabetes Association.

University of Chicago Medicine. (2021). *Neonatal Diabetes*. The University of Chicago Kovler Diabetes Center. http://monogenicdiabetes.uchicago.edu/for-healthcare-professionals/neonatal-diabetes/

CHAPTER 2 Metabolic Syndrome

Metabolic syndrome is actually a group of risk factors that increases risks for diabetes mellitus, heart disease, stroke, and other health problems. There must be at least three of the following metabolic risk factors in order for metabolic syndrome to be diagnosed: A larger than normal waist circumference, high triglyceride level, low HDL cholesterol level, hypertension, and high fasting blood sugar. The risk of having metabolic syndrome is closely linked to obesity and lack of physical activity, as well as insulin resistance. Metabolic syndrome is becoming more common because of increased obesity rates. Conditions that play a role in the development of metabolic syndrome include fatty liver disease, polycystic ovarian syndrome, and respiratory conditions such as obstructive sleep apnea. Metabolic syndrome is treated with a combination of lifestyle improvements and medications.

DEFINITION

Metabolic syndrome involves inflammation and hypercoagulability, along with oxidative stress, endothelial dysfunction, and hyperinsulinemia. It is also referred to as *MetSyn* and *Syndrome X*. At least three of the following conditions must be present for metabolic syndrome to be diagnosed: Abdominal obesity, *atherogenic dyslipidemia* (decreased HDL cholesterol and increased triglycerides), hypertension, insulin resistance, increased plasminogen activator inhibitor, and a proinflammatory state. Fibrinogen increases in response to high levels of cytokines. It is an acute-phase reactant. Importantly, metabolic syndrome may predispose patients to even more serious complications, such as type 2 diabetes mellitus, heart attack, and stroke. The *National Cholesterol Education Program Adult Treatment Panel III Report* is summarized in Table 2.1.

Metabolic syndrome has greatly increased globally, and in the United States alone, about 33% of the population has the condition. It increases with aging and higher body mass index (BMI) levels. Over 35% of all adults in the United States and over 50% of adults over age 60 are estimated to have metabolic syndrome. Prevalence was 18.3% among people 20–39 years of age, but 46.7% in people aged 60 or older. In people over age 60, more than 50% of females and Hispanics had metabolic syndrome. For example, Mexican-Americans had the highest overall prevalence of metabolic syndrome (31.9%).

ETIOLOGY

The causes of metabolic syndrome include obesity, excessive amounts of adipose tissue, glucose intolerance, hypercholesterolemia, hyperinsulinemia, hypertension, hypertriglyceridemia, older age, and an elevated estrogen-to-testosterone ratio. Adipocytes packed with stored fat secrete **adipokines**. These are inflammatory substances that cause damage to the insulin-driven glucose transport system. **Leptin** and **resistin** are important adipokines believed to be involved in **insulin resistance**, which is a condition involving body tissues having lowered response levels to insulin. They likely increase because of both obesity and insulin resistance. The various adipokines that are involved in insulin resistance are shown in Figure 2.1

Metabolic syndrome, in 50% of cases, is caused by genetic factors. Related mitochondrial defects are totally inherited from the mother. Therefore, type 2 diabetes is much more common on the maternal side of a family. Because of aging, a genetic predisposition to insulin resistance, in voluntary muscle and the liver, is worsened by a loss of muscle mass. It is made worse by abdominal obesity, anxiety, corticosteroids, depression, hypogonadism, infection, lack of aerobic exercise, sleep deprivation, and smoking. Metabolic syndrome is related to male patterns of fat distribution, with fat mostly being abdominal instead of on the buttocks and thighs. In obese women, fat is mostly deposited in the buttocks and thighs instead of the abdomen. Buttock and thigh fat is subcutaneous and is mostly stored fat with low metabolic activity.

Table 2.1: ATP III Report Identifying the Features of Metabolic Syndrome

Risk Factors	Identifying Levels
Abdominal obesity – Men	Over 40 inches (102 cm)
Abdominal obesity – Women	Over 35 inches (88 cm)
Blood pressure	Systolic 130 or higher, diastolic 85 or higher (both measured in mm Hg)
Fasting glucose	110 mg/dL or higher
HDL cholesterol – Men	Less than 40 mg/dL
HDL cholesterol – Women	Less than 50 mg /dL
Triglycerides	150 mg/dL or higher

DOI: 10.1201/9781003226727-3

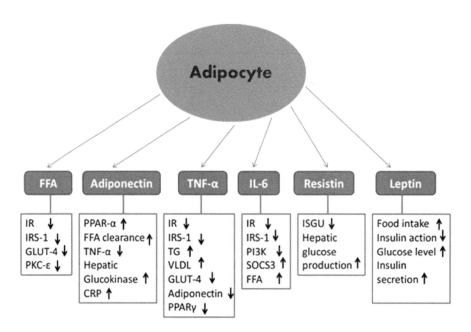

Figure 2.1 Adipokines involved in insulin resistance. (With permission from Kumar and Kumar (2020). *Diabetes: Epidemiology, Pathophysiology and Clinical Management*, 1st Edition, CRC Press/Taylor & Francis.)

With metabolic syndrome, abdominal fat must be excessively deposited in the peritoneal cavity. Here, the adipocytes of the mesenteric, **omental**, perinephric, and retroperitoneal fat are much more metabolically active. Not all obese patients have increased peritoneal fat and metabolic syndrome, and even some thin patients have excessive peritoneal fat with the syndrome. This is why 40% of patients with a BMI over 35 do not have the syndrome, and also why 6% of patients with a BMI under 25 do have the syndrome. Peritoneal fat makes up 20% of male total body fat, but only 6% of female total body fat. Peritoneal fat in females is increased by higher testosterone levels, the same way that testosterone replacement therapy in hypogonadal males increases the levels. The resulting increase in peritoneal fat is due to increased amounts of androgen receptors in the nuclei of peritoneal adipocytes, compared to subcutaneous adipocytes. Increased metabolic activity of peritoneal fat is because of higher densities of beta-adrenergic receptors and lower densities of alpha-1 adrenergic receptors on peritoneal adipocyte surfaces. This results in more catecholamine-induced lipolysis and greater release of free fatty acids (FFAs) into the portal circulation. Increased inflammation is linked to infiltration of peritoneal and hepatic fat with macrophages.

For some reason, Asian people that are thin, yet have type 2 diabetes and metabolic syndrome, are common. In India, the syndrome is extremely prevalent – especially in people that move from rural to urban areas and changed their lifestyles accordingly. With increased peritoneal fat, a BMI above 23 and a waist circumference greater than 34 inches (86 cm), metabolic syndrome develops early because of a genetically predisposed insulin resistance, even though they remain relatively thin.

It is believed that the genetic defect in relation to metabolic syndrome is within the mitochondria. This is where oxidative phosphorylation is reduced by 30% because of decreased expression of peroxisome proliferator-activated receptor (PPAR) gamma coactivator (PGC-1). This a coactivator of the PPAR gamma receptor. Because of decreased PGC-1 expression, the mitochondria are smaller than normal and less efficient on a physiological level. This decreased function allows for accumulation of triglycerides within the cytoplasm. They also build up in the voluntary muscles, liver, and myocardium, as well as the pancreatic beta cells. When a person is insulin-resistant, activity of carnitine palmotransferase-1 (CPT-1) is decreased. The triglycerides are then able to accumulate in the cytoplasm, resulting to conditions such as cardiomyopathy, fatty liver disease, and diabetes mellitus. Even so, only 40% of individuals actually develop type 2 diabetes, at least until greatly decreased secretion of insulin has developed. Eight of the ten identified genes related to type 2 diabetes are linked to defective secretion of insulin, while the remaining two genes are related to insulin resistance. However, patients with insulin-resistant metabolic syndrome that do not actually develop diabetes still have higher risks for cardiovascular events and disease.

Proportional to the number of peritoneal adipocytes, macrophages are recruited from the bone marrow. The more peritoneal adipocytes, the more macrophages recruitment to the peritoneal fat. The adipocytes produce excessive inflammatory adipocytokines as macrophages infiltrate in a **corona** around the peritoneal and liver adipocytes. There is "crosstalk" between adipocytes and macrophages. Due to the excessive adipocytokine production, metabolic syndrome is linked with chronic low-grade inflammation. The crosstalk also causes increased insulin resistance on the adipocytes, more lipolysis, and release of FFAs into the portal circulation. Inflammation in the peritoneal fat causes more release of inflammatory cytokines. Tumor necrosis factor-alpha (TNF-α) that is produced by the peritoneal adipocytes increases free fatty acid release. When they reach the systemic circulation, they decrease insulin sensitivity while increasing coagulability, potentially leading to cardiac arrhythmias.

Interleukin-6 is also excessively produced by the peritoneal adipocytes as well as other tissues. However, about 33% of it is from the adipocytes – mostly the peritoneal adipocytes. With increased production and release, IL-6 that enters the portal circulation results in increased production of C-reactive protein (CRP) in the liver. A chronic low-grade increase of CRP is linked to increased cardiovascular disease. The elevation is a marker of low-grade systemic inflammation as well as inflammation in the atheromatous plaque. This makes the plaque more likely to rupture and cause a cardiac event. Also, CRP may actively help atheromatous plaques to form. In autopsy studies, CRP is present within atheromatous plaques of all sizes and ages, but not in healthy endothelium of the coronary arteries.

Due to a surface CRP receptor, monocytes are attracted to the arterial wall endothelium and can easily penetrate it if CRP is present. This means that CRP may help actively form and rupture atheromatous plaques. Levels of CRP can be greatly lowered if metabolic syndrome is treated with thiazolidinedione (TZD) along with a statin. Since one or more TZDs can slow increase in the volume of coronary and carotid artery atheromas as well as reduce cardiac events, the lowering of CRP and inflammation by using a TZD for a metabolic syndrome patient is helpful with regard to positive cardiovascular drug effects. **Interleukin-6** (IL-6) is prothrombotic. It stimulates fibrinogen production in the liver and increases tissue factor expression in endothelial cells and monocytes. This helps activate the coagulation cascade. Endothelial function is harmed by IL-6, which causes deposition of atheroma, thrombosis, and vasoconstriction. This means that excessive IL-6 directly and indirectly causes endothelial dysfunction, inflammation, and atherogenesis.

The peritoneal adipocytes also excessively produce plasminogen activator inhibitor (PAI$_1$), which directly opposes **tissue plasminogen activator** (TPA), decreasing formation of **plasmin** from plasminogen. In the systemic circulation, less plasmin means that fibrin breaks down slower, decreasing clot lysis and increasing thromboembolic events as well as making them more severe. Plasmin is also needed in vessel walls to degrade and remove collagen from atheromatous plaques, so that vascular smooth muscle cells can enter and replace collagen tissues. This entry stabilizes plaques, making rupture and cardiovascular events less likely. Elevated PAI$_1$ in vessel walls occurs in metabolic syndrome and type 2 diabetes. However, TZDs can reduce PAI$_1$ levels in metabolic syndrome patients. This partly explains reduced cardiovascular events seen when the TZD called pioglitazone is used.

Angiotensinogen is also produced by the peritoneal adipocytes. It is a substrate that renin acts upon to form angiotensin I and eventually angiotensin II. Excessive angiotensinogen may be implicated in the increased hypertension occurrence as part of metabolic syndrome. Increased angiotensin II levels are related to increased inflammation, endothelial dysfunction, oxidative stress, atheroma formation, and cardiac events.

Even though excessive production of leptin is more often of the subcutaneous adipocytes, leptin levels are also increased in metabolic syndrome. Increases are linked in most studies to increased insulin resistance, poor endothelial function, and hypertension because of increased sympathetic nervous system activity. Lowering leptin levels improves metabolic syndrome. Leptin increases appetite and hyperphagia as well as activation of the pancreatic islet alpha cells, increasing release of glucagon. When this release is combined with insulin resistance, risks for type 2 diabetes are increased. Glycemic control is worsened in patients with established diabetes. Leptin is also linked with hematopoiesis, angiogenesis, and vascular endothelial proliferation. On an immune system level, leptin causes T lymphocytes to proliferate.

Currently, **adiponectin** is the only known adipocytokine that is beneficial. If adiponectin is low in the serum, this is linked to metabolic syndrome, obesity, coronary artery disease, and type 2 diabetes. Decreases in adiponectin levels occur before metabolic syndrome. With treatment of the syndrome, adiponectin levels increase quickly. Adiponectin may speed up metabolism of FFAs and decrease oxidative stress. All features of metabolic syndrome are partly based on and associated with the IL-6:adiponectin ratio. With increased IL-6 and decreased adiponectin, insulin sensitivity weakens. Oppositely, insulin sensitivity improves with decreased Il-6 and increased adiponectin. Women have higher adiponectin levels than men, as do people with type 1 diabetes, those using insulin sensitizers, and those that are thinner. Adiponectin levels are lower in obese people, those with **lipodystrophy**, and in men who have type 2 diabetes. Improved insulin sensitivity with increased adiponectin is linked to activation of the enzyme called *glycogen synthase*. Its activation increases glucose uptake in the cells, and free fatty acid oxidation – while decreasing triglycerides in the cytoplasm and glucose production in the liver.

Adiponectin has antiatherogenic effects. These are regulated by reduced adhesion molecules, monocyte adhesion to the endothelium, migration, and proliferation of vascular smooth muscle cells into the endothelium, production of cytokines by infiltrating monocytes, formation of **foam cells**, and uptake of oxidized LDL by macrophages. Adiponectin levels often become elevated in congestive heart failure, renal failure, and acute cardiovascular events. This adiponectin paradox may indicate greater release of adiponectin because of tissue damage, as well as advanced, severe underlying disease progression. On a metabolic level, adiponectin decreases secretion of metalloproteinase tissue inhibitors, thus decreasing adipocyte hypertrophy and the number of peritoneal adipocytes.

DIABETES AND METABOLIC SYNDROME

The cluster of hypertension, obesity, dyslipidemia, and insulin resistance defines metabolic syndrome with diabetes. Diagnostic criteria are somewhat under debate and there is much overlap between the definitions of the syndrome between various international organizations. When a person has metabolic syndrome, he or she is five times more likely to develop type 2 diabetes. Even so, only about 35% of people with metabolic syndrome develop type 2 diabetes. People with a parent or other close relative with type 2 diabetes are also at greater risk for developing metabolic syndrome, even if they are not obese. When insulin resistance is present, there are increased risks for metabolic syndrome, prediabetes, and type 2 diabetes. Addressing metabolic syndrome in its early stages is very important regarding reducing risks of developing type 2 diabetes.

Patients that have metabolic syndrome also have higher blood viscosity than patients without it. Blood viscosity scores are able to predict diabetes mellitus as well as a tendency to develop diabetes. There is a direct relationship between blood viscosity and blood glucose levels. According to the *American Journal of Epidemiology*, elevated blood viscosity may predispose to insulin resistance and type 2 diabetes. This may be by limited delivery of glucose, insulin, and oxygen to metabolically active tissues.

Metabolic syndrome is also referred to as *insulin-resistant syndrome*, *cardiometabolic syndrome*, **syndrome X**, and **Reaven syndrome**. Currently, the International Diabetes Federation (IDF) defines metabolic syndrome as central obesity of more than 37 inches (94 cm) in men and more than 31.5 inches (88 cm) in women. Patients have slightly different qualifying waist measurements based on various ethnicities, plus two of the following four factors:

- Triglycerides over 150 mg/dL (1.7 mmol/L), or specific treatment for this.

- HDL cholesterol under 40 mg/dL (1.03 mmol/L) in men, and under 50 mg/dL (1.29 mmol/L) in women, or specific treatment for this.

- Systolic BP of 130 mm Hg or more, and diastolic BP of 85 mm Hg or more, or treatment of diagnosed hypertension.

- Fasting blood glucose of 100 mg/dL (5.6 mmol/L) or higher, or diagnosed diabetes; if above these levels, an oral glucose tolerance test is recommended, but is not required to define metabolic syndrome as being present.

According to the IDF, as many as 25% of adults throughout the world have metabolic syndrome. Risk factors increasing the likelihood of metabolic syndrome include **acanthosis nigricans**, BMI over 25 kg/m^2 or waist circumference over 40 inches in men and over 35 inches in women, cardiovascular disease, family history of type 2 diabetes or glucose intolerance, hypertension, nonalcoholic fatty liver disease, non-Caucasian ethnicity, polycystic ovary syndrome, and a sedentary lifestyle. Metabolic syndrome predicts cardiovascular and heart disease deaths. Fasting blood glucose is a strong predictor of metabolic syndrome. Diabetes with metabolic syndrome is more likely when a patient is obese. Metabolic syndrome increases the risk for diabetes independently of other risk factors.

Impaired glucose tolerance, via the 2-hour glucose tolerance tests, is signified by levels between 140 and 200 mg/dL. Diabetes is present if the 2-hour glucose level is higher than 200 mg/dL. This is irrespective of the fasting glucose level. Also, two fasting glucose levels of 126 mg/dL or higher, or one random glucose level of over 200 mg/dL along with hyperglycemic symptoms signifies diabetes. The disease is also diagnosed if the HbA1c is higher than 6.5%. The production and release of insulin starts to decline as much as 12 years prior to type 2 diabetes being diagnosed. At the time of diagnosis, the pancreatic beta cells function at 50% or less of their normal level. Within 6 years after diabetes is diagnosed, the beta cells are at 25% of normal function, and after 10 years, they are at 10%. Most patients need insulin at this time. The continuing decline in beta cell function is not related to lifestyle changes or use of insulin, metformin, or the sulfonylureas. The only treatments that can slow the decline in beta cell function, or even improve it, are the injectable incretin mimetics, which include exenatide-4 or liraglutide and the TZDs. There are four risk factors for decreasing in beta cell function:

- *Inflammation* – There are increased proinflammatory cytokines in the pancreatic beta cells of people with type 2 diabetes. There are also five times more macrophages per islet cell in comparison to people without diabetes. The macrophages are centrally located instead of being peripherally located as they are in nondiabetic patients. The macrophages cause cytokine levels to rise, resulting in oxidative stress, and faster beta cell apoptosis.

- *Glucotoxicity* – Rising glucose levels result in decreased insulin release. Corrected hyperglycemia improves insulin sensitivity in the adipocytes, hepatocytes, and myocytes. There is improved insulin release from the beta cells. Extremely high glucose levels cause a hyperosmolar coma. Once hyperglycemia is corrected, insulin resistance decreases as insulin secretion increases. Chronic glucotoxicity treated with sulfonylureas decrease levels of the antioxidant *nicotinamide adenine dinucleotide phosphate (NAPDH)*, speeding up beta cell dysfunction.

- *Lipotoxicity* – Aging and declining of mitochondrial function cause triglycerides in the cytoplasm of most cells to increase. Pancreatic duct cells and alpha cells contain higher levels of lipids while the beta cells have twice as much cytoplasmic lipid in comparison. This indicates that mitochondrial function in the beta cells decreases more than in other cells because of aging. The beta cells are more affected by the mitochondrial dysfunction that is related to metabolic syndrome.

- *Amyloid deposition* – The inflammatory *amyloid* protein is secreted along with insulin. Amyloid precipitates because of toxic amyloid oligomers, mostly in the later stages of type 2 diabetes. It is deposited in the beta cells, interfering with secretion and release of insulin. Amyloid deposition may be related to metabolic syndrome. The toxic oligomers cause stress in the endoplasmic reticulum. They disrupt cell coupling, and the result is apoptosis.

Metabolic syndrome causes more cytoplasmic fat to accumulate in muscle, liver, and heart cells as well as pancreatic beta cells. The mitochondrial oxidative phosphorylation of FFAs decreases. The acids cannot enter the mitochondria for oxidation. They are stored as triglycerides in the cytoplasm. Mitochondrial function decreases more and more with aging, and there is a larger amount of cytoplasmic lipid accumulation. Likely due to a lack of adiponectin, metabolic syndrome is also related to more lipolysis of peritoneal adipocytes and hepatic fat. This increases serum free fatty acid levels, causing higher levels of beta cell cytoplasmic triglycerides. **Ceramide** has the greatest effect upon apoptosis out of all these metabolites. Loss of beta cells mass is linked to accelerated apoptosis.

CENTRAL NERVOUS SYSTEM MANIFESTATIONS OF METABOLIC SYNDROME

Central nervous system manifestations of the metabolic syndrome include dementias, **Alzheimer's disease**, and peripheral neuropathy. There is a strong link between major depression and metabolic syndrome. There is a four times higher risk for premature death, primarily from cardiovascular disease, in relation to major depression. Metabolic syndrome appears to act as a mediator between depression and cardiovascular disorder (CVD). It may share alterations of stress management with depression, including actions of the autonomic nervous system, hypothalamus-pituitary-adrenal axis, immune system, and even the functions of platelets and the endothelium. Both metabolic syndrome and depression cause a low-grade chronic inflammatory state. This leads to more oxidative and nitrosative damage of the endothelium, neurons, and pancreatic cells. Peripheral hormones such as leptin and ghrelin play roles in mood regulation.

In the parts of the brain where amyloid plaque collects, positron emission tomography (PET) scans show reduced uptake of glucose in patients with metabolic syndrome. During cerebral stimulation with insulin, thinner patients show improved information processing, increasing the beta and theta bands of spontaneous activity in the cortex. In obese patients, cerebral stimulation does not increase the beta activity, and decreases the theta activity. There is apparently a specific cerebral insulin resistance occurring. If the patient carries the *arginine* (*ARG*) *allele*, linked to genetic insulin resistance, there is a more extreme insulin-resistance pattern, and decreased beta activity as well as zero theta activity when the cerebrum is stimulated with insulin. The cerebrocortical insulin resistance associated with genetic or acquired metabolic syndrome may be caused by defective glucose transport across the **blood-brain barrier**, an intraneuronal insulin signaling defect, or both. Cerebrocortical insulin resistance may cause higher cerebral insulin levels along with triggering accumulation of beta-amyloid. This will eventually form the amyloid plaques seen in Alzheimer's disease. With cerebrocortical insulin resistance and cerebral hyperinsulinemia, excessive amounts of beta-amyloid accumulates, aggregating into amyloid plaques. This impairs memory and increases risks for neurodegenerative disease. Beta-amyloid accumulation causes cerebrocortical insulin resistance because of oligomers of amyloid-removing insulin receptors from neuronal dendritic plasma membranes – primarily in the **hippocampus**. Use of insulin or TZDs may protect against the insulin receptors from being removed.

Metabolic syndrome impacts the central nervous system to cause neurodegenerative and neurological diseases. If the blood-brain barrier is broken down for any reason, there can be release of **cytokines** and inflammatory mediators, **diapedesis** across the endothelium, and destruction of the cells of the blood-brain barrier. Inflammation is closely linked with neuropathologies. There can be various types of CNS dysfunction, memory deficits, **visuospatial deficits**, executive function deficits, slowed processing speed, and reduced intellectual function. Autopsy studies show that diabetic patients with dementia have more microvascular lesions than diabetic patients without dementia. The lesions are not the primary reason for cognitive deficits, but they are related to

widespread vascular dysfunction, while contributing to cerebral dysfunction. Treatment of metabolic syndrome and insulin resistance may improve memory as well as slow down age-related declines in cognition.

Symptomatic peripheral neuropathy is also commonly present along with type 2 diabetes. The likely cause of this neuropathy is metabolic syndrome that proceeds the diabetes. Patients with over three features of metabolic syndrome are twice as likely to develop neuropathy. Idiopathic neuropathy is also linked to metabolic syndrome. There is also a higher prevalence of hyperlipidemia. Hypertriglyceridemia is also independently related to neuropathy. Endothelial dysfunction is probably implicated in the connection between metabolic syndrome and neuropathy. The nerves have asymmetrical demyelination, which is linked to occlusions of the **vasa nervorum**.

Metabolic syndrome is a risk factor for intracranial arteriosclerosis, ischemic stroke, periventricular white matter hyperintensity, and subcortical white matter lesions. In fact, metabolic syndrome itself is an independent risk factor for stroke. The incidence of nonhemorrhagic stroke is increased. This type of stroke includes atherosclerotic extracranial and intracranial stroke, as well as embolic and lacunar infarcts. The lacunary infarcts are caused by fibrinoid necrosis within the microvascular circulation, resulting in subcortical infarcts, and occasionally silent infarcts. They are linked to diabetes, hypertension, or both – which are often related to metabolic syndrome. Increased carotid intima-medial thickening is also related to metabolic syndrome. In Caucasians, extracranial large artery atherosclerosis is also related, and in other racial groups there is intracranial large vessel atherosclerosis. Embolic strokes from extracranial areas make up most of the strokes related to metabolic syndrome. Often after revascularization of the coronary and carotid arteries, embolic strokes occur because of metabolic syndrome. Since atrial fibrillation is also more common with metabolic syndrome, emboli often come from the left atrium.

Obesity is directly related to impaired cognitive function and increased risk of dementia. Generally, BMI is inversely related to cognitive functioning. Obesity can also affect brain structures, resulting in atrophy. The first area of the brain to be affected is the hypothalamus. As part of metabolic syndrome, hyperglycemia has the strongest association with risks for cognitive deterioration. **Neurotrophins** have an important role in metabolic syndrome, affecting glucose, lipids, and energy.

CARDIAC RISK FACTORS WITH METABOLIC SYNDROME

Cardiac risk factors with metabolic syndrome include hypertension, dyslipidemia, albuminuria, coagulopathy, endothelial dysfunction, and inflammation. Metabolic syndrome is often associated with heart failure and peripheral artery disease. Dyslipidemia involves increased triglycerides and low-density lipoprotein (LDL) cholesterol, and decreased high-density lipoprotein (HDL) cholesterol. In various studies, age-adjusted mortality rates between metabolic syndrome and coronary heart disease have ranged between 2.47 and 2.96 times higher than without metabolic syndrome. Hyperinsulinemia has been shown to be a predictor of cardiovascular disease as well. Insulin resistance is positively correlated to atherosclerosis, a known cardiac risk factor.

Metabolic syndrome increases the risks for CVD, cardiac arrhythmias, heart failure, and thrombotic events. The six major factors related to the development of cardiovascular disease from metabolic syndrome include the following:

- Abdominal obesity

- *Atherogenic dyslipidemia* – Increased serum triglycerides, presence of small LCL cholesterol particles, and a low HCL cholesterol level

- Hypertension

- Insulin resistance with or without glucose intolerance

- *A proinflammatory state* – Elevation of CRP, tumor necrosis factor-alpha, plasma resistin, and interleukins 6 and 18

- *A prothrombotic state* – Abnormalities in procoagulant factors, antifibrinolytic factors, platelet alterations, and endothelial dysfunction

Obesity and insulin resistance are the main risk factors for development of CVD. Other primary risk factors include an atherogenic diet, physical inactivity, cigarette smoking, family history of premature coronary heart disease, and increased age.

Normally, people experience a drop in blood pressure while they sleep, but hypertensive patients with metabolic syndrome do not. This "nondipping" of BP is related to more cardiovascular events, especially those that occur between midnight and 6:00 a.m. Hypertension and sleep apnea are highly linked with metabolic syndrome, and are primary causes of atrial fibrillation. Therefore, most patients with atrial fibrillation also have metabolic syndrome. Hyperinsulinemia with metabolic syndrome stimulates the sympathetic nervous system through the renin-angiotensin-aldosterone system (RAAS). This occurs by direct activation of angiotensin II type 1 receptors and by indirect stimulation of the RAAS by increased catecholamines. Because of insulin, the body retains salt and water. When diabetes develops, hyperglycemia worsens sodium retention, with one sodium molecule being absorbed for every glucose molecule filtered and reabsorbed in the renal tubule. While reducing serum glucose lowers systolic BP, reducing insulin levels cause more lowering of BP.

Hypertension often causes left ventricular hypertrophy (LVH). However, metabolic syndrome potentiates this, partly due to high insulin levels, since insulin is a growth factor. Metabolic syndrome is linked to increased ventricular mass and thickness of the walls. More increases in LVH occur if type 2 diabetes develops. In African American patients, LVH is associated with increased mortality than those from left ventricular systolic dysfunction or multiple-vessel coronary artery disease.

As well as high triglycerides and low HDL, metabolic syndrome features increases LDL particles with elevated apolipoprotein B cholesterol levels. The small size of the LDL and HDL particles is mostly due to presentation of very-low-density lipoprotein (VLDL) particles to increased liver lipase activity. The VLDL particles are rich in triglycerides. This causes formation of additional small, dense LDL and HDL particles. Increased atherogenesis is linked to increased amounts of smaller, denser LDL particles. Their small size allows penetration of the arterial endothelium along with entry into the subendothelial space. Here, the particles are easily oxidized. If they are glycosylated, they are more easily picked up by macrophage scavenger receptors, beginning and allowing atherogenesis.

Small and dense HDL particles are not as protective to the heart as larger HDL particles, due to less capacity for reverse cholesterol transportation. The small particles also have fewer antioxidant and antiinflammatory effects. Endothelial function cannot be improved as much, and there is lower protection from oxidation of LDL particles. The liver more quickly metabolizes smaller, denser HDL particles. They do not exist for as long a time and are therefore lower in number. With metabolic syndrome, activity of hepatic lipase upon triglyceride-rich VLDL particles is higher.

With hypertriglyceridemia, the non-HDL cholesterol level is used to assess risks, instead of the calculated LDL cholesterol level. The HDL cholesterol level is subtracted from the total

17

cholesterol level, based on a fasting or nonfasting specimen. Non-HDL cholesterol should be 30 mg/dL above the goal for calculated LDL cholesterol. However, in diabetic patients with or without metabolic syndrome, the non-HDL cholesterol is very important since it provides the sum of LDL, intermediate-density lipoprotein (IDL), and small dense VLDL particles.

Metabolic syndrome is a risk factor for cardiac events even with other risk factors such as dyslipidemia, coagulopathy, and hypertension. This may be due to the link with endothelial dysfunction. Nitric oxide production is sufficient when the endothelium is healthy. It allows the arteries to vasodilate, provides surfaces that are not sticky so that clots do not attach, and suppresses atheromas from forming due to stopping leukocytes from breaching the endothelium. With metabolic syndrome's inflammation, excessive superoxide is produced, leading to increased atheroma formation, thrombosis, and vasoconstriction.

Endothelial dysfunction causes the glomerulus of the kidney to allow larger molecules to enter, and excessive albumin leaks into the tubules. Not all of it is reabsorbed, so albumin can be found in the urine as microalbuminuria or macroalbuminuria. The presence of albuminuria is well related to other endothelial dysfunction tests. Albuminuria is also a marker for atherosclerosis. When the glomerulus is more permeable to albumin, the endothelium will be more permeable to lipoproteins. Microalbuminuria is an independent risk factor for cardiac events as well as highly predictive for coronary artery disease, likely due to the link between metabolic syndrome as well as endothelial dysfunction. The lower the albumin: creatinine ratio in the urine, the lower the risks for cardiovascular events. The cutoff point is 30 mg albumin:1 g creatinine. However, for cardiovascular risks, the threshold is not as high, only 7 mg albumin:1 g creatinine. Albuminuria in metabolic syndrome can be decreased by TZDs, carvedilol (a beta blocker), and RAAS inhibitors.

The risk of heart failure is 66% higher if metabolic syndrome is present. If a myocardial infarction is present, risks for heart failure with metabolic syndrome increase to 80%. Microalbuminuria is also a marker for diastolic dysfunction, since it is linked to increased permeability of the myocardial microcirculation, leading to myocardial fibrosis. There is vasoconstriction in the myocardium that leads to reperfusion injury, additional myocardial fibrosis, and diastolic dysfunction. Metabolic syndrome is also related to mitochondrial dysfunction in myocardiocytes. The fat: water ratio

of the myocardium increases with body weight and decreased glucose tolerance. Metabolism of triglycerides and FFAs forms lipotoxic compounds such as ceramide. These lead to oxidative stress, increased myocardial apoptosis, and more myocardial fibrosis. With chronic metabolic syndrome, valve calcification, mostly of the aortic leaflets is another heart failure risk factor. It may result in stenosis or regurgitation, which can cause or intensify heart failure. In women, metabolic syndrome is related to an increased risk of future peripheral artery disease, but this is mostly regulated via effects of inflammation and endothelial damage.

RESPIRATORY MANIFESTATIONS OF METABOLIC SYNDROME

Metabolic syndrome has also been linked with a variety of respiratory manifestations. There is a close relationship between the metabolic syndrome and chronic obstructive pulmonary disease (COPD). Though not fully understood, much higher C-peptide levels are seen in patients with metabolic syndrome and COPD. There is also a positive link between C-peptide and the amount of years patients may have smoked cigarettes. There is a negative link between C-peptide and vitamin D in people who still smoke. The prevalence of metabolic syndrome in people with COPD is estimated as being between 21% and 53%.

Other respiratory manifestations of metabolic syndrome include lung function impairment, pulmonary hypertension, asthma, tuberculosis, and obstructive sleep apnea. However, it is not clear as to whether metabolic syndrome affects the respiratory system independent of obesity. While tuberculosis is most prevalent in third world countries, it is important to understand if metabolic syndrome is also present, since treatment modalities can be affected. Some tuberculosis medications cause greater insulin resistance, worsening metabolic syndrome. Diabetic medications can also interact with tuberculosis treatments, cause treatment failure, and even result in drug-resistant tuberculosis. Also, asthma is individually related to diabetes mellitus, insulin resistance, and obesity – all of which are components of metabolic syndrome. Younger patients with severe asthma and metabolic syndrome often experience severe asthma symptoms as they grow. Mechanisms of action include alterations of the immune system of the lungs due to inflammatory cytokines from abdominal visceral fat. The insulin resistance from of repeated insulin increases due to overeating on a regular basis commonly occurs as a link between metabolic syndrome and obstructive sleep apnea. This apnea results in a decrease in oxygen levels in the blood, causing dysfunction of the beta cells that produce insulin.

METABOLIC SYNDROME AND THE LIVER

Metabolic syndrome is linked to nonalcoholic fatty liver disease as well as nonalcoholic **steatohepatitis**. Nonalcoholic fatty liver disease (NAFLD) is the primary hepatic manifestation of metabolic syndrome. It is one the most common liver disease, and is estimated (in the United States) to be present in 38% of obese children, 34% of adults, and 9.6% of nonobese children. Ultrasound studies show that up to 78% of type 2 diabetes patients have a fatty liver. There is accumulation of triglycerides and various amounts of liver injury, inflammation, and repair. Appearance of this condition mostly depends on increased fatty acid flow from excessive lipolysis from insulin-resistant adipose tissue. About 90% of patients with NAFLD have more than one feature of metabolic syndrome, and about 33% have three or more criteria. Lipotoxicity results in accumulation of triglycerides in the liver, because of imbalances between uptake, synthesis, export, and oxidation of fatty acids. The presence of NAFLD is seen in more than 66% of obese patients. Hepatitis C virus (HCV) infection is more common along with type 2 diabetes, and often coexists along with NAFLD. Hepatic steatosis exists in 50% of people infected with HCV. Combined steatosis with HCV infection leads to more fibrosis and a higher likelihood of the patient not responding to antiviral therapies.

With extreme hepatocellular injury and inflammation, nonalcoholic steatohepatitis (NASH) is present. This condition can progress to advanced fibrosis and cirrhosis of the liver. This occurs in 33% or more of patients, reduces life expectancy because of liver-related death and cardiovascular events. Development of NASH is from lipotoxicity, influenced by signaling from outside of the liver, as well as from the intrahepatic activation of fibrogenic and inflammatory pathways. When metabolic syndrome is present, prognosis is worse if cirrhosis is present, due to any cause. There are also complex interactions with the HCV infection. Metabolic syndrome also increases risks for hepatocellular carcinoma. Overall, metabolic syndrome causes higher risks of deaths due to liver-related and unrelated reasons.

Excessive aldehyde production in the liver speeds up apoptosis of hepatocytes, along with necrosis and scarring of the liver. Most patients with NASH have elevated transaminases, a ballooning degeneration of the hepatocytes, **Mallory hyaline bodies**, and polymorphonuclear leukocyte infiltration. These features indicate that there is a chance of developing cirrhosis, and a chance of death within 10 years, either due to liver failure or hepatocellular carcinoma.

Fat accumulation in the liver, like metabolic syndrome, is caused by consuming excessive amounts of refined and processed carbohydrates. These include sugar, high-fructose corn syrup, and refined grains and starches. All of them are quickly converted in the liver to VLDL and triglycerides. Foods and drinks that contain fructose, and other sugars may overwhelm the liver's ability for processing, resulting in excessive fat storage and fatty liver disease. Sometimes, this leads to liver damage, failure, and death. It is also the primary factor involved in insulin resistance. Therefore, fatty liver disease is an important marker for metabolic syndrome. Fortunately, fatty liver disease is reversible, meaning that metabolic syndrome can be treated or prevented.

CANCER AND METABOLIC SYNDROME

Cancers of the breasts (in postmenopausal women), colon, endometrium, esophagus, gallbladder, kidneys, liver, pancreas, and stomach are linked to metabolic syndrome. In men, metabolic syndrome is linked to 67% higher risks of colorectal-related cancer deaths. In women, this risk is only 29% higher. There are many modifiable risk factors that exist between cancer and metabolic syndrome. These include age, genetics, obesity, physical inactivity, alcohol use, smoking, unhealthy diet, endocrine disorders, air pollution, and circadian clock disturbances. Metabolic syndrome increases risks for cancer and related deaths. Also, cancer survivors have an increased risk of developing metabolic syndrome. Links between metabolic syndrome and cancer may include hyperinsulinemia, changes to the insulin-like growth factor system, abnormalities of adipokines and the metabolism of sex hormones, chronic subclinical inflammation, alterations of gene expression and hormone profiles by air pollution or endocrine disruptors, hyperglycemia, and abnormal circadian rhythms. The *common soil hypothesis* explains that metabolic syndrome may be a marker for dietary risk factors of cancer, as well as a warning sign for susceptible people that are exposed to an unhealthy diet. Following healthy dietary patterns reduces risks for metabolic syndrome, and improved diet is always related to reductions in cancer-related deaths.

The inflammation seen in metabolic syndrome is also related to cancer because it influences the growth, apoptosis, and proliferation of tumor and **stromal cells**. The actual mechanisms are not fully understood. Diabetes mellitus and cancer are related to abnormal metabolism of lactate. High lactate levels are important biological features of both diseases. High lactate results in higher insulin resistance as well as greater malignancy in the phenotype of cancer cells. Metabolic syndrome is associated with a 20%–60% estimated increase in risks of colorectal, endometrial, liver, pancreatic, and postmenopausal breast cancers. With prostate cancer and metabolic syndrome, tumors are more likely to be aggressive and recurrent. In patients with metabolic syndrome, once cancer of any type is diagnosed, there are higher risks for postsurgical complications, recurrences, and death. For survivors of childhood cancers, metabolic syndrome is a common late effect, and there may be years of latency before it appears.

Increased leptin levels, seen in obesity and metabolic syndrome, are linked to breast, colon, endometrial, and prostate cancers. Leptin increases production of metalloproteinases and promotes angiogenesis. Therefore, it is related to increased metastatic activities. Vascular endothelial growth factor (VEGF) is produced in greater quantities because of the effects of estrogen, hypoxia, insulin-like growth factor 1, insulin, tumor necrosis factor-alpha, and leptin. Metabolic syndrome increases VEGF levels, increasing angiogenesis, tumor progression, and metastases. Because of high metabolism, cancer cells have increased needs for glucose. The cells speed up the activity of glucose transporters. Therefore, energy restriction inhibits tumor development and progression. In diabetic or glucose-intolerant patients, increased supply of glucose may explain increased risks for some types of cancer and related deaths.

FACTORS THAT WORSEN METABOLIC SYNDROME

About half of all cases of metabolic syndrome are related to genetics, the environment present during intrauterine development, or both. At important points in intrauterine development, the fetus is insulin-resistant in order to conserve energy and survive. This type of insulin resistance may protect against starvation to some degree later in life. Low birth weight is another major predictor for metabolic syndrome. Babies born to smaller women have more subscapular fat, which is proportional to the volume of peritoneal fat. This means the babies have a neonatal form of metabolic syndrome when they are born. By the age of 8 years, most of these babies have features of metabolic syndrome as well. Genetics, the environment in the mother's uterus, and the amount of postnatal growth work together to predispose individuals to later development of metabolic syndrome.

Lifestyle is highly implicated in the development and worsening of metabolic syndrome. Cigarette smoking increases risks for the development of cardiovascular disease and worsens MetSyn. Individuals who smoke more than a pack of cigarettes per day may develop more than 70% type 2 diabetes. Hormone imbalances in smokers promotes accumulation of abdominal fat, leading to insulin resistance. Lack of exercise is another primary factor that worsens metabolic syndrome, along with family history and increased aging. A poor diet is definitely a contributing factor to metabolic syndrome, including excessive alcohol consumption. Carbohydrates are the most important dietary factor to reduce. There should be very limited consumption of sugary foods and drinks, including candy, white flour and rice, carbonated soda, frozen pizza, fried foods, margarine, pastry, potato chips, and nondairy coffee creamer. Also, excessive salt should be avoided since it increases risks for hypertension and other heart diseases. Foods that are high in sodium include potato chips, canned vegetables, cottage cheese, other types of cheese, buttermilk, canned soup, cured meat, bottled salad dressings, soy sauce, and large amounts of ketchup and mustard. Other factors that worsen metabolic syndrome include low-fiber foods, fatty meats, and saturated fat.

Risk factors that worsen metabolic syndrome include aging, loss of muscle mass, obesity, and insufficient exercise. Increased levels of catecholamines worsen anxiety and metabolic syndrome. Diabetic patients with depression may require major increases in insulin dosages to alleviate the depressed mood, and then decreases in insulin once depression subsides. Often, antidepressants are the only method to obtain glycemic control in diabetic patients that are depressed. Infection worsens metabolic syndrome by increasing levels of cytokines, catecholamines, and cortisol. An asymptomatic urinary tract infection or a tooth abscess can cause hyperglycemia in a diabetic patient. Glycemic control is quickly improved by treatment with antibiotics, or by abscess drainage. Illnesses that are acute or severe also worsen metabolic syndrome. Examples include clinically silent myocardial infarctions and various malignant cancers. Other factors that may worsen metabolic syndrome include depletion of testosterone, use of androgen-deprivation therapy, a postmenopausal state, as well as high doses of thiazide diuretics and other agents such as glucocorticoids, and antiretroviral drugs.

FACTORS THAT IMPROVE METABOLIC SYNDROME

There are preventive measures for metabolic syndrome, as well as measures to improve the condition. Prevention is a primary goal. Abdominal obesity must be decreased or prevented as a key factor in relation to metabolic syndrome. There must be an improved-quality diet and increased physical activity for weight loss, as well as prevention of hyperglycemia and insulin resistance. Blood pressure must be lowered to less than 140/90 mm Hg ideally. The **DASH diet**, meaning *dietary approaches to stop hypertension*, helps assist in this process, along with lifestyle modifications.

A variety of diets have been successful for metabolic syndrome. Each individual's meal plan should be designed by a registered dietitian nutritionist, so that energy intake can be decreased. Diets that protect against metabolic syndrome include those balanced in carbohydrate intake, low in saturated fats, high in dietary fiber, high in fruits and vegetables, and those that include low-fat dairy foods. Foods with simple sugars and refined grains must be reduced. These include candy, desserts, juices, soda, sweetened breakfast cereals, and white bread. Whole grain and high-fiber foods must be increased. These include fruits, legumes, oatmeal, vegetables, and whole-grain bread. Omega-3 fatty acid is very important, and is found in fish and flax seed – these should be consumed at least two times per week.

A Mediterranean-style diet has been proven to reduce risks for metabolic syndrome. This includes beans, fruits, grains, nuts, and vegetables. Olives and olive oil are important components. Sweet foods are only used occasionally, such as for birthdays and relatively rare events. *Healthy carbohydrates* should make up 40%–50% of the daily energy intake. *Healthy fats* should make up 30%–5%, and *healthy proteins* should make up the remainder. Losing just 5%–% of body weight helps reduce insulin levels. In comparative studies between the Mediterranean diet a general low-fat diet, 44% of the Mediterranean diet group still had metabolic syndrome over 2.5 years, but an outstanding 86% of the general low-fat diet still had the syndrome. Other features of this study included four times more weight loss in the Mediterranean diet group, and greatly reduced inflammatory markers and insulin resistance. Foods that are rich in antioxidants help to combat levels of free radicals and oxidate stress that are related to meals that are high in calories and contain refined carbohydrates. Also, one glass of red wine with an evening meal reduces postprandial glucose by about 30% in a healthy adult – including those with metabolic syndrome or type 2 diabetes. Other types of alcohol lower the postprandial glucose by about 20%.

For adults, just 60 minutes or more every day in moderate-to-vigorous physical activity reduces abdominal obesity, hypertriglyceridemia, and improves HDL cholesterol levels. People that spend less than 30 minutes per day in this type of activity have much higher rates of metabolic syndrome and its related conditions. Regular physical activity improves metabolic syndrome, regardless of gender, age, education, alcohol use, smoking, and amount of time spent being inactive. Vigorous physical activity reduces risks of metabolic syndrome by 33%, while moderate activity only provides a small risk reduction. In patients that already had impaired glucose tolerance, regular participation in resistance training is proven to have improved metabolic syndrome. Examples of vigorous and moderate physical activities are listed in Table 2.2.

Management of metabolic syndrome, between patients and healthcare providers, includes controlling BP, lowering LDL cholesterol, increasing HDL cholesterol, and lower triglycerides. Treatment is also designed to prevent onset of type 2 diabetes mellitus. Medications can be added when lifestyle changes are completely effective. These include metformin, statins, and antihypertensives. Allopurinol may also reduce insulin resistance and symptoms of metabolic syndrome. Supplements include alpha lipoic

Table 2.2: Examples of Vigorous and Moderate Physical Activities

Vigorous Physical Activities	Moderate Physical Activities
Aerobic dancing	Ballroom dancing
Bicycling at 10 miles/hour or more	Bicycling at less than 10 miles/hour
Heavy gardening – continuously digging	General gardening
Hiking uphill, while wearing a heavy backpack	Tennis
Jumping rope	Walking briskly (3 miles/hour or faster, but not race-walking)
Running, jogging, or race-walking	Water aerobics

acid, green tea or green tea extract, glycine powder, raspberry ketone, bitter melon extract, potassium, and omega-3 fatty acids.

Smoking cessation or avoidance means that risks for metabolic syndrome are lowered. Another factor linked to metabolic syndrome is sleep deprivation. There is evidence supporting a link between metabolic syndrome and nonalcoholic fatty liver disease. Gallstones are also related to metabolic syndrome. Overall, the global population needs to be counseled about lifestyle modifications, include better diets and increased physical activity. Cardiovascular disease risks should be emphasized.

KEY TERMS

- Acanthosis nigricans
- Adipokines
- Adiponectin
- Alzheimer's disease
- Angiotensinogen
- Blood-brain barrier
- Ceramide
- Corona
- Cytokines
- DASH diet
- Diapedesis
- Foam cells
- Hippocampus
- Insulin resistance
- Interleukin-6
- Leptin
- Lipodystrophy
- Mallory hyaline bodies
- Neurotrophins
- Omental
- Plasmin
- Reaven syndrome
- Resistin
- Steatohepatitis
- Stromal cells
- Syndrome X
- Tissue plasminogen activator
- Vasa nervorum
- Visuospatial deficits

REFERENCES

Ahima, R.S. (2016). *Metabolic Syndrome: A Comprehensive Textbook*. Springer Reference.

American Diabetes Association – Diabetes Care. (2003). *The Metabolic Syndrome as Predictor of Type 2 Diabetes – The San Antonio Heart Study*. American Diabetes Association. https://care.diabetesjournals.org/content/26/11/3153

Bagchi, D., and Sreejayan, N. (2012). *Nutritional and Therapeutic Interventions for Diabetes and Metabolic Syndrome*. Academic Press.

Cambridge University Press – Cambridge Core. (2013). *Metabolic Syndrome and Major Depression*. Cambridge University Press. https://www.cambridge.org/core/journals/cns-spectrums/article/abs/metabolic-syndrome-and-major-depression/33155DD83C8758ED4EF83274575794D7

Challem, J., Berkson, B., and Smith, M.D. (2000). *Syndrome X: The Complete Nutritional Program to Prevent and Reverse Insulin Resistance*. Wiley.

CommunityBulkSupplements.com – Conditions. (2019). *Metabolic Syndrome: Risk Factors, Diagnosis & Treatment*. BulkSupplements.com. https://community.bulksupplements.com/metabolic-syndrome/

DeFronzo, R.A., Ferrannini, E., Zimmett, P., and Alberti, G. (2015). *International Textbook of Diabetes Mellitus*, 2 Volume Set, 4th Edition. Wiley-Blackwell.

Diabetes Care Community. (2021). *What Is the Link between Diabetes and Metabolic Syndrome?* Diabetes Care Community. https://www.diabetescarecommunity.ca/diabetes-overview-articles/link-diabetes-metabolic-syndrome/

Diabetes Education Services. (2008). *Diabetes Mellitus and Metabolic Syndrome by Beverly Thomassian*. Diabetes Education Services. https://www.diabetesed.net/page/_files/Diabetes-Mellitus-and-Metabolic-Syndrome.PDF

Duarte, C.B., and Tongiorgi, E. (2019). *Brain-Derived Neurotrophic Factor (BDNF) (Neuromethods, 143 – Springer Protocols)*. Humana Press.

Ekoe, J.M., Rewers, M., Williams, R., and Zimmet, P. (2008). *The Epidemiology of Diabetes Mellitus*, 2nd Edition. Wiley-Blackwell.

Farrell, G.C., McCullough, A.J., and Day, C.P. (2013). *Non-Alcoholic Fatty Liver Disease: A Practical Guide*. Wiley-Blackwell.

Frontiers in Cell and Developmental Biology – Cellular Biochemistry. (2021). *From Metabolic Syndrome to Neurological Diseases: Role of Autophagy*. Frontiers Media S.A. https://internal-journal.frontiersin.org/articles/10.3389/fcell.2021.651021/full

Garg, A. (2015). *Dyslipidemias: Pathophysiology, Evaluation and Management (Contemporary Endocrinology)*. Humana Press.

George, A., Augustine, R., and Sebastian, M. (2021). *Diabetes Mellitus and Human Health Care*. Apple Academic.

Gonzalez-Campoy, J.M., Hurley, D.L., and Garvey, W.T. (2019). *Bariatric Endocrinology: Evaluation and Management of Adiposity, Adiposopathy and Related Diseases*. Springer.

Hindawi – Mediators of Inflammation, Yong Wu et al. (2017). *Metabolic Syndrome, Inflammation, and Cancer*. https://www.hindawi.com/journals/mi/2017/8259356/

Holt, R.I.G., Cockram, C., Flyvbjerg, A., and Goldstein, B.J. (2016). *Textbook of Diabetes*, 4th Edition. Wiley-Blackwell.

Holt, R.I.G., and Hanley, N.A. (2021). *Essential Endocrinology and Diabetes*, 7th Edition. Wiley-Blackwell.

Jesse Santiano M.D. (2019). *Lung Diseases Associated with Metabolic Syndrome*. https://drjessesantiano.com/diseases-related-to-the-metabolic-syndrome-part-2/

Joshi, S.R. (2020). *RSSDI Textbook of Diabetes Mellitus*, 4th Edition. Jaypee Brothers Medical Publishers, Ltd.

Litwack, G. (2017). *Neurotrophins (ISSN Book 104)*. Academic Press.

Myerson, M. (2018). *Dyslipidemia: A Clinical Approach*. Wolters Kluwer.

National Cholesterol Education Program. (2002). *Third Report of the NCEP Expert Panel on Detection, Evaluation, and Treatment of High Blood Cholesterol in Adults (Adult Treatment Panel III) Final Report*. NCEP. https://www.nhlbi.nih.gov/files/docs/resources/heart/atp-3-cholesterol-full-report.pdf

NCBI – PMC – U.S. National Library of Medicine – National Institutes of Health. (2017). *Prevalence of Metabolic Syndrome and Metabolic Syndrome Components in Young Adults: A Pooled Analysis*. National Center for Biotechnology Information – U.S. National Library of Medicine. https://www.ncbi.nlm.nih.gov/pmc/articles/PMC5540707/

NIH – National Library of Medicine – National Center for Biotechnology Information. (2018). *Metabolic Syndrome and Cancer: "The Common Soil Hypothesis"*. National Library of Medicine. https://pubmed.ncbi.nlm.nih.gov/29807099/

NIH – National Library of Medicine – National Center for Biotechnology Information. (2017). *Metabolic Syndrome and Chronic Obstructive Pulmonary Disease (COPD): The Interplay among Smoking, Insulin Resistance and Vitamin D*. National Library of Medicine. https://pubmed.ncbi.nlm.nih.gov/29065130/

NIH – National Library of Medicine – National Center for Biotechnology Information. (2016). *Metabolic Syndrome and the Lung*. National Library of Medicine. https://pubmed.ncbi.nlm.nih.gov/26836925/

NIH – National Library of Medicine – National Center for Biotechnology Information. (2014). *The Metabolic Syndrome and Chronic Liver Disease*. National Library of Medicine. https://pubmed.ncbi.nlm.nih.gov/24320032/

NIH – National Library of Medicine – National Center for Biotechnology Information. (2009). *Metabolic Syndrome and Non-Alcoholic Fatty Liver Disease*. National Library of Medicine. https://pubmed.ncbi.nlm.nih.gov/19381120/

Poretsky, L. (2017). *Principles of Diabetes Mellitus*, 3rd Edition. Springer Reference.

Proctor Joslin, E. (2017). *The Treatment of Diabetes Mellitus: With Observations upon the Disease Based upon Thirteen Hundred Cases*. Andesrite Press.

Rolla, A.R., and Agarwal, S. (2019). *Clinical Atlas of Diabetes Mellitus*. Jaypee Brothers Medical Publishers, Ltd.

Rygiel, K.A. (2013). *Atherogenic Dyslipidemia Index: A Helpful Marker for Detecting Primary Care Patients with High Cardiometabolic Risk*. Lap Lambert Academic Publishing.

ScienceDirect – Nutrition, Metabolism and Cardiovascular Diseases. (2021). *Metabolic Syndrome and the Risk of COVID-19 Infection: A Nationwide Population-Based Case-Control Study*. Elsevier B.V. https://www.sciencedirect.com/science/article/pii/S0939475321002398

Semantic Scholar. (2008). *Blood Viscosity and Hematocrit as Risk Factors for Type 2 Diabetes Mellitus*. Semantic Scholar. https://www.semanticscholar.org/paper/Blood-Viscosity-and-Hematocrit-as-Risk-Factors-for-Tamariz-Young/5163f75ce0f9ee351ba1a9f201893da873c54d34

Sies, H. (2007). *Oxidative Stress and Inflammatory Mechanisms in Obesity, Diabetes, and the Metabolic Syndrome (Book 22)*. CRC Press.

Southwestern Vermont Health Care. (2020). *Fatty Liver Disease and Metabolic Syndrome*. Southwestern Vermont Health Care. https://svhealthcare.org/Wellness-Connection/fatty-liver-disease-and-metabolic-syndrome

Tantuzzi, G., and Braunschweig, C. (2014). *Adipose Tissue and Adipokines in Health and Disease (Nutrition and Health)*, 2nd Edition. Humana Press.

Thomas, N. (2018). *A Practical Guide to Diabetes Mellitus*, 8th Edition. Jaypee Brothers Medical Publishers, Ltd.

Today's Dietitian. (2020). *Cancer Nutrition: Metabolic Syndrome and Cancer – Insights on Their Intersection*. Great Valley Publishing Company. https://www.todaysdietitian.com/newarchives/1020p14.shtml

Umpierrez, G.E. (2014). *Therapy for Diabetes Mellitus and Related Disorders*, 6th Edition. American Diabetes Association.

U.S. Department of Health and Human Services, Agency for Healthcare Research and Quality. (2014). *Effects of Omega-3 Fatty Acids on Lipids and Glycemic Control in Type II Diabetes and the Metabolic Syndrome and on Inflammatory Bowel Disease, Rheumatoid Arthritis, Renal Disease, Systemic Lupus Erythematosus, and Osteoporosis. (Report/Technology Assessment #89)*. CreateSpace Independent Publishing Platform.

U.S. Department of Health & Human Services – NIH – National Heart, Lung, and Blood Institute. (2021). *Metabolic Syndrome*. NIH – National Heart, Lung, and Blood Institute. https://www.nhlbi.nih.gov/health-topics/metabolic-syndrome

U.S. Pharmacist – Cardiovascular. (2009). *Metabolic Syndrome and Cardiovascular Risk Factors*. Jobson Medical Information LLC. https://www.uspharmacist.com/article/metabolic-syndrome-and-cardiovascular-risk-factors

Wallach, J.D., and Lan, M. (2005). *Hell's Kitchen: Causes, Prevention and Cure of Obesity, Diabetes and Metabolic Syndrome*, 3rd Edition. Wellness Publications.

Watson, R.R., and Zibadi, S. (2018). *Lifestyle in Heart Health and Disease*. Academic Press.

White, Jr., J.R. (2020). *The 2020–21 Guide to Medications for the Therapy of Diabetes Mellitus*. American Diabetes Association.

CHAPTER 3 Prevalence, Mortality, and Risk Factors

INCIDENCE

Incidence is the occurrence of new cases of a disease in a population, over a specific time period. It is based on three key factors. These are the new occurrences of the disease, the population in which it occurs, and the amount of time that the population is monitored until the disease develops. For recurrent diseases, incidence usually defines the *first occurrence*. A **candidate population** is the group of people at risk for the disease. While incidence is measurable in people that are not "at risk," it is not as important. Since incidence assesses a transition from good health to a disease state, time is required for its measurement.

Cumulative Incidence

Cumulative incidence is the number of people in a candidate population that develops a disease over a specific amount of time. This is expressed as the number of new cases, divided by the amount in the candidate population, over a certain time period. The possible value of cumulative incidence ranges between 0 and 1. If it is thought of as a percentage, the cumulative incidence ranges between 0% and 100%. For example, if there were 3,055 new cases of diabetes in a candidate population of 28,000 people over a study period of 1 year, the cumulative incidence would be 10.9% for that time period. Another way to understand this is that cumulative incidence illustrates the average risk of developing a disease over a certain period of time. A *risk* is the likelihood of the disease being developed. The *lifetime risk of diabetes mellitus* is about 40% of the global population. Generally, cumulative incidence is higher over a lifetime or many years than for only a few years.

Incidence Rate

The **incidence rate** is the amount of new cases of a disease during an observation of *person-time*. It is calculated by dividing the number of new cases by the person-time within a candidate population. Since time (t) is a component here, the incidence rate is a *true rate*. The dimension used to calculate this is *1 over t*, also written as t^{-1}. The possible values do not range from 0 to 1, but instead range from zero to **infinity**. An incidence rate of infinity would only be present if all members of the population died at once. **Person-time** is more difficult to understand. It adds up in people who are at risk for a disease. Each person contributes time to the incidence rate until being diagnosed with the specific disease. Unlike cumulative incidence, incidence rate is based on all the candidate population being monitored for a certain period. Person-time adds up only during this period. It stops if a person dies or is no longer monitored –

which sometimes happens if he or she moves to another location. Incidence may be calculated for a *fixed population* or a *dynamic population*. Since it considers population changes from births, deaths, and migration, incidence rate is helpful in measuring transitions between health and disease in dynamic populations.

PREVALENCE

Prevalence calculates the actual frequency of a disease. It is the proportion of a total population with the disease. **Point prevalence** is the proportion of the population with the disease at *one point in time*. The *point* can be an actual date, or a specific occurrence in an individual's life. Point prevalence is expressed as the number of existing cases, divided by the number in the total population, at a specific point in time. Therefore, the prevalence of diabetes mellitus refers to the existing cases or deaths, expressed as proportions of the population, over certain times. The amounts are divided by the number of people in the specific population, to calculate the percentages. *Point prevalence* refers to *all cases or deaths*. It is calculated by dividing the number of cases by the size of the same population, then multiplied by a certain value. If 100 is the value used to multiply, a percentage is created. So, if there were 5,000 existing cases of diabetes within a total population of 160,000, the point prevalence now the study was performed would be 3.1%.

Period prevalence is the proportion of a population with the disease during a *period of time*, such as a certain year. It includes the cases that were present over the course of that year. Period prevalence is expressed as the number of existing cases, divided by the number in the total population, during a specific time period. If a 1-year study was done, with 35,000 existing cases of diabetes, within a total population of 265,000, the period prevalence over 1 year would be 13.2%. *Lifetime prevalence* refers to cases of a disease diagnosed at any time during a person's lifetime.

USES OF INCIDENCE AND PREVALENCE

Incidence is important in evaluating the effectiveness of methods tried, to prevent a disease from occurring. New cases are preferred to be studied, compared to existing cases (prevalence). This is true because prevalence combines incidence with survival. Incidence is also preferred since the timing of causative factors related to development of the disease can be determined more accurately. *Prevalence* is effective for estimating needs of healthcare providers in treating people who have developed a disease. It is required to study conditions such as diabetes,

DOI: 10.1201/9781003226727-4

birth defects and arthritis, since it is difficult to ascertain exactly when these conditions were caused.

GLOBAL PREVALENCE OF DIABETES

Diabetes is the most diagnosed noncommunicable disease throughout the world, and is also the fastest growing chronic disease. According to the International Diabetes Federation, cases of diabetes increased from 108 million in 1980 to 463 million in 2019. They are predicted to increase to 700 million by the year 2045. Proportions of people with type 2 diabetes are increasing in most countries. Most adults with diabetes (about 79%) live in low- or middle-income countries. Over 20% of people over age 65 have diabetes, and 50% of people with diabetes have not been diagnosed. In 2019, there were about 4.2 million global deaths attributed to diabetes. Healthcare costs were equivalent to 760 billion US dollars, which was 10% of the total spending of adult health care in 2019. Type 1 diabetes is present in over 1.1 million children and teenagers. Over one of every six live births is affected by diabetes during pregnancy. Approximately 374 million people are at increased risk of eventually developing type 2 diabetes sometime in their lives. *Diabetes UK* published a 2013 study that summarized a list of countries regarding incidence of type 1 diabetes in children up to age 14. The list was updated by the International Diabetes Federation in 2019. Though the United Kingdom ranks very low on other incidence lists concerning diabetes, they placed sixth in this list.

Over decades, due to more widespread Westernized lifestyles and diet, there has been a global epidemic of type 2 diabetes. Adult cases of diabetes will more than double by the year 2030. Most increases will occur in developing countries, especially Asia. By 2030, India may have 79–87 million people with type 2 diabetes, and China may have 42–63 million. This means that the complications of diabetes will also increase. In the United States, for all body mass index (BMI) categories, Asian Americans have an overall 60% higher prevalence of diabetes than Caucasians. Interventions concerning diabetes must focus on advertising, patient education, workplaces, availability and pricing of healthy foods, and taxation policies.

DISTRIBUTION OF DIABETES BY HOST FACTORS

Diabetes is distributed globally based on a variety of host factors. Prevalence of diabetes increases greatly by age. Approximately 14% of adults 80 years of age or older have the disease. There is a similar prevalence between men and women, though rates are about 1% higher in elderly women compared to elderly men. This difference is believed to be because there are simply more elderly women than men in most populations, due to life expectancy.

Age

Older age increases risks for type 2 diabetes, heart disease, and stroke. Healthy diets, sufficient physical activity, and weight management are important in helping to prevent type 2 diabetes from developing. Cholesterol, blood pressure, and blood glucose control are also required. Globally, patients that follow medical advice in these areas are more likely to stop diabetes progression and resulting complications. About half of all people with diabetes are over 60 years of age. The highest prevalence is in people over 80. In the United States alone, this number is expected to reach 40 million by the year 2050.

Sex

Men are at a slightly higher risk of developing diabetes than women. This may be in relation to lifestyle, weight, and the locations of the weight on their bodies. For example, abdominal weight is more often linked to type 2 diabetes than when weight is located around the hips. More men have also been shown to become sedentary as they age compared to women. Also, men develop diabetes when they have a lower degree of obesity than women. Generally, men have more abdominal fat, while women have more peripheral fat. Men often have more visceral and hepatic fat, but women have more subcutaneous fat. Better insulin sensitivity occurs with more subcutaneous fat compared to more visceral fat. Therefore, men developing diabetes at a lower BMI is because of their higher amounts of visceral fat.

Gender differences in body fat distribution are related to different **insulin resistance**. Men usually have more insulin resistance than women, and also have elevated fasting glucose levels. However, more women have elevated 2-hour glucose concentrations. Differences in glucose concentrations during fasting are probably due to physiological differences linked to male or female sex hormones. After menopause, decreased insulin sensitivity may mean that *estrogen* has beneficial effects in women. Estrogen also affects distribution of adipose tissue. Oppositely, *testosterone* levels are obviously higher in men than women, and are related to central fat accumulation in both genders. Low amounts of *sex hormone binding globulin* are linked to increased risk of insulin resistance and type 2 diabetes. This occurs regardless of the amounts of circulating sex hormones.

Genetic Susceptibility

Diabetes mellitus is made up of a **heterogeneous** group of disorders. Type 1 diabetes is less inheritable than other forms of the disease. The concordance rate of type 1 diabetes, even in monozygous twins, is only 30%. For dizygous twins, the rate is just 10%. First-degree relatives have a higher risk for type 1 diabetes than unrelated people. More than 20 regions of the **genome** may be implicated in genetic susceptibility to the disease. This region contains several hundred genes involved in immune responses.

Type 1 diabetes is not totally genetically determined. Environmental risk factors are more important, acting as initiators or accelerators of beta cell autoimmunity. They may also precipitate symptoms when there already has been beta cell destruction. Viruses such as Coxsackie virus B (CVB), cytomegalovirus, mumps, rotavirus, and rubella play larger roles in development of type 1 diabetes than genetics. Though genetics do not currently play a role in the management or prevention of the disease, it is hoped that genetic testing will be able to identify individuals at high risk, before type 1 diabetes actually develops. Predictive genetic testing could be preventive. It would be offered to families that already have an affected individual before being made available to the general public.

For type 2 diabetes mellitus, the situation is different. First-degree relatives of people with this type are about three times more likely to develop type 2 diabetes than people with no family history of the disease. Concordance rates for monozygotic twins are 60%–90%. This is much higher than for dizygotic twins (20%–30%). Type 2 diabetes obviously has genetic susceptibility, based on identification of **candidate genes**. These genes may be involved in pancreatic beta cell function, energy intake, energy expenditure, glucose metabolism, insulin action, and lipid metabolism.

Race and Ethnicity

As of 2021, diabetes *incidence (new cases)* based on population is highest in China, India, the United States, Indonesia, Pakistan, Brazil, Nigeria, Bangladesh, Russia, and Mexico. However, the countries with the highest diabetes *prevalence (actual frequency)* included the Marshall Islands (30.5%), Kiribati (22.5%), Tuvalu (22.1%), Sudan (22.1%), Mauritius (22%), New Caledonia (21.8%), Pakistan (19.9%), French Polynesia (19.5%), the Solomon Islands (19%), and Guam (18.7%). The Marshall Islands, Kiribati, and Tuvalu are also among the most obese populations in the entire world.

According to the Centers for Disease Control and Prevention (CDC) *2020 National Diabetes Statistics Report*, all nonwhite racial and ethnic groups were more likely to have diabetes and its complications in comparison to Caucasians. Black, non-Hispanic individuals had the highest percentage of diabetes (16.4% of their population). This was followed by Native Americans/Alaska Natives (15.9%), Asian non-Hispanics (14.9%), Hispanics (14.7%), and Caucasian non-Hispanics (11.9%). Black patients were two times as likely to have diabetic-related kidney problems, vision loss, and amputations. Black and Hispanic patients were diagnosed at slightly younger ages than other groups. Hispanics had higher rates of diabetes-related kidney failure and loss of vision than other groups. Hispanics have specific genes that increase their chances of developing the disease. Also, in some Hispanic or Latino cultural groups, foods are high in fat and calories. There are higher rates of obesity and lower rates of physical activity. These general facts do not apply to some Hispanic or Latino cultural groups.

Socioeconomic Factors

Lower income may be related to a higher prevalence of diabetes and its complications. The lowest socioeconomic group has the most cases of diabetes mellitus per their population, and the most hospitalizations for the disease. The highest socioeconomic group has the least cases and hospitalizations. Factors include employment insecurity, low income, less education, and poor living conditions. Access to quality food sources is a major problem. People with lower income and less education are two to four times more likely to develop diabetes than those in higher socioeconomic groups. Lower socioeconomic groups often have chronic stress because of difficulties in simply surviving. This may result in poor choices such as use of tobacco and alcohol, and the consumption of inexpensive, unhealthy foods. Chronic stress increases blood pressure, cortisol, and blood glucose. These factors combine to increase the likelihood of obesity and development of type 2 diabetes.

Once diabetes develops, a poorer individual may not be able to afford proper care for the disease. There may be lack of access to health care, nutrition, and adequate housing. The situation then is able to continually worsen, and complications of the disease multiply. Diabetes can reduce work productivity or college study, leading to more deprivation, poverty, and social exclusion. In people of lower socioeconomic status, there is usually less **glycemic control** and more complications that otherwise should be avoidable.

MORTALITY ATTRIBUTABLE TO DIABETES AND ITS COMPLICATIONS

According to the World Health Organization, in 2020, an estimated 4.2 million deaths occurred globally in relation to diabetes and its complications. There was a 5% increase in premature deaths from diabetes between the years 2010 and 2016. Almost 50% of deaths attributed to high blood glucose occur before the age of 70 years. Diabetes will likely become the seventh leading cause of death by the year 2030. In 2018, rural areas of America were found to have a much higher number of diabetes-related hospital deaths compared to urban areas. Most hospitalizations because of diabetes occurred in the South and Midwest. In a rural area, the likelihood of dying during a diabetes-related hospitalization was 3.4% higher than in an urban area. Rural residents have longer distances to travel, and therefore, a more difficult time accessing health care. Approximately 62% of nonmetropolitan counties do not have diabetes self-management programs. Mortality rates were 21 per 100,000 in the South and 15 per 100,000 in the Midwest. In the Northeast, deaths were 11 per 100,000 and in the West, 10.8 per 100,000.

RISK FACTORS OF DIABETES MELLITUS

The risk factors of diabetes mellitus are different between the various forms of the disease. Known risk factors for type 1 diabetes include family history of the disease in a parent or sibling, younger patient age, and the Caucasian racial group. Risk factors for type 2 diabetes include prediabetes, being overweight or obese, age of 45 years or older, family history of the disease in a parent or sibling, being physically active fewer than three times per week, previous gestational diabetes, having given birth to a baby heavier than 9 pounds at delivery, and being from one of the racial or ethnic groups that have higher incidence. These groups include African American, Hispanic/Latino American, American Indian, Alaska Native, and some subgroups of Pacific Islanders and Asian Americans. Another risk factor is nonalcoholic fatty liver disease. Risk factors for prediabetes are almost identical to the risk factors for type 2 diabetes. When a woman is pregnant, the risk factors for gestational diabetes include previously diagnosed gestational diabetes, being overweight or obese, age above 25 years, family history of type 2 diabetes, **polycystic ovary syndrome**, and being from the same racial or ethnic groups as in type 2 diabetes.

DISABILITY ADJUSTED LIFE YEARS FOR DIABETES AND ITS COMPLICATIONS

Disability adjusted life years (DALYs) lost are measurements of *years of life lost* (YLL) due to premature death, plus *years lost to severe disability* (YLD). The formula for DALYs is:

$$DALY = YLL + YLD$$

The burden of disease is expressed in DALYs per 1,000 population, and rates are increasing in most countries. This is especially the case in developing nations of Asia, Africa, the Middle East, Central America, South America, and the Southwest Pacific. According to WHO, a DALY indicates the loss of an equivalent *one year of full health*. For countries with high DALYs for diabetes, populations are moving from more rural areas to cities. There are lifestyle changes that often include a more sedentary lifestyle and a high calorie diet.

Diabetes shortens life expectancy by increasing risks for many severe conditions. Poorly controlled diabetes increases risks of bacterial and fungal skin infections. It also increases chances of retinopathy, glaucoma, and cataracts. About half of all diabetic patients have resultant neuropathy. High blood glucose levels increase demands placed on the kidneys, leading to nephropathy. It also damages the cardiovascular system, increasing risks for heart disease and stroke. According to *The Lancet – Diabetes & Endocrinology*, excess body weight is associated with risk factors for cardiovascular disease and type 2 diabetes. Effects of excess weight upon YLL are highest for young individuals, decreasing with aging. YLL for obese males range from 0.8 years in the 60–79 age group, to 5.9 years in the 20–39 age group. For greatly obese males, years lost range from 0.9 years (60–79 years) to 8.4 years (20–39 years). Similar results exist for women. Healthy life years lost were up to four times higher than total YLL for all age groups and weights.

GLOBAL BURDEN OF DIABETES AND ITS COMPLICATIONS

The global burden of diabetes and its complications has greatly increased between past decades and today. In 1995, the global prevalence of diabetes in adults was estimated to be at 4%, but is predicted to reach 5.4% by the year 2025. Diabetes has a higher burden in developed countries than in developing countries. By 2025, the amount of adults with diabetes is expected to more than double. There is a predicted 42% increase in developed countries, but a 170% increase in developing countries. By 2025, most diabetic individuals will live in developing countries. The countries with the greatest diabetes burden in 2025 are predicted to be India, China, and the United States. In the United States, just 1% of the population had diabetes in 1960. As of 2020, 10.5% of the population had diabetes. This is more than 34.2 million Americans. Approximately 21.4% of the population actually has diabetes but has not yet been diagnosed.

The global burden of diabetic retinopathy is of immense significance, since the complication affects about one of every three people with diabetes and is the leading cause of blindness in adults of working age. Overall, blindness from diabetic retinopathy has decreased in higher income countries, including the United States and United Kingdom, because of better public health education, screening, control of risk factors, and treatments. However, increased cases of diabetic retinopathy-induced blindness are being seen in lower- and middle-income countries, including China, India, and Indonesia. There must be a shift toward primary and secondary prevention measures. Diabetes-related blindness costs may exceed $500 million per year in the United States alone.

The increase in the global burden of diabetes mellitus is also reflected in increased cases of diabetic neuropathy. Treatments include intensive glycemic control, pathogenetic therapies, and treatment of symptoms. Diabetic neuropathy is resulting in increased complications and healthcare costs. The total median healthcare costs were nearly $17,000 within the first year after diagnosis. Painful diabetic neuropathy costs nearly $5,200 per year for its treatment, while nonpainful diabetic neuropathy costs nearly $2,800 per year.

Diabetic patients have a two to four times greater chance of having a heart attack or stroke than nondiabetic patients. Cardiovascular conditions cause 69% of the medical cost burden globally. Cardiovascular disease is the principal cause of morbidity and death in diabetic patients – especially in those with type 2 diabetes mellitus. Diabetes-related cardiovascular complications include cerebrovascular disease, coronary heart disease, heart failure, peripheral vascular disease, and cardiovascular autonomic neuropathy. About 43% of patients with type 2 diabetes mellitus have some form of cardiovascular disease. Heart failure occurs in 50.1% of cases, followed by coronary artery disease (37.4%), myocardial infarction (18.2%), angina (17.3%), and stroke (10.5%). Atherosclerotic cardiovascular disease is the leading cause of morbidity and mortality in type 2 diabetes, and accounts for the majority of direct and indirect diabetes costs.

In adults aged 20 or older with diagnosed diabetes, nephropathy is estimated to affect 36.5%. Average expenditures for diagnosed diabetes were approximately $13,700 per year, of which $7,900 was attributed directly to diabetes. Average medical expenditures with diagnosed diabetes were about 2.3 times higher than for people without diabetes. Cost burdens also focus on insulin, which increased in price by almost two times between the years 2012 and 2016. Global costs of all types of diabetes and its complications will greatly increase by 2030, according to *Clinical Endocrinology News*. The total economic burden will increase from $1.3 trillion in 2015 to $2.1 trillion by 2030 in the United States alone.

Diabetic foot complications are among the most disabling of all outcomes. Estimated costs of amputations range between $5,000 and $70,000 based on individual studies in various countries. According to the World Diabetes Foundation, estimated costs for treatment of diabetic foot complications without amputation average nearly $18,000 per patient. Foot complications cause emotional, physical, productivity, and financial losses. Long-term costs include prosthetic devices, special footwear, rehabilitation, and costs related to chronic disability. Costs for home care and social services must also be considered.

Despite treatment options, diabetic patients face difficult challenges that reduce their quality of life and cause less productivity. They complete fewer days at work, and often, unemployment. To change this, related comorbidities must be addressed. Nearly 90% of diabetic patients have two or more underlying conditions. These include hyperlipidemia, cardiovascular disease, retinopathy, and nephropathy. More than 50% of type 2 diabetic patients die from cardiovascular disease.

According to the CDC, lifetime risks for type 2 diabetes currently stands at 40% in the United States. For some ethnic groups, risks are higher. This is a 20% increase for men and a 13% increase for women since 1985. Currently, Hispanic men and women, and African American women are at the highest risk for developing the disease. In these groups, more than 50% of people aged 20 or older are expected to develop it at some point. However, the number of life years lost in a typical patient, at age 40, declined from 7.7 years lost (in 1990–1999) to 5.8 years lost (in 2000–2011). This is because of the improvements in diabetes treatments.

KEY TERMS

- Candidate genes
- Candidate population
- Cumulative incidence
- Genome
- Glycemic control
- Heterogeneous
- Incidence

- Incidence rate
- Infinity
- Insulin resistance
- Period prevalence
- Person-time
- Point prevalence
- Polycystic ovary syndrome
- Prevalence

REFERENCES

Afroz, A. (2012). *Economic Burden of Type 2 Diabetes Mellitus: Direct Cost, Indirect Cost, and Nutritional Cost.* Lap Lambert Academic Publishing.

American Diabetes Association. (2011). *American Diabetes Association Complete Guide to Diabetes: The Ultimate Home Reference from the Diabetes Experts*, 5th Edition. American Diabetes Association.

American Diabetes Association – Diabetes Care. (2012). *Type 2 Diabetes: An Epidemic Requiring Global Attention and Urgent Action.* American Diabetes Association. https://care.diabetes-journals.org/content/35/5/943

American Diabetes Association – Diabetes Care. (2002). *Diabetes-Related Morbidity and Mortality in a National Sample of U.S. Elders.* American Diabetes Association. https://care.diabetesjournals.org/content/25/3/471

Centers for Disease Control and Prevention. (2013). *Diabetes State Burden Toolkit – Estimated Years of Life Lost (YLL) Due to Diabetes, United States, 2013.* U.S. Department of Health & Human Services – HHS/Open – USA.gov. https://nccd.cdc.gov/toolkit/diabetesburden/yll

Centers for Disease Control and Prevention. (2021). *Diabetes Risk Factors.* U.S. Department of Health & Human Services – USA.gov – CDC. https://www.cdc.gov/diabetes/basics/risk-factors.html

Centers for Disease Control and Prevention – Diabetes – National Diabetes Statistics Report. (2017). *Estimates of Diabetes and Its Burden in the United States.* U.S. Department of Health & Human Services – USA.gov – CDC. https://www.cdc.gov/diabetes/data/statistics-report/index.html

Centers for Disease Control and Prevention – National Center for Chronic Disease Prevention and Health Promotion (NCCDPHP). (2020). *Division of Diabetes Translation At A Glance.* U.S. Department of Health & Human Services – USA.gov – CDC. www.cdc.gov/chronicdisease/resources/publications/aag/diabetes.htm

Centers for Disease Control and Prevention – National Center for Chronic Disease Prevention and Health Promotion (NCCDPHP). (2017a). *Diabetes 2017 Report Card.* CDC. www.cdc.gov/diabetes/pdfs/library/diabetesreportcard2017-508.pdf

Centers for Disease Control and Prevention – National Center for Chronic Disease Prevention and Health Promotion (NCCDPHP). (2017b). *Diabetes and Prediabetes.* U.S. Department of Health & Human Services – USA.gov – CDC. https://www.cdc.gov/chronicdisease/resources/publications/factsheets/diabetes-prediabetes.htm

Centers for Disease Control and Prevention – National Center for Health Statistics. (2018). *Diabetes.* U.S. Department of Health & Human Services – USA.gov – CDC. https://www.cdc.gov/nchs/fastats/diabetes.htm

Centers for Disease Control and Prevention – National Health Interview Survey (NHIS). (2018). *Diagnosed Diabetes.* CDC. https://gis.cdc.gov/grasp/diabetes/diabetesatlas.html

Cryer, P.E. (2013). *Hypoglycemia in Diabetes: Pathophysiology, Prevalence, and Prevention*, 2nd Edition. American Diabetes Association.

Davis, B., and Barnard, T. (2013). *Defeating Diabetes: A No-Nonsense Approach to Type 2 Diabetes and the Diabesity Epidemic*, 16th Edition. ReadHowYouWant.

Diabetes.org.uk. (2013). *List of Countries by Incidence of Type 1 Diabetes Ages 0 to 14.* The British Diabetic Association. https://www.diabetes.org.uk/about_us/news_landing_page/uk-has-worlds-5th-highest-rate-of-type-1-diabetes-in-children/list-of-countries-by-incidence-of-type-1-diabetes-ages-0-to-14

Friedell, G.H., and Joyner, J.I. (2014). *The Great Diabetes Epidemic: A Manifesto for Control and Prevention.* Butler Books.

Funnell, M.M. (2014). *Life with Diabetes: A Series of Teaching Outlines*, 5th Edition. American Diabetes Association.

Healthline. (2020). *Type 2 Diabetes Statistics and Facts.* Healthline Media. https://www.healthline.com/health/type-2-diabetes/statistics

Healthline. (2019). *How Type 2 Diabetes Affects Life Expectancy.* Healthline Media. https://www.healthline.com/health/allergic-to-electricity#are-wi-fi-allergies-real

Index Mundi. (2019). *Diabetes Prevalence (% of Population 20 to 79) – Country Ranking.* Index Mundi. https://www.index-mundi.com/facts/indicators/sh.sta.diab.zs/rankings

International Diabetes Federation. (2020). *About Diabetes – Diabetes Facts & Figures.* International Diabetes Federation. https://www.idf.org/aboutdiabetes/what-is-diabetes/facts-figures.html

Marmarelis, V., and Mitsis, G. (2014). *Data-driven Modeling for Diabetes: Diagnosis and Treatment (Lecture Notes in Bioengineering).* Springer.

Mary Ann Liebert, Inc., Publishers – Population Health Management. (2017). *Diabetes 2030: Insights from Yesterday, Today, and Future Trends.* Mary Ann Liebert, Inc., Publishers. https://www.dogpile.com/serp?q=clinical+endocrinology+news+global+costs+of+diabetes+and+its+complications+will+greatly+increase+by+2030&sc=L9SZADSEfBqv10

McCulley, D. (2012). *Death to Diabetes – The 6 Stages of Type 2 Diabetes Control & Reversal.* Amazon Digital Services LLC.

MDedge Endocrinology – ClinicalEdge. (2018). *Diabetes Costs Likely to Increase Greatly by 2030.* Frontline Medical Communications Inc. https://www.mdedge.com/endocrinology/clinical-edge/summary/diabetes/diabetes-costs-likely-increase-greatly-2030

Melmed, S., Polonsky, K.S., Larsen, P.R., and Kronenberg, H.M. (2015). *Williams Textbook of Endocrinology*, 13th Edition. Elsevier.

Montana Public Radio – National Native News. (2015). *The Thrifty Gene Hypothesis And Its Offspring.* MTPR. https://www.mtpr.org/post/thrifty-gene-hypothesis-and-its-offspring

National Institute of Diabetes and Digestive and Kidney Diseases, et.al. (2012). *The Burden of Digestive Diseases in the United States.* CreateSpace Independent Publishing Platform.

NHIC. (2013). *Diabetes in America: A Geographic & Demographic Analysis of an Epidemic (Health in America).* Grey House Publishing.

Patterson, M. (2015). *The Diabetes Report Type 1 Global Prevalence.* Amazon Digital Services LLC.

ScienceDaily – Science News. (2017). *Diabetes Accounts for More US Deaths than Previously Thought, Study Shows.* ScienceDaily. www.sciencedaily.com/releases/2017/01/170125145848.htm

ScienceDaily - Science News. (2016). *True Impact of Global Diabetes Epidemic Is Vastly Underestimated.* ScienceDaily. https://www.sciencedaily.com/releases/2016/07/160711121513.htm

ScienceDirect - Diabetes Research and Clinical Practice. (2019). *Mortality Attributable to Diabetes in 20-79 Year Old Adults, 2019 Estimates: Results from the International Diabetes Federation Diabetes Atlas,* 9th edition. Elsevier B.V. https://www.sciencedirect.com/science/article/pii/S016882272030139X

ScienceDirect - The Lancet Diabetes & Endocrinology. (2015). *Years of Life Lost and Health Life-Years Lost from Diabetes and Cardiovascular Disease in Overweight and Obese People: A Modelling Study.* Elsevier B.V. https://www.sciencedirect.com/science/article/abs/pii/S2213858714702293

United States Congress et al. (2017). *Diabetes Research: Reducing the Burden of Diabetes at All Ages and Stages.* CreateSpace Independent Publishing Platform.

Warren, J., and Smalley, K.B. (2014). *Rural Public Health: Best Practices and Preventive Models.* Springer.

Wass, J., and Owen, K. (2014). *Oxford Handbook of Endocrinology and Diabetes (Oxford Medical Handbooks),* 3rd Edition. Oxford University Press.

Watson, R.R., and Dokken, B. (2014). *Glucose Intake and Utilization in Pre-Diabetes and Diabetes: Implications for Cardiovascular Disease.* Academic Press.

World Health Organization. (2021). *Diabetes.* World Health Organization. https://www.who.int/news-room/fact-sheets/detail/diabetes

World Health Organization – Global Health Observatory (GHO). (2004). *Age Standardized Disability-Adjusted Life Year (DALY) Rates, by Country.* World Health Organization. https://www.who.int/gho/mortality_burden_disease/countries/situation_trends_dalys/en/

World Health Rankings. (2018). *Diabetes Mellitus – Death Rate Per 100,000 – Age Standardized.* World Health Rankings. https://www.worldlifeexpectancy.com/cause-of-death/diabetes-mellitus/by-country/

Yamagishi, S. (2018). *Diabetes and Aging-Related Complications.* Springer.

PART II

MICROVASCULAR COMPLICATIONS OF DIABETES

CHAPTER 4 Diabetic Neuropathy

Diabetic neuropathy is a disease process associated with diabetes. It affects sensory axons, autonomic axons, and later, to a less extent, motor axons. How diabetes affects neurons/axons remains debated. Progressive diabetic neuropathy involves retraction and dying back of terminal sensory axons in the periphery. Data suggest that dysfunction of key plasticity molecules promotes abnormal protein processing, oxidative damage, and mitochondrial dysfunction, leading to the loss of peripheral nerve function. Diabetes is associated with a wide range of neuropathies, including mononeuritis multiplex, compression and entrapment mononeuropathies, cranial neuropathies, and autonomic neuropathies. It can also cause amyotrophy and dysautonomia. When diabetic neuropathy is severe, it can lead to ulcerations, infections, and eventual amputations of the affected areas of the body. Differential diagnosis is difficult because not all sensorimotor neuropathies are caused by diabetes. The classifications of the various types of diabetic neuropathy are shown in Figure 4.1.

CRANIAL NEUROPATHY

Cranial neuropathy is not a common manifestation of diabetes. The cranial nerves most affected are the oculomotor (III) nerve, followed by the trochlear (IV) nerve and then the facial (VII) nerve. Third nerve palsy with pupillary sparing is the hallmark of a diabetic oculomotor palsy and is believed to be a result of nerve infarction. The pupillary fibers are peripherally located, and therefore escape being affected in a diabetic oculomotor palsy.

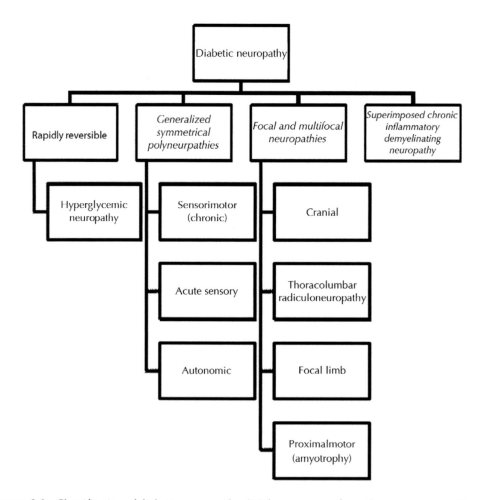

Figure 4.1 Classification of diabetic neuropathy. (With permission from George, A., Augustine, R., and Sebastian, M. (2014). *Diabetes Mellitus and Human Health Care a Holistic Approach to Diagnosis and Treatment*. CRC Press/Taylor & Francis.)

DOI: 10.1201/9781003226727-6

Epidemiology

Since cranial neuropathy is a rare outcome of diabetes, there is insufficient data on the amount of people that are affected. There is no documentation of whether there are any gender, age, or racial differences in predilection.

Etiology and Risk Factors

Palsies that affect the third cranial nerve are commonly due to diabetes mellitus. High blood glucose injures nerves throughout the body, and though the nerves of the legs and feet are most often damaged, cranial neuropathy may also occur. Additional risk factors for cranial neuropathy include hypertension, head injury, infections, strokes, and brain tumors.

Pathophysiology

The pathophysiology of cranial neuropathy, as with other forms of diabetic neuropathy, involves an increased **polypol** pathway, nonenzymatic glycation of proteins that results in advanced glycation end products (AGE), activation of protein kinase C, and increased **hexosamine pathway flux**.

Clinical Manifestations

Common signs and symptoms of cranial neuropathy depend on the nerve affected. In an oculomotor palsy, there will be double vision on lateral and upward gaze with drooping of the eyelid of the affected eye. If the cell body of the third nerve has been affected, bilateral ptosis may also be appreciated. Involvement of the trochlear nerve leads to double vision on vertical gaze and a compensatory head tilt. A diabetic facial nerve palsy leads to loss of the ability to raise the eyebrow, close the eye, raise the corner of the mouth, change in hearing on the affected side, and a loss of taste.

Diagnosis

Diagnosis of a cranial neuropathy is mainly a clinical diagnosis. An MRI or CT scan of the brain is useful to rule out other potential causes of the cranial neuropathy. Electromyography (EMG) is sometimes performed on the facial nerve to help determine prognosis.

Treatment

Sometimes, diabetic cranial neuropathies resolve on their own without treatment. In the case of a facial palsy, lubrication for the eye and an eye patch are used until the patient is able to close the eyelid and avoid any corneal laceration.

Prevention

The only preventive measure of diabetic cranial neuropathy is to properly manage diabetes mellitus so that the neuropathy can be as limited as possible.

Prognosis

While most patient do have meaningful recovery of their deficit, there is occasionally a permanent loss of eye movement resulting in chronic double vision in some patients.

CLINICAL CASE

1. Which cranial nerves are most often affected by cranial neuropathy?
2. In this patient's case, which complication of diabetes is likely present?
3. What diagnostic methods are used for cranial neuropathies?

A 56-year-old woman was taken by her husband to their family physician because of acute onset of left eye ptosis and binocular double vision. She had been diagnosed with diabetes mellitus 10 years previously, and had been taking oral antihyperglycemic agents. Over the past 2 years, the patient experienced transient right- and left-sided facial palsies. The patient had 3 mm ptosis of the left upper eyelid. There was limitation of left eye movement except for lateral gaze. Clinically, multiple diabetic-related cranial neuropathies were present, involving the left oculomotor, and trochlear, nerves.

ANSWERS

1. Cranial neuropathy most often affects cranial nerves III (oculomotor), IV (trochlear), and VII (facial).
2. Because of this patient's ptosis and double vision, cranial mononeuropathy III is the complication of diabetes that is likely present. It may occur along with diabetic peripheral neuropathy. It is the most common cranial nerve disorder caused by diabetes, due to damage to the small blood vessels feeding cranial nerve III.
3. Diagnosis of diabetic cranial neuropathy is a diagnosis of exclusion and other potential causes must be ruled out.

ISCHEMIC OPTIC NEUROPATHY

Ischemic optic neuropathy occurs when blood does not flow normally to the optic nerves, causing long-term damage. Vision is lost in one or both eyes. This disease can affect central or peripheral vision – or both. Vision loss is usually permanent, though many affected individuals still retain some amount of peripheral vision. Diabetes is one of the common causes of ischemic optic neuropathy. There are two general subtypes of this disease: Arteritic and nonarteritic. The arteritic form is caused by temporal arteritis, also known as **giant cell arteritis**. The more common nonarteritic form is caused by cardiovascular risk factors that include diabetes mellitus, hypertension, and high cholesterol. It usually occurs in slightly younger patients and is less likely to cause total loss of central vision. The arteritic form usually involves complete or nearly complete vision loss.

Epidemiology

The nonarteritic form of ischemic optic neuropathy is more common than the arteritic form. The nonarteritic form affects people that are 50 years or older. Over 10,000 people in the United States are affected annually, but global statistics are not well documented. Incidence is about 10 cases per 100,000 people. The arteritic form affects people that are over 70 years of age. Approximately 8,000 people in the United States are affected annually. The disease, in both forms, is more common in males. There appears to be no racial predilection for this disease.

Etiology and Risk Factors

Acute ischemia results in optic nerve edema, which then makes the ischemia worse. No medical condition is an apparent cause of the nonarteritic form of the disease. Risk factors may include diabetes, hypertension, smoking, obstructive sleep apnea, hypercoagulable disorders, and drugs such as amiodarone or the phosphodiesterase-5 inhibitors. Risk factors for giant cell arteritis include age between 70 and 80, female gender, Caucasian racial group, polymyalgia rheumatica, and family history.

Pathophysiology

Atherosclerotic narrowing of the posterior ciliary arteries may result in nonarteritic optic nerve infarction – especially after an episode of hypotension. The arteritic form may follow giant cell arteritis, also known as **Horton's disease**, or other inflammatory conditions such as periarteritis nodosa, systemic **lupus erythematosus**, chickenpox, and **amyloidosis**. The nonarteritic form is linked to acute ischemia of the optic nerve that is secondary to low blood flow in the posterior ciliary arteries.

Clinical Manifestations

Vision loss with both forms of ischemic optic neuropathy usually occurs quickly over minutes to days, and is painless. With giant cell arteritis, additional symptoms include general malaise, headaches over the temples, muscle aches and pains, jaw claudication, pain when combing the hair, and tenderness over the temporal artery. These symptoms sometimes do not occur until vision is already lost. There is reduced visual acuity and an afferent pupillary defect. The optic disk swells and becomes elevated. Swollen nerve fibers obscure the thin surface vessels of the optic nerve. Hemorrhages may surround the optic disk in many cases. The disk is often pale in the arteritic form, but hyperemic in the nonarteritic form. With both forms, a visual field examination often reveals a central defect, an altitudinal defect, or both.

Diagnosis

Diagnosis of optic nerve infarction is usually clinical, though ancillary testing may be required. It is important to exclude the arteritic form since the unaffected eye is at risk without prompt treatment. Immediate tests include CBC, C-reactive protein (CRP), and erythrocyte sedimentation rate (ESR). The CBC is performed to identify thrombocytosis of more than 400×103 per μL. This test offers better predictability than when ESR is used alone. The ESR is usually highly elevated with the arteritic form – often above 100 mm per hour, yet normal in the nonarteritic form.

Changes in the CRP level help to monitor the course of the disease and the response to treatment. For nonarteritic disease, other tests may be needed, based on causes and risk factors. If the patient is obese, snores, or has excessive daytime sleepiness, **polysomnography** may be needed to diagnose obstructive sleep apnea. If the patient has vision loss upon awakening, 24-hour BP monitoring can be performed.

Treatment

Treatment of the arteritic form is with oral corticosteroids – usually once daily prednisone, which is tapered based on the ESR – to protect the unaffected eye from the disease. IV corticosteroids are considered if vision loss is happen quickly. Even while awaiting biopsy or its results, treatment should not be delayed. Tocilizumab is a drug that appears to improve glucocorticoid-free remission, in comparison to corticosteroids, only if giant cell arteritis is present. Aspirin or corticosteroids have not been effective for the nonarteritic form.

Prevention

Controlling the risk factors associated with the nonarteritic form of this disease is considered an important preventive measure. People with risk factors must avoid BP-lowering medications or erectile dysfunction drugs prior to bedtime. These drugs, combined with the normal drop in BP while asleep, could interrupt the blood supply to the optic nerve. For the arteritic form, continual corticosteroid use can prevent further loss of vision, but this must be closely followed up with a rheumatologist.

Prognosis

Though there is no treatment that is effective for the nonarteritic form of ischemic optic neuropathy, as many as 40% of patients recover some amount of vision spontaneously. In the arteritic form caused by giant cell arteritis, there are usually greater losses of the visual field and acuity. Without sufficient treatment, there may be relapses and more vision loss.

DISTAL SYMMETRIC SENSORIMOTOR PERIPHERAL NEUROPATHY

Distal symmetric sensorimotor peripheral neuropathy is a common form of polyneuropathy. This is a process that affects many nerves in a length-dependent manner. It is usually bilateral and symmetrical. Diabetes mellitus is one of the most common causes of this neuropathy. The sensory fibers are affected first, with less effect upon motor fibers. The subtypes of distal symmetric sensory peripheral neuropathy include large fiber predominant, small fiber predominant, or mixed.

Large Fiber Predominant

Large fiber predominant peripheral neuropathy impairs somatosensory feedback and leads to a sense on imbalance. Both motor and sensory fibers are large, myelinated fibers. The large, myelinated motor fibers are responsible for motor control. Large myelinated sensory fibers perceive touch, **proprioception**, and vibration.

Epidemiology

It is estimated that at least 8% of the world population has some form of peripheral neuropathy. In the United States alone, there are more than

CLINICAL CASE

1. What are the risk factors for giant cell arteritis, a primary cause of arteritic ischemic optic neuropathy?
2. What other conditions may cause arteritic ischemic optic neuropathy?
3. What is the general outlook for this form of the disease?

An 84-year-old man with suspected giant cell arteritis was scheduled for a temporal artery biopsy, which showed no inflammation. He also had polymyalgia rheumatica and seronegative rheumatoid arthritis. Type 2 diabetes mellitus was also present. The patient complained of a headache that had been persistent, with the pain localized behind his left eye. He stated that his scalp felt tender when he combed his hair. His rheumatologist performed tests that revealed the patient's ESR and CRP levels were elevated – indicating that giant cell arteritis was likely. The patient was started on prednisone therapy. In 1 week, the patient's visual acuity was nearly normal and his headache had somewhat improved. Seven months later, the patient's left eye vision had become cloudy, but there were no other abnormalities. He had been tapered to a much lower dose of prednisone in the months since his first visit. Final diagnosis was arteritic anterior ischemic optic neuropathy, with posterior ciliary artery occlusion of the left eye.

ANSWERS

1. Risk factors for giant cell arteritis include age between 70 and 80, female gender, Caucasian racial group, polymyalgia rheumatica, and family history.
2. Besides giant cell arteritis, other conditions that may cause arteritic ischemic optic neuropathy include periarteritis nodosa, systemic lupus erythematosus, Churg-Strauss disease, chickenpox, and amyloidosis.
3. In the arteritic form caused by giant cell arteritis, there are usually greater losses of the visual field and acuity. Without sufficient treatment, there may be relapses and more vision loss.

40 million people affected with neuropathy. At least 10% of people over age 40 develop the condition, along with 20% of cancer chemotherapy patients, and 50% of diabetics. There are no distinct epidemiological predilections for this condition – anyone that is diabetic or has any other underlying cause may develop it – regardless of age, gender, or race.

Etiology and Risk Factors

Diabetes mellitus accounts for 75% of distal symmetrical neuropathies. The aging process is also causative and can result in the same loss of large fiber nerve function. Risk factors include alcohol abuse, autoimmune diseases, toxins, family history, infections, kidney or liver disease, repetitive motion injuries, thyroid disorders, and deficiency of vitamin B complex.

Pathophysiology

There are three primary pathophysiological mechanisms that cause this disease. They include distal axonopathy, myelinopathy, and neuronopathy. Distal axonopathy involves a metabolic abnormality, causing failure of protein synthesis and axonal transport, resulting in degenerated distal axonal regions – this affects the smaller fibers more often than the larger fibers, however. With myelinopathy, the larger fibers are more often affected. With neuronopathy, there is selective involvement of the cell bodies of motor, sensory, and autonomic nerves. The smaller and larger fibers can be affected.

Clinical Manifestations

Large fiber peripheral neuropathy can cause loss of proprioception, vibration, touch, and pressure sensation. Muscle stretch reflexes may be lost in a length-dependent fashion. These losses commonly cause falling because of reduced balance and postural control. Falling is a major healthcare factor in elderly and diabetic patients. Large fiber neuropathy can lead to gait instability and contribute to muscle wasting. This would be seen more notably in the legs and in later stages affects the hands.

Diagnosis

Diagnosis of large fiber peripheral neuropathy is based on loss of joint position, vibration sense, and loss of ankle reflexes. Electrodiagnostic tests include motor and sensory nerve conduction, and needle electromyography. These tests help document the extent of sensorimotor deficits, and differentiate demyelinating and axonal pathology. Demyelinating effects include slowed nerve conduction velocity, and dispersion and conduction blocks. Axonal effects include slight slowing of nerve conduction as well as reduced or loss of compound muscle or sensory action potentials. Denervation may be seen on EMG in the affected distal muscles.

Treatment

Treatments for large fiber peripheral neuropathy include insulin and medications for achieving good glycemic control. If there are other causative conditions, these should be addressed. Patients with paresthesia or painful sensations may be treated with anticonvulsants such as gabapentin, pregabalin or carbamazepine. Antidepressants such as amitriptyline or duloxetine are also used. Physical therapy and balance training are important.

Prevention

Prevention of large fiber peripheral neuropathy involves managing underlying conditions and limiting risk factors. Alcohol use, as well as use of tobacco products, should be stopped or reduced. Patients should avoid exposures to toxins, limit activities that could cause physical trauma or injury, have good sleep hygiene, engage in healthy and safe exercise regimens, eat a balanced diet rich in vitamins and minerals, and take vitamin B 12 supplements if eating a vegetarian or vegan diet.

Prognosis

Prognosis for large fiber predominant peripheral neuropathy is varied, based on the cause, the nerves involved, and the extent of nerve damage. Treatment may improve prognosis for some patients, but for others, permanent damage may worsen the outlook over time.

Small Fiber Predominant

Small fiber predominant peripheral neuropathy occurs when small fibers in the peripheral nervous system are damaged. In the skin, these fibers normally relay pain and temperature. In body organs, they regulate heart rate, breathing, and other automatic functions. Small fiber peripheral neuropathy can signify diabetes mellitus, or may have no underlying cause. It may be one of the earliest signs of prediabetes. Small fiber neuropathy causes pain, burning, and tingling that usually begin in the feet and progress upwards, potentially becoming severe.

Epidemiology

Small fiber predominant neuropathy is less common than other types of diabetic neuropathies. It is seen more often in people over the age of 65, and is also more common in men than in women. There is no significant racial or ethnic predilection.

Etiology and Risk Factors

Besides diabetes mellitus, other conditions that can cause small fiber neuropathy include endocrine or metabolic disorders, hypothyroidism, hereditary diseases, metabolic syndrome, **Fabry disease**, hereditary amyloidosis, hereditary sensory autonomic neuropathy, immune system disorders, **Tangier disease**, celiac disease, **Guillain-Barre syndrome**, inflammatory bowel disease, *lupus erythematosus*, mixed connective tissue disease, psoriasis, rheumatoid arthritis, **sarcoidosis**, scleroderma, **Sjögren's syndrome**, infectious diseases, vasculitis, viral hepatitis C, human immunodeficiency virus (HIV), and **Lyme disease**. Additional causes include chemotherapy, certain medications, alcoholism, and vitamin B 12 deficiencies. Sometimes, small fiber neuropathy is of unknown cause. Risk factors for small fiber neuropathy include all of these conditions, but primarily diabetes mellitus. Age is another risk factor.

Pathophysiology

In small fiber neuropathy, the unmyelinated and myelinated nerve fibers are affected. The condition occurs in prediabetes, diabetes, and metabolic syndrome without diabetes.

Clinical Manifestations

Symptoms of small fiber predominant neuropathy most often include pain, with or without burning, **paresthesia**, tingling, and loss of sensation. The pain sometimes occurs in short "bursts." Pain can be triggered by touching objects, including bedding or clothing. Early symptoms are often mild. Sometimes, small fiber neuropathy disrupts autonomic functions, including regulation of BP, digestion, and urinary function. Balance and strength are not affected. If autonomic nerve fibers are affected, symptoms may include constipation, inability to sweat normally, dizziness, dry eyes or mouth, incontinence, sexual dysfunction, and skin discoloration.

Diagnosis

Diagnostic examination may reveal loss of cold perception and decreased pinprick sensation. Electromyography and nerve conduction studies are normal. The best test is a skin biopsy, to compare epidermal nerve fiber density samples to control values, matched for biopsy location and patient age. Sudomotor testing include sweat gland density in skin biopsies and tests to evaluate sweating function.

Treatment

Treatment is based on the underlying condition. If prediabetes or diabetes is the cause, good blood glucose and weight management must occur. If the cause is unknown, treatment is focused on symptom management and include analgesics, corticosteroids, anticonvulsants, antidepressants, angiotensin-converting enzyme (ACE) inhibitors, and topical pain creams.

Prevention

The prevention of diabetic small fiber neuropathy requires blood glucose control, good foot care to prevent any infections, and exercise only in physician-approved regimens. Other methods of prevention include treating any underlying causes.

Prognosis

There is usually a slow progression of small fiber neuropathy. Diagnosis of the condition does not mean that larger fiber neuropathy will occur later. Pain can become worse over time or resolve on its own. Most patients with small fiber neuropathy need to manage their continuing pain. Prognosis is improved with proper treatment of the underlying cause.

CLINICAL CASE

1. Is distal symmetric sensorimotor peripheral neuropathy in relation to diabetes mellitus more sensory or motor in its impairments?
2. What do the large fibers perceive?
3. What are the three primary pathophysiological mechanisms that cause this disease?

A 68-year-old man had been diagnosed with impaired glucose tolerance 3 years ago and was currently receiving treatment with an ACE inhibitor for his hypertension. The patient quit smoking 20 years previously and did not drink alcohol. However, he had recently noticed burning and tingling in his feet. Physical examination revealed hyperesthesia of both feet and decreased vibratory sensation. The patient had been keeping a blood glucose log, which he showed to his physician. It revealed fasting and premeal blood glucose of less than 130 mg/dL and postmeal glucose levels higher than 150 mg/dL. Laboratory studies showed a high fasting blood glucose of 146 mg/dL. The patient was started on repaglinide, twice per day, and encouraged to increase his exercise. Within a few weeks, the patient's blood glucose was at near-normal levels. Two months later, he had lost 9 pounds, but his feet had become more painful, and he exhibited slight ataxia. The patient was started on vitamin B 12 treatments, which slightly improved his neurological symptoms.

ANSWERS

1. Distal symmetric sensorimotor peripheral neuropathy is usually bilaterally symmetrical, and with diabetes, mostly sensory fibers are affected, with less effect upon motor fibers. Subtypes include large fiber predominant, small fiber predominant, and a combination of both types.
2. The large fibers are myelinated motor fibers responsible for motor control. Myelinated sensory fibers perceive touch, proprioception, and vibration.
3. Distal axonopathy, myelinopathy, and neuronopathy are implicated. Distal axonopathy involves a metabolic abnormality, causing failure of protein synthesis and axonal transport, resulting in degenerated distal axonal regions – this affects the smaller fibers more often. With myelinopathy, larger fibers are more often affected. With neuronopathy, there is selective involvement of the cell bodies of motor, sensory, and autonomic nerves.

AUTONOMIC NEUROPATHY

Autonomic neuropathy is a peripheral nerve disorder, but with the autonomic fibers being disproportionately involved. The most common autonomic neuropathies accompany peripheral neuropathy caused by diabetes mellitus, amyloidosis, or autoimmune conditions. Diabetic autonomic neuropathy is a common, serious complication of diabetes. There is an increased risk for cardiovascular problems, which can be fatal. Approximately 20% of patients with autonomic neuropathy have abnormal cardiovascular autonomic function. Diabetic autonomic neuropathy may be an isolated disease, or coexist with other peripheral neuropathies as well as other complications of diabetes.

Epidemiology

The prevalence of diabetic autonomic neuropathy is about 27% of diabetic patients globally. In various studies, the prevalence of cardiovascular autonomic neuropathy was seen in 25.3% of type 1 diabetes cases and in 34.3% of type 2 diabetes cases. If more strict criteria is used and there are abnormalities in 50% of all autonomic function tests, the prevalence is lower – 16.8% for type 1 cases and 22.1% for type 2 cases. Cardiovascular autonomic neuropathy is detected in about 7% of all diabetic patients at the time of diagnosis. The average age of patients that develop diabetic autonomic neuropathy is 62 years. Males are slightly more affected than

females. There appears to be no predilection for any racial or ethnic group.

Etiology and Risk Factors

Diabetic autonomic neuropathy is caused by long-term high blood glucose and high levels of triglycerides and other fats in the blood. The nerves become damaged as well as the small blood vessels that nourish them, and autonomic neuropathy results. Risk factors include poor glycemic control and concurrent amyloidosis, porphyria, hypothyroidism, kidney disease, obesity, smoking, and cancer. Other risk factors certain drugs and paraneoplastic syndromes.

Pathophysiology

The theorized pathophysiology of diabetic autonomic neuropathy includes metabolic insults upon nerve fibers, neurovascular insufficiency, autoimmune damage, and neurohormonal growth factor deficiency. Hyperglycemic activation of the **polyol pathway** leads to accumulation of **sorbitol**. There may be changes in the *nicotinamide adenine dinucleotide* (NAD) to *nicotinamide adenine dinucleotide hydrogen* (NADH) ratio, resulting in direct neuronal damage, decreased nerve blood flow, or both. Protein kinase C activation causes vasoconstriction and reduces neuronal blood flow. Increased oxidative stress and free radical production causes vascular endothelium damage while reducing the bioavailability of nitric oxide. Also, excessive production of nitric oxide can cause the formation of *peroxyni-trite*, while there is damage to the endothelium and neurons. This process is called **nitrosative stress**. Immune mechanisms are sometimes involved. Endoneurial blood flow reduction and nerve hypoxia along with altered nerve function are linked to reductions in neurotrophic growth factors, insufficient essential fatty acids, and the formation of advanced glycosylation end products in the endoneurial blood vessels.

Clinical Manifestations

Autonomic neuropathy is signified by neurogenic bladder, orthostatic hypotension, erectile dysfunction, retrograde ejaculation, gastroparesis, and constipation that is difficult to control. Gastroparesis must be suspected if there is inconsistent glucose control. If the somatic fibers are affected, there can be loss of sensation in a stocking-and-glove distribution (see Figure 4.2). Clinical manifestations also include resting tachycardia, exercise intolerance, sudomotor dysfunction, impaired neurovascular function, **brittle diabetes**, and hypoglycemic autonomic failure. Gastrointestinal disturbances include esophageal enteropathy, diarrhea (alternating with the constipation), and fecal incontinence.

All sections of the GI tract can be affected. Neurovascular dysfunction may cause loss of skin integrity and abnormal vascular reflexes. There may be dry skin, reduced sweating, or developing cracks or fissures that allow entry of pathogens. Ulcers, gangrene, and loss of limbs may result.

Diagnosis

The diagnosis of autonomic neuropathy occurs when autonomic failure is discovered and there is a specific cause such as diabetes mellitus or amyloidosis. Diagnostic approaches should exclude autonomic dysfunction and neoplasia. Evaluation of bladder dysfunction is required if the patient is diabetic and has recurring urinary tract infections, incontinence, a palpable bladder, or pyelonephritis. Heart rate variability (HRV) should be measured when autonomic neuropathy is diagnosed and within 5 years after a diagnosis of type 1 diabetes – unless the patient has symptoms suggesting autonomic dysfunction earlier. Therefore, regular HRV testing allows for early detection and better diagnostic and therapeutic outcomes. It may allow for the symptoms to be attributed to autonomic dysfunction, and encourage the improvement of metabolic control or use

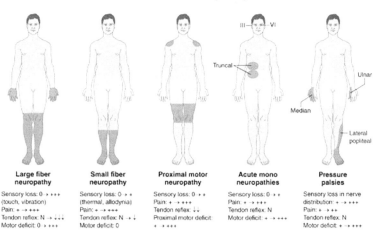

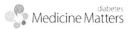

Figure 4.2 Stocking-and-glove distribution of autonomic neuropathy. (With permission from Vinik, A.I. (2012). Diabetic Neuropathies. In Skyler, J. (eds.), *Atlas of Diabetes*. Springer, Boston, MA. https://doi.org/10.1007/978-1-4614-1028-7_14.)

of therapies such as ACE inhibitors and beta-blockers – effective for cardiovascular autonomic neuropathy.

Treatment

To resolve autonomic neuropathy, the underlying cause must be treated. Patients should follow physician instructions about managing their diabetes – the blood glucose, BP, and cholesterol. This can stop the nerve damage from progressing. Measures used for treatment include more physical activity, increased salt in the diet if there is orthostatic hypotension, increasing hydrating fluids, raising the head of the bed, wearing elastic stockings to improve blood flow, rising up from sitting to standing slowly, and avoiding hypoglycemia. Medications may be prescribed to help the body retain salt, increase BP, and regulate the heart rate. Dietary changes may be needed, and some patients require OTC medications to treat constipation, diarrhea, and fecal incontinence. For bladder problems, prescription medications may be needed, such as antibiotics for bladder infections.

For men, there may be a need for medications or devices to treat erectile dysfunction. Vaginal lubricants may be required for some women if neuropathy is causing dryness. For any patient experiencing excessive sweating, excessive heat and humidity should be avoided, and sometimes prescription antiperspirants are needed. If neuropathy is causing the patient to be unaware of hypoglycemia, more regular blood glucose monitoring is needed, using a *continuous glucose monitor*. These devices check blood glucose several times throughout the day and night, and inform the patient if the glucose is lowering quickly. When a patient becomes unconscious due to severe hypoglycemia, a glucagon injection is required, and 911 should be contacted. *Glucagon emergency kits* may be needed, and affected patients should wear a diabetes medial alert ID bracelet.

Prevention

The prevention of diabetic autonomic neuropathy is achieved by managing the patient's diabetes mellitus. This is accomplished by management of blood glucose, BP, and cholesterol. It is important that every patient stays close to the ideal numbers of each of these in order to prevent nerve damage from worsening.

Prognosis

Diabetic autonomic neuropathy may eventually cause a *silent myocardial infarction*, which leads to the death of 25%–50% of affected patients within 5–10 years. Some studies have revealed that nearly 66% of all diabetic patients have autonomic neuropathy. Therefore, prognosis is based on the management of diabetes mellitus.

DIABETIC AMYOTROPHY

Diabetic amyotrophy is also called *proximal diabetic neuropathy*. It occurs most often in type 2 diabetic patients. Symptoms usually develop quickly on one side of the body, though both sides are sometimes affected. The leg weakness often results in the patient having difficulty standing from a sitting position. Canes or crutches are often needed.

Epidemiology

Diabetic amyotrophy affects about 1 of every 100 people with type 2 diabetes, and 3 of every 1,000 people with type 1 diabetes. It is much less common than peripheral neuropathy. Diabetic amyotrophy mostly affects men over the age of 50, though younger patients are sometimes affected. There is no racial or ethnic predilection for the disease.

Etiology and Risk Factors

Diabetic amyotrophy may be caused by an immune system abnormality that damages small blood vessels supplying the leg nerves – microvasculitis. Development of diabetic amyotrophy is not likely related to the duration of diabetes or its severity. However, amyotrophy only rarely occurs without diabetes. Increased blood glucose may not directly cause nerve damage, but somehow contributes to the damage process.

Pathophysiology

Diabetic amyotrophy generally starts on one side of the body and spreads to the other side in a series of pathophysiological steps. The process can be very quick, but some patients develop it relatively slowly, with about half of those affected also having distal symmetrical polyneuropathy of the feet and toes.

Clinical Manifestations

Signs and symptoms of diabetic amyotrophy include weakness in the buttocks, hips, and legs as well as muscle wasting within weeks of onset – usually in the front of the thighs. Pain is sometimes severe and can even affect the back. Some patients have altered sensation and tingling, which is usually less severe than the weakness and pain. Distal neuropathy is present in about 50% of patients with this condition, and there is concurrent weight loss. The two sides of the body are usually not affected equally. The condition can become severe enough to cause the patient to require a wheelchair. Some patients do not fully recover, and mild or moderate weakness may continue throughout life. Some patients may develop pain or weakness in the upper back, chest, and arms.

Diagnosis

Electrodiagnostic testing is used to diagnose diabetic amyotrophy. Nerve conduction studies and needle electromyography may also be required. If peripheral neuropathy is also present, leg sensations may be greatly reduced. Diagnosis is also based on blood tests for vitamin B deficiencies, assessment of blood glucose, lumbar puncture to check for inflammation in the cerebrospinal fluid, and MRI scans of the lower back to rule out nerve compression.

Treatment

Diabetic amyotrophy usually improves over time and self-resolves. However, physical therapy and careful management of blood glucose are required, and some patients require pain medications. It is important to exercise the affected muscles as much as possible. A healthy diet and avoiding smoking are other factors that are helpful. Antidepressants and anticonvulsants may also be prescribed. To increase recovery time, corticosteroids and immunosuppressants may be needed, but they are not always effective. Length of treatment is based on the disease course and the amount of nerve damage.

Prevention

Prevention of diabetic amyotrophy is based on control of blood glucose, avoiding or stopping smoking, eating a healthy diet, maintaining a healthy weight, and close management of diabetes.

Prognosis

The prognosis of diabetic amyotrophy is good since most patients recover fully or almost fully. The condition can relapse, so maintaining control of blood glucose is essential.

CLINICAL CASE

1. How common is diabetic amyotrophy?
2. How does diabetic amyotrophy generally develop?
3. What treatments are possible for diabetic amyotrophy?

An 83-year-old woman was hospitalized because of abdominal distention and swelling of her left leg, even though she was on furosemide therapy – a diuretic. She was previously diagnosed with type 2 diabetes. The patient was fatigued and experiencing diffuse arthralgias. Her appetite was poor and her temperature was slightly elevated. Five years before, she was successfully treated with chemotherapy for diffuse B cell lymphoma. A musculoskeletal exam revealed muscle tenderness upon palpation. There was proximal muscle weakness, mostly of the hip flexors, but also of the upper arms. A large amount of tests were performed to exclude a variety of musculoskeletal conditions, including polymyalgia rheumatica, myopathy, vasculitis, and muscle infarction. A lumbar puncture yielded clear cerebrospinal fluid, and an MRI revealed bilaterally symmetric muscle edema. A surgical biopsy of the left quadriceps muscle excluded myositis, and the final diagnosis was diabetic amyotrophy.

ANSWERS

1. Diabetic amyotrophy affects about 1 in every 100 people with type 2 diabetes and 3 in every 1,000 people with type 1 diabetes. It is much less common than peripheral neuropathy.
2. Diabetic amyotrophy generally starts on one side of the body and spreads to the other side in a series of pathophysiological steps. It can be quick or slow, with about half of those affected also having distal symmetrical polyneuropathy of the feet and toes.
3. The condition usually improves over time and self-resolves. However, physical therapy and careful management of blood glucose are required. Some patients require pain medications. It is important to exercise the affected muscles as much as possible. A healthy diet and avoiding smoking are helpful. Nerve pain medications include amitriptyline, and antidepressants or anticonvulsants may be prescribed. Corticosteroids and immunosuppressants are used, but not always effective.

ADDITIONAL TYPES OF NEUROPATHY

There are additional types of neuropathy that are related to diabetes mellitus. These include Charcot's joint, compression mononeuropathy, femoral neuropathy, focal neuropathy, thoracic/lumbar radiculopathy, and **unilateral foot drop**.

Charcot's Joint

Charcot's joint is also known as *neuropathic arthropathy*. It occurs when a joint breaks down due to a nerve abnormality. This occurs in the feet, but not always. Usually, most of the normal sensation is lost. The patient cannot feel foot pain and becomes unable to sense the position of the joint. The muscles of the affected foot lose the ability to support the joint and the foot becomes unstable. Walking worsens the condition. If the patient twists his or her ankle or experiences another foot injury, the condition worsens as joints grind directly on bones. Inflammation develops, causing more instability, and eventually a dislocation. Ultimately, the foot's bone structure collapses. Though the foot will eventually heal, the breakdown of bone results in deformity. People at risk for Charcot's joint are those that already have neuropathy. To prevent bone destruction and help with proper healing, they must be aware of any excessive foot warmth, lack of sensation, redness, swelling, or an extremely strong pulse.

Epidemiology

Charcot's joint has varying prevalence, based on the severity of diabetes mellitus. It affects about 30% of patients that also have peripheral neuropathy, about 15% of high-risk diabetic patients, and about 0.1% of the general diabetic population. The average global incidence of Charcot's joint is 8.5 cases per every 1,000 people, per year. Most patients that also have type 1 diabetes are over the age of 40 years, while most patients that also have type 2 diabetes are over the age of 50 years. Males and females are affected nearly equally. For unknown reasons, Caucasians are affected more than any other racial or ethnic group.

Etiology and Risk Factors

Diabetes mellitus is the most common cause of Charcot's joint, and the condition usually affects the feet and ankles. The primary predisposing factors are sensorimotor and autonomic neuropathies. Other causes of Charcot's joint include **syringomyelia**, neurosyphilis with **tabes dorsalis**, traumatic spinal cord injury, alcoholism, compressive tumors of the peripheral nerves or spinal cord, pernicious anemia, **leprosy**, and multiple sclerosis.

Pathophysiology

The pathophysiology of Charcot's joint is believed to involve an inflammatory response caused by a minor injury, resulting in osteolysis. With peripheral neuropathy, the initial injury and inflammatory response may not be fully realized, and continuing inflammation and further injury can occur. Usually, Charcot's joint is unilateral, though it may occur bilaterally in about 20% of cases. The two patterns of pathophysiology are *atrophic* and *hypertrophic*. The atrophic form is most common and occurs earlier. Joint destruction occurs along with resorption of fragments. There is a lack of osteophytes or osteosclerosis. The atrophic form mainly occurs in nonweight bearing joints of the arms. In the hypertrophic form, only the sensory nerves are affected, and the condition progresses slowly. The joint space first widens, and then narrows. **Osteophytes** and osteosclerosis are present.

Clinical Manifestations

Charcot's joint may be insidious or incidentally discovered. The swollen joint or joints do not feel warm when palpated, unlike the features of septic arthritis. There are no elevated inflammatory markers, and no pain.

Diagnosis

Diagnosis may be made if deformity of the foot is being assessed. On plain X-rays and CT scans, the disease appears destructive, causing disorganization of affected joints and surrounding bones. The earliest finding is subchondral osteopenia. This is followed by bone fragmentation and joint malalignment. Debris form that appear as intraarticular loose bodies. Because of **ligamentous laxity**, subluxation or dislocation occurs. Bony consolidation begins, with subchondral sclerosis, periosteal bone formation, and then fusion of large fragments with absorption of small fragment. Remodeling occurs as fragments become rounded. As ankylosis develops, the deformity becomes permanent. On T1-weighted MRI with gadolinium contrast, areas of inflammation show enhancement, with central necrotic areas that do not enhance. Differential diagnoses may include advanced osteomyelitis, chondrosarcoma, osteoarthritis, and **Pott's disease**.

Treatment

Nonsurgical treatments for Charcot's joint include protective splinting, walking braces, protective orthotics, casting, and avoidance of weightbearing. Surgical treatments include open reduction and internal fixation and fusion in early stages of the disease. Diabetic patients will heal more slowly than those without the disease. For Charcot foot and ankle, healing after fusion may need 6 months of protection and orthotics. The condition can recur or flare. If both feet are affected, which is common, impairment may be permanent. Regular follow-up with a specialist is required throughout life.

Prevention

Prevention of Charcot's joint involves good diabetic control, avoiding excessive weight bearing or injury, wearing supportive shoes, checking the feet regularly, daily bathing, use of diabetic foot soap, and always wearing socks with shoes.

Prognosis

If joint stability, protection to the affected area, and proper bracing are used, the overall prognosis is good. Should ulceration or infection occur, the prognosis is worsened. Outcomes from surgery are poorer than when surgical intervention is not needed. The worst prognosis is given if ulcers, infections, or treatment failure result in amputation.

Compression Mononeuropathy

Compression mononeuropathy develops with damage to a single nerve and is fairly common. Two different types of damage may occur: Compression of nerves where they pass through a constricted "tunnel" in the body, or over a mass of bone, and with blood vessel disease due to diabetes mellitus, which limits blood flow to part of the nerve. The first type of damage is also more common along with diabetes mellitus. The most common type of compression mononeuropathy is carpal tunnel syndrome.

Epidemiology

Carpal tunnel syndrome has a prevalence of about 1 in every 25 people. Incidence is between 1.5 and 3.5 per 1,000 person-years. People between 40 and 60 years of age are mostly affected. Women develop the condition more often than men. There is no racial or ethnic predilection. Peroneal nerve palsy is most common in bedridden patients that are emaciated, or in thin people that cross their legs habitually. It affects between 3.2% and 23.6% of these individuals, but actual prevalence and incidence are not well documented. There is no age or gender difference in occurrence, and no racial or ethnic predilection. Radial nerve palsy is of unknown prevalence, except for when it is associated with fractures of the shaft of the humerus (occurring in 11.8% of cases). Incidence ranges between 2% and 17% of the global population. The condition is most common in adults of all ages. It is

slightly more common in men. There is no racial or ethnic predilection. Ulnar nerve palsy is second only to carpal tunnel syndrome in prevalence. It affects up to 40% of the population at least once during life, though actual statistics on prevalence and incidence are not well documented. Men are slightly more affected. There is no age, racial, or ethnic predilection.

Etiology and Risk Factors

Carpal tunnel syndrome may be unilateral or bilateral and is caused by compression of the median nerve within the volar aspect of the wrist. This is between the transverse superficial carpal ligament and the flexor tendons of the muscles of the forearm muscles. Risk factors include diabetes mellitus, pregnancy, rheumatoid arthritis, repeated forceful movements with the wrist extended, and possibly, use of a poorly positioned computer keyboard. Most cases are idiopathic. Peroneal nerve palsy is usually caused by compression of the peroneal nerve against the lateral aspect of the neck of the fibula. Risk factors for peroneal nerve palsy include obesity and fibular head fracture. Radial nerve palsy is also known as Saturday night palsy, and is due to compression of the radial nerve against the humerus, such as when the arm is laid over the back portion of a chair for a long period of time – often during deep sleep or because of intoxication. Risk factors for radial nerve palsy include the male gender, jobs that require repetitive motion, or awkward postures or positions, and injuries to the bones and joints. Ulnar nerve palsy, near the elbow, is usually caused by trauma to the nerve within the ulnar groove, from leaning repeatedly on the elbow. It is also caused by asymmetric bone growth after a childhood fracture has occurs – known as tardy ulnar palsy. The ulnar nerve may be compressed along its length, under the medial epicondyle, through the tissues of the cubital tunnel. This sometimes results in cubital tunnel syndrome. Risk factors for ulnar nerve palsy include smoking, male gender, elbow fracture or subluxation, obesity, excessive alcohol consumption, repetitive arm motions, diabetes mellitus, and hypertension.

Pathophysiology

In carpal tunnel syndrome, the compression of the median nerve causes paresthesias within the radial-palmar aspect of the hand, plus pain in the palm and wrist. The pain can be referred to the forearm and shoulder, and may be worse at night. The muscles controlling thumb abduction and opposition may be weakened and atrophied. In peroneal nerve palsy, paralysis of the common peroneal nerve, also called the fibular nerve, affects movement of the ankle, making walking difficult. Nerve damage from injury to the knee or fibula starts the pathophysiological process. Radial nerve palsy progresses to paralysis of all extensors of the wrist and digits, along with the forearm muscles. Extremely proximal lesions may affect the triceps. Ulnar nerve palsy progresses as the lack of control and sensation causes the hand muscles to tighten, resulting in a claw-like deformity in severe cases.

Clinical Manifestations

With carpal tunnel syndrome, there is a sensory deficit in the palmar aspect of the first three fingers that follows the development of paresthesias, pain, numbness, swelling, or prickling of the fingers. The symptoms are often felt in a variety of situations, including during rest, performing activities with the hands such as typing on a computer keyboard, or when driving a vehicle. Peroneal nerve palsy causes footdrop, which is weakened dorsiflexion and eversion of the foot, and sometimes a sensory deficit within the anterolateral aspect of the lower leg, dorsum of the foot, or in the webbed space between the first and second metatarsals. While L5 radiculopathy causes similar abnormalities, it usually weakens hip abduction by affecting the gluteus medius and weak foot inversion (tibialis posterior). Common symptoms of radial nerve palsy include wristdrop, which is weakness of the wrist and finger extensors, plus loss of sensation in the dorsal aspect of the first dorsal interosseous muscle. Similar motor abnormalities are caused by C7 radiculopathy. Compression of the ulnar nerve near the elbow may cause paresthesias, plus a sensory deficit in the fifth digit and the medial half of the fourth digit. There may be weakness and atrophy of the thumb adductor, fifth digit abductor, and the interosseous muscles. If chronic ulnar palsy is severe, a **clawhand deformity** will occur. Sensory symptoms are similar to those caused by C8 root dysfunction that is secondary to cervical radiculopathy. The difference is that radiculopathy usually affects more proximal aspects of the C8 **dermatome**.

Diagnosis

Diagnosis of carpal tunnel syndrome is based on patient medical history, physical examination, positive **Tinel's sign**, electromyography, and nerve conduction studies. Diagnosis of peroneal nerve palsy requires patient medical history, and a comprehensive clinical and neurological examination. Electromyography and nerve conduction studies may be needed. Imaging techniques include CT and ultrasound. Diagnosis of radial nerve palsy requires physical examination, electromyography, X-rays,

ultrasound, MRI, and nerve conduction studies. Ulnar nerve palsy is diagnosed via physical examination, electromyography, and nerve conduction studies. High-resolution ultrasound is being used to diagnosis compression neuropathies of the arm and leg.

Treatment

Carpal tunnel syndrome should be treated as early as possible. Prior to treatment, patients can take breaks from work to rest the hands, avoid activities that worsen symptoms, and use ice packs to reduce inflammation. Other options include wrist splinting, medications, and surgery. Patients are advised to see their physician if there is numbness in the hands. Medications include NSAIDs and injected corticosteroids. For severe or nonresponsive symptoms, there are two surgical techniques. In endoscopic surgery, an endoscope allows visualization of the inside of the carpal tunnel, and the ligament is cut via one or two small incisions. Endoscopic surgery causes less pain than the other technique, which is open surgery.

Treatments for peroneal nerve palsy include resting from any activities that worsen the condition, ice packs, anti-inflammatory medications, bracing of the ankle and foot, strengthening and stretching exercises, and surgery. Surgical procedures include peroneal nerve decompression via an incision made over the neck of the fibula. The fascia surrounding the nerves to the lateral side of the leg is released. The early surgery is performed, the better will be the recovery. Physical therapy interventions include a range of motion exercises. Other treatment methods involve cold therapy, electrical stimulation, ultrasound, and **iontophoresis**. Treatment of radial nerve palsy includes OTC drugs or prescription analgesics, physical therapy, splinting or casting, transcutaneous electrical nerve stimulation, and surgery to remove compressive cysts, tumors, or broken bones. Treatment of ulnar nerve palsy includes OTC analgesics, corticosteroids, splinting, physical therapy, physical therapy, and surgery.

Prevention

Prevention of carpal tunnel syndrome involves keeping the wrists straight while working and not keeping them lower than the hands. Hand positions should be changed often, and the wrists should not be put onto the desk top while the hands are moving. Body position must incorporate good posture and back support. Other preventive measures include losing weight if you are overweight or obese, and treating diabetes mellitus, hypothyroidism, and rheumatoid arthritis. For older people, it is very important to take care of and protect the wrists. When sleeping, it is important to try to avoid putting the hands under the body, especially if they are flexed. Wrist braces can be worn while sleeping to keep the hands in a neutral position. When gripping objects during the day, try to avoid holding them very tightly. Jobs in which carpal tunnel syndrome most often develops include housecleaning, food processing, and manufacturing. Wrist stretching, grip strengthening, and yoga are all helpful for carpal tunnel syndrome.

For peroneal nerve palsy, preventive measures include warming up and stretching properly before physical activity, wearing properly fitted and padded protective equipment, avoiding crossing the legs treating leg or knee injuries immediately, and alerting your physician if casts, splints, or dressings on the lower leg cause it to feel tight or numb. Most cases of radial nerve palsy cannot be prevented. Good ergonomics and work postures can reduce the likelihood of developing the condition. Pillows can be used to correct awkward positions while sleeping. Prevention of ulnar nerve palsy involves requesting medical treatment as soon as symptoms are noticed. Affected individuals should contact their physician immediately if they have pain, numbness, or tingling in the fourth and fifth fingers. Occupational therapy can also prevent the condition. Some patients require braces, casts, or splints for support.

Prognosis

Carpal tunnel syndrome usually has a good prognosis with prompt, adequate treatment. However, when left untreated for too long, the condition's outlook is worsened and the pain is more severe. In peroneal nerve palsy, prognosis is usually good since nonsurgical treatments are often curative, and symptoms often self-resolve. After surgery to relieve pressure from the nerve, prognosis is very good. Prognosis for radial nerve palsy is usually good with adequate treatment. The prognosis for ulnar nerve palsy is usually good as long as diagnosis and treatment are done early.

Femoral Neuropathy

Femoral neuropathy occurs most often because of type 2 diabetes. Pain develops in the front portion of one thigh, followed by muscle weakness and then wasting. It is similar to diabetic amyotrophy except that femoral neuropathy is always on one side of the body and is always painful.

Epidemiology

Femoral neuropathy is relatively uncommon, and exact prevalence and incidence is not clear. It is estimated that about 60% of all femoral nerve injuries are **iatrogenic**. Femoral neuropathy is most common in older adults with diabetes. There is no gender, racial, or ethnic predilection.

Etiology and Risk Factors

The femoral nerve controls the muscles that help to straighten the leg and move the hips, while providing sensation in the lower leg and front of the thigh. When damaged, the ability to walk is compromised, and there may be problems with leg and foot sensation. Damage may result from diabetes, direct injury, tumors, prolonged nerve pressure, pelvic fracture, pelvic radiation, bleeding into the retroperitoneal space, and catheters placed into the femoral artery. Diabetes is able to cause widespread nerve damage, but femoral neuropathy is believed by some to be a form of diabetic amyotrophy and not a true peripheral neuropathy.

Pathophysiology

Decreased blood flow due to chronic pressure to the femoral nerve can cause tissue damage. Nerve damage may be accompanied by damage to the femoral artery or vein, leading to internal hemorrhage. Injuries and hemorrhage can compress the femoral nerve.

Clinical Manifestations

Signs and symptoms of femoral neuropathy include leg or knee weakness, inability of weight bearing, leg numbness or tingling, a dull ache in the genital region, muscle weakness, difficulty extending the knee because of weakness of the quadriceps, and a feeling like the leg or knee is going to collapse. Often, the condition is initially very painful, but spontaneously resolves over time.

Diagnosis

Diagnosis of femoral neuropathy involves patient medical history, comprehensive physical examination, reflex tests, nerve conduction studies, electromyography, and imaging studies such as CT and MRI.

Treatment

Treatment of femoral neuropathy begins with the underlying cause or condition. Management of blood glucose may alleviate nerve dysfunction. Other treatments include injected corticosteroids, analgesics, gabapentin, pregabalin, amitriptyline, physical therapy, orthotics, occupational therapy, and surgery.

Prevention

Managing diabetes is an excellent way to prevent femoral neuropathy. Other preventive measures are focused on different causes. One overall method of prevention is to remain active, keeping the leg muscles strong and improving stability.

Prognosis

Once the underlying cause or condition is treated, the prognosis is very good since many patients are cured. Prognosis is worsened if treatments fail or if the nerve damage is severe, resulting in permanent loss of sensation or inability to make normal movements.

Focal Neuropathy

Focal neuropathy can affect one nerve or a group of nerves. It causes sudden pain and weakness. In most cases, focal neuropathies occur in the head, torso, hands, or legs.

Epidemiology

Focal neuropathy is less common than peripheral or autonomic neuropathy, but many different focal neuropathies occur along with diabetes mellitus. Approximately 25% of diabetic patients have some amount of focal neuropathy. The focal neuropathies that do not involve trapped nerves mostly affect older adults. There is no gender, racial, or ethnic predilection.

Etiology and Risk Factors

Focal neuropathies develop over time, as high blood glucose and high levels of triglycerides and other fats in the blood damage the nerves and their nourishing blood vessels. Risk factors include high body mass index (BMI) and older age.

Pathophysiology

The most common type of focal neuropathy involves entrapments (entrapment syndromes). These occur when nerves become compressed or trapped where nerves pass through the narrow passages between bones and tissues. Other focal neuropathies are even less common and do not involve trapped nerves.

Clinical Manifestations

Symptoms of focal neuropathies include numbness, pain, tingling, weakness, aches, double vision, and partial paralysis.

Diagnosis

Diagnosis of focal neuropathies is based on patient medical history, physical examination, nerve conduction studies, and electromyography.

Treatment

Treatment of focal neuropathies involves the same medications used for peripheral neuropathies. Other therapies include splints, braces, anti-inflammatories, and when these fail,

surgery. For the focal neuropathies that do not involve trapped nerves, the majority of people recover within weeks to months, even without treatment.

Prevention

The prevention of focal neuropathies is based on control of diabetes mellitus, including weight loss, increased physical activity, and better overall health.

Prognosis

The prognosis is generally good as long as diabetes is controlled and the patient follows physician instructions on improvement of overall health.

Spinal Radiculopathy

This type of **radiculopathy** may affect the lumbar, cervical, and thoracic portions of the torso, and is similar to femoral neuropathy. The lumbar region is most often affected, followed by the cervical region, with the thoracic region being least effected. A band-like area of the chest or abdominal wall may be affected, on one or both sides of the body. It is another example of a condition that is commonly a feature of type 2 diabetes. This neuropathy resolves over time.

Epidemiology

Lumbar radiculopathy is the most common form of spinal radiculopathy, occurring in the lower back. This form is most common in adults between the ages of 30 and 50. Though clear epidemiologic data is lacking, there is an estimated prevalence of 3%–5% of the population affected by lumbar radiculopathy. There is no reported gender, racial, or ethnic predilection. Cervical radiculopathy occurs as the next most common form. It is most prominent between the ages of 40 and 50, affecting about 83 out of every 100,000 people. Cervical radiculopathy affects men more often than women – 107.3 men of every 100,000 are affected, and 63.5 women of every 100,000 are affected. For some reason, cervical radiculopathy occurs most often in Caucasians. The actual epidemiology of thoracic radiculopathy is unknown since the condition's diagnosis is overlooked. The condition has only been reported infrequently and is considered uncommon.

Etiology and Risk Factors

Lumbar radiculopathy is also called **sciatica** since the nerve roots making up the sciatic nerve are often involved. It may be caused by an injury or occur without warning. Often, it is due to a structural abnormality such as a herniated disc or bone spur, or caused by mechanical stretching or trauma. Discs can be damaged by strenuous activity or congenital defects also. Causes of cervical radiculopathy include material from a ruptured disc, degenerative bone changes, arthritis, and injuries that compress the nerve roots. Cervical foraminal stenosis may also be causative. Risk factors include smoking, previous radiculopathy, and lifting heavy items. Thoracic radiculopathy is caused by a compressed nerve root in the thoracic area of the spine. Causative factors include narrowing of the space where the nerve roots exit the spine. This can be due to bone spurs, stenosis, or disc herniation. Radiculopathy is usually a mechanical root compression caused by diabetes mellitus. Diabetic thoracic polyradiculopathy is present in 15% of insulin-dependent patients and in 13% of noninsulin-dependent patients. Other causes include spondylosis, metastatic tumors, trauma, scoliosis, and tuberculosis.

Pathophysiology

When lumbar radiculopathy is due to disc damage, material within the intervertebral disc leaks out, compressing the nerve root. Cervical radiculopathy is marked by nerve compression from herniated disks or arthritic bone spurs. It occurs with pathologies that cause symptoms on the nerve roots such as compression, irritation, traction, and lesions. The pinched nerve may occur in different areas of the thoracic spine. Important structures that are involved in this condition include all of the thoracic vertebrae, the intervertebral discs, the 12 pairs of spinal nerve roots, and the 12 rami. The posterior rami innervate the regional back muscles, while the ventral rami innervate the chest and abdominal skin and muscles.

Clinical Manifestations

In sciatica, pain radiates from the back down the back of the leg and numbness, tingling of the leg or foot, accompanied by weakness and muscle spasms. Cervical radiculopathy causes numbness or tingling in the hands or figures as well as muscle weakness, lack of coordination, and loss of reflexes in the arms or legs. Often, symptoms of thoracic radiculopathy follow a dermatomal distribution. There is pain and numbness that wraps around to the front of the body. The pain is often described as burning or "shooting." There are usually no related motor deficits.

Diagnosis

Diagnosis of lumbar radiculopathy starts with physical examination and is supported by electromyography, MRI, CT, and myelography with a contrast agent. Diagnosis of cervical radiculopathy involves X-rays, MRI, electromyography, and nerve conduction studies. Root compression on MRI may confirm the condition, though *spiral CT* is the best method to detect foraminal stenosis that causes bony compression upon the nerve. Because of its rareness, thoracic radiculopathy is often misdiagnosed as **shingles**, or complications of heart, abdominal, or gallbladder conditions. The condition is often not diagnosed for months or years after symptoms begin. Diagnostic methods include X-rays, MRI, CT, and electromyography. The most important diagnostic step is to exclude other causes of pain. A sensory examination is important. Differential diagnoses include chronic abdominal wall pain, intervertebral disc compression, spinal cord tumors, spondylosis, spinal stenosis, **facet syndrome**, osteoporosis, kyphosis, scoliosis, and peripheral polyneuropathy.

Treatment

Treatments for lumbar radiculopathy are varied, including back supports, medications, physical therapy, spinal corticosteroid injections, and surgery. For cervical radiculopathy, surgical options are varied. Techniques include anterior cervical discectomy to achieve decompression, anterior cervical discectomy and fusion, total disc arthroplasty, laminotomy, and **corpectomy**. Physiotherapy and surgery together provide better results. Epidural corticosteroid injections are also helpful. These injections often are sufficient, and surgery can be avoided. Thoracic radiculopathy can often be treated nonsurgically, though minimally invasive surgery is often helpful. Medications include NSAIDs, oral or injected corticosteroids, narcotic analgesics, physical therapy, and application of ice or heat.

Prevention

The only methods of prevention for lumbar radiculopathy involve avoiding the causes and risk factors of the condition. Cervical radiculopathy can be prevented by decreasing risk factors, utilizing good **ergonomics** when working, always maintaining good posture, limiting repetitive activities, taking frequent breaks from repetitive activities, and weight control. The best methods of prevention for thoracic radiculopathy include staying physically fit and maintaining a healthy weight. Good posture and learning proper exercise techniques are also preventive.

Prognosis

Fortunately, most patients about 85% with lumbar radiculopathy and sciatic recover without having to have surgery. For cervical radiculopathy, a better prognosis is possible if the patient is under 54 years of age, the dominant arm is not affected, symptoms are not worsened when the patient looks downward, and treatments include cervical traction, deep neck flexor strengthening, and manual therapy. The prognosis for thoracic radiculopathy is generally good since the condition is usually reversible when managed adequately.

KEY TERMS

- Amyloidosis
- Brittle diabetes
- Charcot's joint
- Clawhand deformity
- Corpectomy
- Dermatome
- Diabetic amyotrophy
- Ergonomics
- Fabry disease
- Facet syndrome
- Giant cell arteritis
- Guillain-Barre syndrome
- Hexosamine pathway flux
- Horton's disease
- Iatrogenic
- Iontophoresis
- Leprosy
- Ligamentous laxity
- Lupus erythematosus
- Lyme disease
- Nitrosative stress
- Osteophytes
- Paresthesia
- Polyol pathway
- Polypol
- Polysomnography
- Pott's disease
- Proprioception
- Radiculopathy
- Sarcoidosis
- Sciatica
- Shingles
- Sjögren's syndrome
- Sorbitol
- Syringomyelia
- Tabes dorsalis
- Tangier disease
- Tinel's sign
- Unilateral foot drop

REFERENCES

American Academy of Ophthalmology. (2021). *What Is Ischemic Optic Neuropathy?* American Academy of Ophthalmology. https://www.aao.org/eye-health/diseases/what-is-ischemic-optic-neuropathy

American Association of Neuromuscular & Electrodiagnostic Medicine. (2021a). *Diabetic Amyotrophy.* AANEM. https://www.aanem.org/Patients/Muscle-and-Nerve-Disorders/Diabetic-Amyotrophy

American Association of Neuromuscular & Electrodiagnostic Medicine. (2021b). *Lumbar Radiculopathy.* AANEM. https://www.aanem.org/Patients/Muscle-and-Nerve-Disorders/Lumbar-Radiculopathy

American Diabetes Association. (2021a). *Neuropathy – Steps to Prevent or Delay Nerve Damage.* American Diabetes Association. https://www.diabetes.org/diabetes/complications/neuropathy/steps-prevent-or-delay-nerve-damage

American Diabetes Association. (2021b). *Neuropathy – Additional Types of Neuropathy.* American Diabetes Association. https://www.diabetes.org/diabetes/complications/neuropathy/additional-types-neuropathy

American Diabetes Association – Diabetes Care. (2003). *Diabetic Autonomic Neuropathy.* American Diabetes Association. https://care.diabetesjournals.org/content/26/5/1553

American Family Physician. (2018). *Charcot Foot: Clinical Clues, Diagnostic Strategies, and Treatment Principles.* American Academy of Family Physicians. https://www.aafp.org/afp/2018/0501/p594.html

American Stroke Association. (2021). *Foot Drop.* (A division of the) American Heart Association. https://www.stroke.org/en/about-stroke/effects-of-stroke/physical-effects-of-stroke/physical-impact/foot-drop

Ankle Foot Orthosis. (2018). *Peroneal Nerve Palsy – Peroneal Neuropathy.* Ankle Foot Orthosis. http://anklefootorthosis.org/peroneal-nerve-palsy-peroneal-neuropathy/

AOFAS – FootCareMD. (2021). *Charcot Arthropathy (Neuroarthropathy).* American Orthopaedic Foot & Ankle Society / Orthopaedic Foot & Ankle Foundation. https://www.footcaremd.org/conditions-treatments/the-diabetic-foot/charcot-arthropathy

Babu, S.C., and Jackson, N.M. (2019). *Cost-Effective Evaluation and Management of Cranial Neuropathy.* Thieme.

Baptist Health. (2021). *Radial Nerve Palsy – Neurology Care.* Baptist Health. https://www.baptisthealth.com/services/neurology-care/conditions/radial-nerve-palsy

Basu, D., and Bahrus, K. (2018). *Diabetes and Musculoskeletal Disorders.* Jaypee Brothers Medical Publishing Ltd.

Bilbao, J.M., and Schmidt, R.E. (2015). *Biopsy Diagnosis of Peripheral Neuropathy,* 2nd Edition. Springer.

BMJ Best Practice. (2021). *Carpal Tunnel Syndrome.* BMJ Publishing Group. https://bestpractice.bmj.com/topics/en-gb/380

Cedars Sinai. (2021). *Cranial Neuropathies – What Are Cranial Neuropathies?* Cedars-Sinai. https://www.cedars-sinai.org/health-library/diseases-and-conditions/c/cranial-neuropathies.html

Cheng, J. (2019). *Neuropathic Pain: A Case-Based Approach to Practical Management.* Oxford University Press.

Cleveland Clinic. (2021). *Prevention – How Can Anterior Ischemic Optic Neuropathy Be Prevented?* Cleveland Clinic. https://my.clevelandclinic.org/health/diseases/15770-anterior-ischemic-optic-neuropathy#prevention

Cleveland Clinic – Indian River Hospital. (2021). *Cranial Mononeuropathy III.* Cleveland Clinic Indian River Hospital. https://ccirh.org/articles/1228/

Diabetic Microvascular Complications Today. (2021). *Large, Small Fiber Neuropathy: Know the Signs and Symptoms.* DiabeticMCToday.com. http://www.diabeticmctoday.com/HtmlPages/DMC1105/DMC1105_Neuro_LaFontaine.html

Eleftheriadou, I., Kokkinos, A., Liatis, S., Makrilakis, K., Tentolouris, N., Tentolouris, A., and Tsapogas, P. (2019). *Atlas of the Diabetic Foot,* 3rd Edition. Wiley-Blackwell.

Gries, F.A., Cameron, N.E., Low, P.A., and Ziegler, D. (2011). *Textbook of Diabetic Neuropathy.* Thieme.

Hayreh, S.S. (2012). *Ischemic Optic Neuropathies.* Springer.

Healthline. (2021a). *Small Fiber Neuropathy – Treatment Depends on the Underlying Condition.* Healthline Media. https://www.healthline.com/health/small-fiber-neuropathy#treatment

Healthline. (2021b). *What Are the Symptoms of Ulnar Nerve Palsy?* Healthline Media. https://www.healthline.com/health/ulnar-nerve-dysfunction#symptoms

Healthline. (2019). *Ulnar Nerve Palsy (Dysfunction).* Healthline Media. https://www.healthline.com/health/ulnar-nerve-dysfunction#treatment

Healthline. (2018a). *Femoral Neuropathy.* Healthline Media. https://www.healthline.com/health/femoral-nerve-dysfunction

Healthline. (2018b). *What Is Small Fiber Neuropathy?* Healthline Media. https://www.healthline.com/health/foot-problems#see-a-doctor

HealthPrep. (2021). *Ways to Treat and Prevent Charcot Foot.* HealthPrep.com. https://healthprep.com/articles/diabetes/treat-prevent-charcot-foot/

Herscovici, Jr., D. (2016). *The Surgical Management of the Diabetic Foot and Ankle.* Springer.

Hsieh, S.T., Anand, P., Gibbons, C.H., and Sommer, C. (2019). *Small Fiber Neuropathy and Related Syndromes: Pain and Neurodegeneration.* Springer.

Johns Hopkins Medicine – Health. (2021a). *Peroneal Nerve Injury.* The Johns Hopkins University, The Johns Hopkins Hospital, and Johns Hopkins Health System. https://www.hopkinsmedicine.org/health/conditions-and-diseases/peroneal-nerve-injury

Johns Hopkins Medicine – Health. (2021b). *Radiculopathy.* The Johns Hopkins University, The Johns Hopkins Hospital, and Johns Hopkins Health System. https://www.hopkinsmedicine.org/health/conditions-and-diseases/radiculopathy

Jozefowicz, R.F. (2021). *Peripheral Neuropathy – Clinical Features.* URMC Rochester. https://www.urmc.rochester.edu/MediaLibraries/URMCMedia/center-experiential-learning/cme/types-of-activities/documents/PERIPHERAL-NEUROPATHY-HANDOUT.pdf

Kaiser, M.G., Haid, R.W., Shaffrey, C.I., and Fehlings, M.G. (2019). *Degenerative Cervical Myelopathy and Radiculopathy: Treatment Approaches and Options.* Springer.

Kalyani, R.R., Corriere, M.D., Donner, T.W., and Quartuccio, M.W. (2018). *Diabetes Head to Toe: Everything You Need to Know about Diagnosis, Treatment, and Living with Diabetes.* Johns Hopkins University Press.

Kelkar, S. (2020). *Diabetic Neuropathy and Clinical Practice.* Springer.

Latov, N. (2006). *Peripheral Neuropathy: When the Numbness, Weakness and Pain Won't Stop.* Demos Medical Publishing.

Levine, T., Saperstein, D., Argoff, C., Gibbons, C., Hendin, H., Pasnoor, M., Walk, D., and Lopate, G. (2017). Small Nerves, Big Problems: A Comprehensive Patient Guide to Small Fiber Neuropathy. Hilton Publishing.

Living Gossip Home Health. (2021). *A Guide on Peripheral Neuropathy.* Living Gossip Home Health. https://livinggossip.com/a-guide-on-peripheral-neuropathy/

Mao Clinic. (2021). *Foot Drop.* Mayo Foundation for Medical Education and Research (MFMER). https://www.mayoclinic.org/diseases-conditions/foot-drop/symptoms-causes/syc-20372628

Mayo Clinic. (2021a). *Carpal Tunnel Syndrome.* Mayo Foundation for Medical Education and Research (MFMER). https://www.mayoclinic.org/diseases-conditions/carpal-tunnel-syndrome/diagnosis-treatment/drc-20355608

Mayo Clinic. (2021b). *Diabetic Neuropathy.* Mayo Foundation for Medical Education and Research (MFMER). https://www.mayoclinic.org/diseases-conditions/diabetic-neuropathy/symptoms-causes/syc-20371580

Mayo Clinic. (2012). *Left Untreated, Carpal Tunnel Syndrome Can Lead to Weakness in Fingers and Thumb.* Mayo Foundation for Medical Education and Research (MFMER). https://newsnetwork.mayoclinic.org/discussion/left-untreated-carpal-tunnel-syndrome-can-lead-to-weakness-in-fingers-and-thumb/

MedicalNewsToday Newsletter. (2021). *The American Academy of Family Physicians Recommend that Peripheral Neuropathy Treatment Address the Underlying Disease Process, Correct Nutritional Deficiencies, and Aim to Provide Relief from Symptoms.* MedicalNewsToday. https://www.medicalnewstoday.com/articles/live-updates-coronavirus-covid-19#31

Medscape. (2018). *What Is the Prevalence of Ulnar Neuropathy in the US?* WedMD LLC. https://www.medscape.com/answers/1141515-82630/what-is-the-prevalence-of-ulnar-neuropathy-in-the-us

Mobile Physiotherapy Clinic. (2017). *Common Peroneal Nerve Injury: Physiotherapy Treatments.* Mobile Physiotherapy Clinic Ahmedabad Gujarat. https://mobilephysiotherapyclinic.in/common-peroneal-nerve-injury-physiotherapy-treatments/

NCBI – PMC – US National Library of Medicine – National Institutes of Health. (2016). *Age as an Independent Factor for the Development of Neuropathy in Diabetic Patients.* National Center for Biotechnology Information, U.S. National Library of Medicine. https://www.ncbi.nlm.nih.gov/pmc/articles/PMC4801151/

NCBI – PMC – US National Library of Medicine – National Institutes of Health. (2008). *Diagnostic Approach to Peripheral Neuropathy.* National Center for Biotechnology Information, U.S. National Library of Medicine. https://www.ncbi.nlm.nih.gov/pmc/articles/PMC2771953/

Nerve and Muscle Center of Texas. (2021). *Diabetic Neuropathy – Questions and Answers.* Nerve and Muscle Center of Texas. https://www.nerveandmuscle.org/diabetic-neuropathy/

NervePainRemedies.com. (2021). *Cranial Neuropathy: Causes, Types, Symptoms, Treatment & Prevention.* NervePainRemedies.com. https://nervepainremedies.com/cranial-neuropathy/

Neuropathy Commons. (2021). *Neuropathy Overview.* Massachusetts General Hospital. https://neuropathycommons.org/neuropathy/neuropathy-overview

Neuropathy Commons. (2017). *Neuropathies Associated with Diabetes and the Metabolic Syndrome.* Massachusetts General Hospital. https://neuropathycommons.org/neuropathy/causes-neuropathy/neuropathies-associated-diabetes-and-metabolic-syndrome

NIH – National Institute of Diabetes and Digestive and Kidney Diseases. (2021a). *Autonomic Neuropathy.* U.S. Department of Health and Human Services – National Institutes of Health – USA.gov. https://www.niddk.nih.gov/health-information/diabetes/overview/preventing-problems/nerve-damage-diabetic-neuropathies/autonomic-neuropathy#causes

NIH – National Institute of Diabetes and Digestive and Kidney Diseases. (2021b). *Focal Neuropathies.* U.S. Department of Health and Human Services – National Institutes of Health – USA.gov. https://www.niddk.nih.gov/health-information/diabetes/overview/preventing-problems/nerve-damage-diabetic-neuropathies/focal-neuropathies

NIH - National Institute of Neurological Disorders and Stroke. (2021). *Foot Drop Information Page – What Research Is Being Done?* National Institutes of Health. https://www.ninds.nih.gov/disorders/all-disorders/foot-drop-information-page

NIH – National Library of Medicine – MedlinePlus. (2021a). *Cranial Mononeuropathy III – Diabetic Type.* U.S. Library of Medicine – U.S. Department of Health and Human Services – National Institutes of Health. https://medlineplus.gov/ency/article/000692.htm

NIH - National Library of Medicine – MedlinePlus. (2021b). *Common Peroneal Nerve Dysfunction*. U.S. National Library of Medicine – U.S. Department of Health and Human Services – National Institutes of Health. https://medlineplus.gov/ency/article/000791.htm

NIH – National Library of Medicine – National Center for Biotechnology Information. (2019). *Constitutional Risk Factors for Focal Neuropathies in Patients Referred for Electromyography*. National Library of Medicine. https://pubmed.ncbi.nlm.nih.gov/31692180/

NIH – National Library of Medicine – National Center for Biotechnology Information. (2012). *Risk Factors for Peroneal Nerve Injury and Recovery in Knee Dislocation*. National Library of Medicine. https://pubmed.ncbi.nlm.nih.gov/21822573/

NIH - National Library of Medicine – National Center for Biotechnology Information. (2010a). *Ischemic Optic Neuropathy: Are We Any Further?* National Library of Medicine. https://pubmed.ncbi.nlm.nih.gov/20802327/

NIH – National Library of Medicine – National Center for Biotechnology Information. (2010b). *The Level of Fibula Osteotomy and Incidence of Peroneal Nerve Palsy in Proximal Tibial Osteotomy*. National Library of Medicine. https://pubmed.ncbi.nlm.nih.gov/22091324/

PainAssist / ePainAssist.com. (2021). *Life Expectancy of Someone with Diabetic Neuropathy*. PainAssist Inc (ePainAssist). https://www.epainassist.com/diabetes/life-expectancy-of-someone-with-diabetic-neuropathy

Patient: Diabetic Amyotrophy. (2020). *Diabetic Amyotrophy Is a Nerve Disorder Complication of Diabetes Mellitus*. Egton Medical Information Systems Limited. https://patient.info/diabetes/diabetes-mellitus-leaflet/diabetic-amyotrophy

PatientsLikeMe. (2021). *Large Fiber Axonal Neuropathy*. PatientsLikeMe. https://www.patientslikeme.com/conditions/large-fiber-axonal-neuropathy

Physiopedia. (2021a). *Cervical Radiculopathy*. Physiopedia. https://www.physio-pedia.com/Cervical_Radiculopathy

Physiopedia. (2021b). *Lumbar Radiculopathy*. Physiopedia. https://www.physio-pedia.com/Lumbar_Radiculopathy

Physiopedia. (2021c). *Thoracic Radiculopathy*. Physiopedia. https://www.physio-pedia.com/Thoracic_Radiculopathy

Preston, D.C., and Shapiro, B.E. (2012). *Electromyography and Neuromuscular Disorders – Clinical-Electrophysiologic Correlations*, 3rd Edition. Elsevier.

Radiopaedia.org. (2021). *Charcot Joint*. Radiopaedia.org. https://radiopaedia.org/articles/charcot-joint

RehabMart.com. (2021). *The Ultimate Guide to Preventing Foot Drop*. Maximtech.com. https://library.rehabmart.com/post/the-ultimate-guide-to-preventing-foot-drop

RCEM Learning. (2021). *Radial Nerve Injuries: Radial Nerve Palsy*. RCEM Learning. https://www.rcemlearning.nl/modules/common-entrapment-syndromes/lessons/radial-nerve-in-the-forearm/topic/radial-nerve-injuries-radial-nerve-palsy/

ScienceDirect. (2020). *Acute Ischemic Optic Nerve Disease: Pathophysiology, Clinical Features and Management*. Elsevier B.V. https://www.sciencedirect.com/science/article/abs/pii/S0181551219305315

ScienceDirect. (2019). *Femoral Neuropathy*. Elsevier B.V. https://www.sciencedirect.com/topics/medicine-and-dentistry/femoral-neuropathy

ScienceDirect. (2013). *Diabetic Neuropathy – Peripheral Nerve Disorders*. Elsevier B.V. https://www.sciencedirect.com/topics/neuroscience/diabetic-neuropathy

ScienceDirect. (2010). *Cranial Neuropathy*. Elsevier B.V. https://www.sciencedirect.com/topics/medicine-and-dentistry/cranial-neuropathy

ScienceDirect. (2008). *Epidemiology of the Charcot Foot*. Elsevier B.V. https://www.sciencedirect.com/science/article/abs/pii/S0891842207000845

SpringerLink. (Originally 1981, Revised 2021). *Prevalence of Diabetic Autonomic Neuropathy Measured by Simple Bedside Tests*. Springer Nature Switzerland AG. https://link.springer.com/article/10.1007/BF00252626

SpringerLink. (2007). *Risk Factors for Ulnar Nerve Compression at the Elbow: A Case Control Study*. Springer Nature Switzerland AG. https://link.springer.com/article/10.1007/s00701-007-1166–5

SpringerOpen – Journal of Orthopaedics and Traumatology. (2019). *Final Outcomes of Radial Nerve Palsy Associated with Humeral Shaft Fracture and Nonunion*. BioMed Central Ltd. https://jorthoptraumatol.springeropen.com/articles/10.1186/s10195-019-0526–2

StatPearls. (2021). *Foot Drop – Continuing Education Activity*. StatPearls. https://www.statpearls.com/articlelibrary/viewarticle/21885/

Strakowski, J.A. (2020). *Ultrasound Evaluation of Peripheral Nerves and Focal Neuropathies – Correlation with Electrodiagnosis*, 2nd Edition. Demos Medical.

Tatva Health-PIE. (2016). *Cervical Radiculopathy: Prevention and Complications*. mTatva. https://www.mtatva.com/en/disease/cervical-radiculopathy-prevention-and-complications/

University of Iowa Health Care – Ophthalmology and Visual Sciences – EyeRounds.org. (2018). *Successive Presentation of Arteritic and Non-arteritic Anterior Ischemic Optic Neuropathy*. The University of Iowa. https://www.eyerounds.org/cases/276-AAION-NAION.htm

VeryWellHealth. (2021). *Prevention of Carpal Tunnel Syndrome*. About, Inc. (Dotdash). https://www.verywellhealth.com/preventing-carpal-tunnel-syndrome-2224091

VeryWellHealth. (2020). *Ulnar Nerve Injury – How Doctors Diagnose and Treat the "Funny Bone"*. About, Inc. (Dotdash). https://www.verywellhealth.com/ulnar-nerve-conditions-overview-4586755

Veves, A., and Malik, R.A. (2008). *Diabetic Neuropathy: Clinical Management*, 2nd Edition. Humana Press.

WebMD. (2020). *Cervical Radiculopathy*. WebMD LLC. https://www.webmd.com/pain-management/pain-management-cervical-radiculopathy

Wiesman, J.F. (2016). *Peripheral Neuropathy: What It Is and What You Can Do to Feel Better*. Johns Hopkins University Press.

CHAPTER 5 Diabetic Retinopathy

Retinal vascular disease (diabetic retinopathy) is one of the most common causes of blindness in the United States. The International Diabetes Federation estimates that the global population with diabetes mellitus will reach 700 million by the year 2045. Diabetic retinopathy is a common complication of diabetes and a leading cause of preventable blindness in adults. The global prevalence of diabetic retinopathy is 22.27% of diabetic patients, and vision-threatening diabetic retinopathy is at 6.17%. Diabetic retinopathy is damage to the retinal blood vessels, which become leaky or blocked. Vision loss most commonly occurs due to swelling in the macula, the central part of the retina, which can lead to vision impairment. Abnormal blood vessels can also grow from the retina, causing bleeding and blindness. Subclassifications include nonproliferative diabetic retinopathy, which may or may not be severe, and proliferative diabetic retinopathy. Complications of diabetes mellitus also include macular edema and retinal detachment. Other outcomes include intraretinal hemorrhage, exudates, macular ischemia, vitreous hemorrhage, and neovascularization.

NONPROLIFERATIVE DIABETIC RETINOPATHY

Nonproliferative diabetic retinopathy (NPDR) involves intraretinal vascular changes. There is no extraretinal fibrovascular tissue present. The subtypes of NPDR are described as mild, moderate, and severe. Another term for NPDR is *background diabetic retinopathy*. It is important to understand that NPDR differs from *proliferative diabetic retinopathy*, in which there is ischemia-related neovascularization from diabetes and its complications. *Clinically significant diabetic macular edema* (CSDME) exists if **macular edema** has progressed past minimal levels. The retinal microvascular changes in NPDR are only within the retina. They do not extend past the *internal limiting membrane*. Microaneurysms, capillary nonperfusion, intraretinal microvascular abnormalities, nerve fiber layer infarcts – also known as *cotton-wool spots* – *dot-and-blot* intraretinal hemorrhages, hard exudates, retinal edema, arteriolar changes, and retinal vein dilation and beading are often seen with NPDR. There are two ways in which NPDR affects vision. These include the following:

- Intraretinal vascular permeability increases, leading to macular edema

- Intraretinal capillary closure occurs, leading to macular ischemia

Diabetic Macular Edema

Diabetic macular edema involves edema of the macula that threatens or involves the fovea, the center of the macula. Vision loss is a common result. Macular edema is an outcome, in diabetic retinopathy, of abnormal retinal vascular permeability (see Figure 5.1).

Epidemiology

There have been a variety of epidemiological studies on diabetic macular edema. Most studies have revealed it to be more common in type 1 diabetics compared to type 2, but there are some studies that reversed this result. Overall prevalence of macular edema ranges from 4.2% to 14.25% in type 1 diabetic patients, and from 1.3% to 12.8% in type 2 diabetic patients. In patients diagnosed with diabetes before age 30, the 10-year incidence of diabetic macular edema is about 20%. If diagnosed with diabetes after age 30, the incidence is about 40%. Another study revealed that about 27% of patients developed signs of macular edema within 9 years of the onset of diabetes. It appears that female patients with diabetic macular edema are diagnosed and treated at stages when visual acuity and **optical coherence tomography** were worse than in males. Therefore, female diabetic patients should be assessed early for this disease. There appears to be no significant racial or ethnic predilection for diabetic macular edema.

Etiology and Risk Factors

The duration of diabetes mellitus strongly influences the development of diabetic macular edema. Chronic hyperglycemia is the primary risk factor for diabetic macular edema. Other risk factors include poorly controlled diabetes with chronically elevated hemoglobin A1c (HbA1c), hypertension, hyperlipidemia, kidney disease, and use of the thiazolidinedione-type drug called pioglitazone.

Pathophysiology

Diabetic macular edema can develop as focal or diffuse retinal thickening. Exudates may or may not be present. There are two basic categories

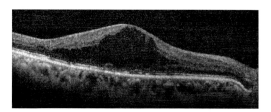

Figure 5.1 Diabetic macular edema.

DOI: 10.1201/9781003226727-7

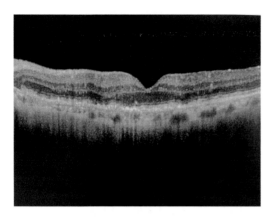

Figure 5.2 Macular degeneration.

of macular edema – focal and diffuse, though these can overlap. There may or may not be hard exudates that are precipitated plasma lipoproteins. The aqueous fluid is resorbed faster than the lipid plasma components. Therefore, lipid residues (hard exudates) accumulate, mostly in the inner and outer plexiform layers. Sometimes the lipid accumulates below the sensory retina. The lipids are yellow to white in color. Age-related macular degeneration may influence the development of macular edema (see Figure 5.2).

Diffuse macular edema involves retinal capillary leakage over wide areas and a large amount of breakdown of the blood-retinal barrier. **Cystoid fluid** often accumulates in the perifoveal macula, known as *cystoid macular edema*. Criteria have also been developed that help determine the clinical significance of either type of macular edema, influencing treatments.

Clinical Manifestations

Signs of diabetic macular edema include macular thickening with or without hard exudates, as seen during **stereobiomicroscopy**. Thickening may occur in focal, multifocal, and diffuse areas. The hard exudates may show different patterns, such as circinate rings. Diabetic macular edema can be asymptomatic, but decreased visual acuity usually occurs. It involves moderate vision loss. Some patients have *metamorphopsia*, a type of distorted vision in which a grid of straight lines appears "wavy." Parts of the grid may actually appear blank. Some patients first notice this condition while looking at the window blinds in their homes.

Diagnosis

Diabetic macular edema is diagnosed when retinal thickening is seen during slit-lamp biomicroscopy or optical coherence tomography. During the diagnostic process, there are three

important observations made, which include the following:

- The location of thickening of the retina, in relation to the center of the fovea
- Exudates being present, and their location
- Cystoid macular edema being present

Fluorescein angiography shows a breakdown of the blood-retinal barrier, via leakage of the retinal capillaries. Even so, angiography is not the best test to evaluate whether macular edema is present or not. Leakage seen on an angiogram can occur without macular retinal thickening, so it is not diagnostic of macular edema.

Treatment

Current treatments for diabetic macular edema were developed from the Early Treatment Diabetic Retinopathy Study. This was a random clinical trial that evaluated photocoagulation in diabetic patients with less than high-risk proliferative diabetic retinopathy in both eyes. The study defined clinically significant macular edema. Treatment with **focal laser photocoagulation** was recommended if the following criteria existed:

- The retinal edema was at or within 500 μm of the macula's center. The hard exudates were at or within 500 μm of the center if related to thickening of the nearby retina
- There was an area of thickening larger than one disc area, if present within one disc diameter of the macula's center

For diabetic macular edema, lifestyle modifications include increased exercise and weight reduction, quitting smoking, and improved control of body mass index as well as blood glucose, blood pressure, and blood lipids. When medical management has reached its most successful levels, eye therapies are considered in order to stop progressive vision loss and achieve the best vision possible. Treatments include ocular pharmacology and **laser photocoagulation**. To manage the condition of the eyes with diabetic macular edema, corticosteroids and antivascular endothelial growth factor drugs have been investigated.

For refractory macular edema, a posterior sub-Tenon injection of triamcinolone acetonide has improved visual acuity at 30 days, as well as stabilizing vision for up to 1 year. Increased intraocular pressure and ptosis only occurred rarely. This type of injection has been studied as an adjunct to macular laser photocoagulation to manage mild macular edema, but did not prove highly beneficial. When intravitreal triamcinolone acetonide was compared with macular laser treatment, the laser provided better visual acuity over 2 and 3 years. Sustained-release implants that contain fluocinolone and dexamethasone are effective, but result in progression of cataracts and glaucoma caused by the use of corticosteroids.

Laser surgery is very effective in managing diabetic macular edema. However, the exact role of **vitrectomy** is evolving. Focal- or grid-pattern macular argon laser photocoagulation treatment is also referred to as *macular laser*. It is proven to be effective for clinically significant macular edema (CSME). *Moderate visual loss (MVL)* is defined as a doubling of the visual angle such as a decrease from 20/20 vision to 20/40, or from 20/50 to 20/100. It is also described as a decrease of 15 or more letters on visual acuity charts used in the Early Treatment Diabetic Retinopathy Study, or a decrease of three or more lines of the Snellen visual acuity test. Laser photocoagulation reduces risks of MVL, increases the likelihood of visual improvement, and is linked to only slight loss of the visual field. Treatment of patients without CSME is usually deferred until edema threatens the center of the macula.

Deciding when to start treatment in CSME patients with normal visual acuity can be difficult, influenced by closeness of the exudates to the fovea, the health of the other eye, any cataract surgery that may be likely, or high-risk proliferative diabetic retinopathy. Photocoagulation for edema is preferred before performing scatter photocoagulation for high-risk proliferative diabetic retinopathy. Also, the edema should be treated before any cataract surgery due to the possible progression of retinopathy and macular edema after surgery. Subretinal fibrosis occurs less often when laser photocoagulation is performed. This fibrosis is linked to hard exudates in the macula and their severity. Adverse effects of laser photocoagulation for macular edema include **paracentral scotomata**, a transient increase of edema and/or a decrease in vision, choroidal neovascularization, subretinal fibrosis, photocoagulation scar expansion, and accidental foveolar burns. There are features linked to worsened visual acuity after photocoagulation, which include the following:

- Diffuse fluorescein leakage
- *Diffuse macular edema* – When there is foveal involvement
- Hard exudates in the fovea
- Macular ischemia
- Significant cystoid macular edema

Prevention

The primary prevention of diabetic macular edema is strict control of diabetes and other systemic diseases.

Prognosis

Prognosis is based on the severity of the edema. Between 25% and 30% of patients with CSME will have MVL within 3 years.

CLINICAL CASE

1. How prevalent is macular edema in type 1 and type 2 diabetic patients?
2. What are the risk factors for diabetic macular edema?
3. What are the three important observations made in the diagnosis of diabetic macular edema?

A 39-year-old diabetic woman began to notice moderate vision loss. Fluorescein angiography was used as part of the diagnosis and focal macular edema was diagnosed. The patient underwent laser photocoagulation and was driven home by her husband. Her eyesight remained hazy and blurry throughout the next day, but then began to improve. The patient reported seeing small spots in her field of vision – a normal result of laser photocoagulation – but these disappeared within 1 week. The patient was counseled about better control of blood glucose and started on a more intensive glucose-monitoring schedule, increased exercise, a more nutritional diet, and follow-up occurred every months for the first 6 months. She then had a thorough ophthalmological examination and was scheduled for another within 1 year.

ANSWERS

1. Overall prevalence of macular edema ranges from 4.2% to 14.25% in type 1 diabetic patients and from 1.3% to 12.8% in type 2 diabetic patients.

2. Chronic hyperglycemia is the primary risk factor for diabetic macular edema. Other risk factors include poorly controlled diabetes with chronically elevated HbA1c, hypertension, hyperlipidemia, kidney disease, and use of the thiazolidinedione-type drug called pioglitazone.

3. During diagnosis of diabetic macular edema, the three important observations include the location of retinal thickening in relation to the center of the fovea, the presence and location of exudates, and the presence of cystoid macular edema.

Diabetic Macular Ischemia

Diabetic macular ischemia involves closure of small blood vessels in the eye, resulting in a lack of blood supply to the macula. It is an important clinical feature of diabetic retinopathy. Selective loss of **pericytes** and thickening of the basement membrane in retinal capillaries may occur due to exposure to hyperglycemia over extended periods of time. There is an enlargement of the *foveal avascular zone* (FAZ) and paramacular areas of capillary nonperfusion. About 41% of patients with diabetic retinopathy have some evidence of macular ischemia. Visual function is affected only in those with moderate to severe macular ischemia.

Retinal capillary nonperfusion is commonly linked with moderate to severe nonproliferative diabetic retinopathy. Fluorescein angiography can reveal the amount of capillary nonperfusion. The FAZ may become irregular due to nonperfusion of the marginal capillaries. Microaneurysms often group together at the margins of areas of capillary nonperfusion. Retinal arteriole closure may cause large areas of nonperfusion, and ischemia that is progressive. If the FAZ is larger than 1,000 μm in diameter, this is generally related to central vision loss. Overall, diabetic macular ischemia is difficult to detect and there is a lack of treatment options. Methods are being studied about achieving revascularization of the retina and macula by guiding new blood vessels into the ischemic tissue, to reduce or prevent additional damage. Preclinical studies are ongoing regarding *ischemia modulator* medications.

Severe Nonproliferative Diabetic Retinopathy

Severe nonproliferative diabetic retinopathy is the most serious form of this disease. It is characterized by the *4:2:1 rule*, which requires at least one of the following factors:

- 4 quadrants of diffuse intraretinal hemorrhages and microaneurysms

- 2 quadrants of venous beading

- 1 quadrant of intraretinal microvascular abnormalities

In the previous decades, the term *preproliferative diabetic retinopathy* was used to describe this condition. The 4:2:1 rule was eventually developed to identify patients that are at the highest risk of developing proliferative diabetic retinopathy as well as *high-risk proliferative diabetic retinopathy*. Severe nonproliferative diabetic retinopathy progresses to high-risk proliferative diabetic retinopathy within 1 year in 15% of cases. *Very severe nonproliferative diabetic retinopathy* is present if there are two of the features listed in the 4:2:1 rule present, with a 45% chance of progression to high-risk proliferative diabetic retinopathy in 1 year. All of these patients must be considered for early panretinal photocoagulation. With disease progression, the amount of capillary damage and nonperfusion is increased. This leads to retinal ischemia and a release of vasoproliferative factors, which include vascular endothelial growth factor. This factor was isolated from vitrectomy specimens, from patients with proliferative diabetic retinopathy, and can stimulate retinal neovascularization as well as neovascularization of the optic nerve head or anterior segment.

CLINICAL CASE

1. How is the 4:2:1 rule used to assess severe nonproliferative diabetic retinopathy?
2. How often does severe nonproliferative diabetic retinopathy progress to proliferative diabetic retinopathy?
3. Which vasoproliferative factor has been found in vitrectomy specimens, in relation to the development of proliferative diabetic retinopathy?

A 61-year-old diabetic woman had started to develop nonproliferative retinopathy in her left eye, which had recently become severe. Examination revealed diffuse intraretinal hemorrhages, hard exudates, microaneurysms, venous beading of two fields, and intraretinal microvascular abnormalities in two fields. Her left eye vision was equivalent to 20/30 on the Snellen eye chart. The patient had been diagnosed with type 2 diabetes 14 years earlier and was receiving insulin and the antidiabetic drug canagliflozin. She also had experienced an ischemic stroke that was currently being treated with aspirin and clopidogrel. Her father also had type 2 diabetes as well as heart disease.

ANSWERS

1. The 4:2:1 rule requires at least one of the following factors to be present: 4 quadrants of diffuse intraretinal hemorrhages and microaneurysms, 2 quadrants of venous beading, and 1 quadrant of intraretinal microvascular abnormalities.
2. Severe nonproliferative diabetic retinopathy progresses to high-risk proliferative diabetic retinopathy within 1 year in 15% of cases.
3. Vascular endothelial growth factor has been found in vitrectomy specimens, from patients with proliferative diabetic retinopathy. It can simulate retinal neovascularization as well as neovascularization of the optic nerve head or anterior segment.

PROLIFERATIVE DIABETIC RETINOPATHY

Proliferative diabetic retinopathy is a severe form of retinopathy that can lead to vitreous hemorrhage and *tractional retinal detachment*. There is abnormal neovascularization – the formation of new blood vessels on the retinal surface. This can continue into the vitreous cavity, where it causes vitreous hemorrhage. Neovascularization is often present with pre-retinal fibrous tissue. Along with the vitreous, it can contract and cause tractional retinal detachments. Neovascularization can occur in the anterior segment of the eye, on the iris, as well as neovascular membrane growth in the anterior chamber angle, at the peripheral margin of the iris. This results in *neovascular glaucoma*. Vision loss can be severe. Extreme macular edema can develop with any form of retinopathy. It is the most common cause of vision loss in relation to diabetic retinopathy.

Epidemiology

Proliferative diabetic retinopathy is a prevalent complication in 23% of insulin-dependent individuals when their diabetes was diagnosed before 30 years of age, and in 10% of insulin-dependent individuals with diabetes diagnosed after 30 years of age. Proliferative retinopathy is also a prevalent complication in 3% of patients that do not take insulin for their diabetes. However, while not always a *prevalent* complication, retinopathy is present in about 75% of patients with type 1 diabetes, and in about 50% of patients with type 2 diabetes. About 25% of diabetic patients develop macular edema. By the year 2038, it is predicted that more than 360 million people throughout the world will have diabetes and complications such as retinopathy. In the United States alone, about 500,000 patients have CSDME, with an annual incidence of 75,000. About 700,000 patients have proliferative diabetic retinopathy, with an annual incidence of 65,000. Diabetic retinopathy is the leading cause of blindness in people between the ages of 20 and 64. According to the World Health Organization, diabetic retinopathy is estimated to account for 4.8% of all cases of blindness worldwide. With type 1 diabetes, retinopathy affects 10%–50% of patients based on the population, screening methods, and disease duration. With type 2 diabetes, overall prevalence is 25.2% of the population. There appears to be no significant male-to-female predilection or any racial or ethnic differences. Fortunately, because of increased awareness of risk factors, better glycemic control, and access to screening, there is a decline occurring in the global prevalence and incidence of diabetic retinopathy in developed countries. The regions of the world with the most cases of diabetic retinopathy include the Western Pacific Region (45 million), Southeast Asia Region (32 million), European Region (22 million), North-Central-South American Region (21 million), Eastern Mediterranean Region (14 million), and African Region (8 million).

Etiology and Risk Factors

Proliferative diabetic retinopathy involves degeneration of the **retinal neuropil**, even in areas that are not close to any vascular lesions. There are **Müller cell** defects present. All retinal cell types are damaged, including the inner retinal neurons and their projections. There is

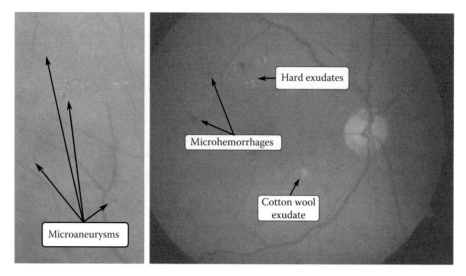

Figure 5.3 Typical retinal lesions of diabetic retinopathy. (With permission from Ng, E. Y. K., Rajendra Acharya, U., Suri, Jasjit S., and Campilho, A. (2014). *Image Analysis and Modeling in Ophthalmology.* CRC Press/Taylor & Francis.)

dysfunction of the Müller cells and astrocytes. Clinical risk factors for proliferative diabetic retinopathy include the severity of the diabetes and its duration, hypertension, other complications, anemia, hyperlipidemia, family history, and insulin resistance and deficiency. One nucleotide polymorphism in the promoter region of the *erythropoietin* gene results in a two times higher risk of proliferative retinopathy as well as end-stage renal disease, compared to patients lacking this mutation. Genetic risk factors include changes in chromosomes 1p, 3 and *insulin-like growth factor 1* (IGF-1) *gene.* Other risk factors concern changes in the *vitamin D receptor* and the *receptor for advance glycation endproducts* (RAGE) *gene.* Aside from hyperlipidemia, other modifiable risk factors include hyperglycemia, hypertension, smoking, pregnancy, and obesity.

Pathophysiology

Along with the causative cellular defects, there is pathophysiological progression from severe nonproliferative to high-risk proliferative retinopathy. The microglia are activated, there are resident immune cells from the nervous system, and the pigment epithelium degenerates. Leakage of the perifoveal capillaries is believed to cause macular thickening. Histology reveals loss of retinal neurons and foveal cysts. Diabetes affects the eyes by causing chronic inflammation, diffuse vascular dilation, leakage, neovascularization, tortuosity, atrophy of the retinal neural parenchyma, macular edema, and eventually, fibrosis. There are often

microaneurysms, microhemorrhages, and exudates that may be hard or described as "cotton-wool" exudates (see Figure 5.3). A maladaptive response occurs, with inflammation damaging the tissues because of edema, and invasion of circulating immune cells. In the retina, the insulin receptor is expressed in every cell, forming heterodimers with the insulin-like growth factor 1 receptor.

Clinical Manifestations

Prior to proliferative retinopathy, macular edema or ischemia begins to cause visual problems. Sometimes, there is no vision loss even if retinopathy becomes advanced. Initial signs of nonproliferative retinopathy include capillary microaneurysms, soft exudates known as *cotton-wool spots*, dot-and-blot hemorrhages of the retina, and hard exudates. Hard exudates suggest that chronic edema is present. Cotton-wool spots are microinfarctions of the retinal nerve fiber layer that result in opacification of the retina. They have fuzzy edges, a white color, and they obscure the blood vessels lying below them. In later states, signs include macular edema, intraretinal microvascular abnormalities, and venous dilation. Macular edema can be seen during slit-lamp biomicroscopy. It appears as elevations and blurring of the retinal layers.

The symptoms of proliferative retinopathy include blurred vision, flashing lights in the visual field, and **floaters**. There can also be painless vision loss that occurs suddenly, which is severe. All of these symptoms are usually due to traction retinal detachment or vitreous hemorrhage. Unlike nonproliferative retinopathy, the proliferative form causes fine preretinal vessel neovascularization. This can be viewed on the retinal surface or optic nerve. **Funduscopy** may reveal macular edema or retinal hemorrhage.

Diagnosis

Diagnosis of proliferative diabetic retinopathy is by funduscopy. The level of the disease may be graded via color fundus photography. To determine extent of the disease, guide treatment, and monitor results of treatment, fluorescein angiography is indicated. Optical coherence tomography is used to assess the severity of macular edema and the response to treatment. Ultra-wide-field imaging is used to screen for and detect diabetic retinopathy, along with ultra-wide-field angiography. All patients with diabetes must have an annual dilated ophthalmologic examination, and pregnant diabetic women must be examined every trimester. An ophthalmologic referral is needed if there is blurred vision or other vision symptoms.

Treatment

The treatment of proliferative diabetic retinopathy is critically based on control of blood pressure and blood glucose. Progression of the disease is slowed with intense control of blood glucose. Cognitive behavioral therapy in combination with self-management and adherence interventions has been successful in slowing or preventing the development of diabetic retinopathy. If there is CSME, this is treated with intraocular injection of antivascular endothelial growth factor (VEGF) drugs. These drugs include *aflibercept* (*Eylea*), *bevacizumab* (*Avastin*), and *ranibizumab* (*Lucentis*). Also, focal laser photocoagulation can be used, with or without the VEGF drugs. For persistent macular edema, there are intraocular corticosteroids such as *dexamethasone* (*Ozurdex*) implants and intravitreal *triamcinolone* (*Triesence*). In various countries, there is an intraocular *fluocinolone* implant available for chronic diabetic macular edema. Trade names for this agent include *Iluvien* and *Retisert*. These corticosteroids reduce inflammation, inhibit VEGF, and increase tight junctions between capillary endothelial cells. They are very effective when used with macular laser therapy.

For recalcitrant diabetic macular edema, vitrectomy may be needed. Sometimes, panretinal laser photocoagulation is used for severe nonproliferative retinopathy, but this is often delayed until proliferative retinopathy has developed. If proliferative retinopathy is of high risk, accompanied with extensive preretinal neovascularization, or there is anterior segment neovascularization with neovascular glaucoma, it must be treated with panretinal photocoagulation (PRP). Intravitreal anti-VEGF drugs are also usually successful. These treatments greatly reduce risks for severe vision loss. Vitrectomy may preserve or restore vision loss if there is extensive preretinal membrane formation, persistent vitreous hemorrhage, recalcitrant diabetic macular edema, or traction retinal detachment.

A "full" PRP includes 1,200 or more 500 μm burns that use argon green or a blue/green laser, which are separated by one-half burn width. Contracture of fibrovascular tissue occurs, so treatment can be followed by additional vitreous hemorrhage, **vitreoretinal traction**, combined tractional-rhegmatogenous retinal detachment, and tractional retinal detachment. Also, the contraction of fibrovascular tissue and additional traction can cause recurring vitreous hemorrhages. The adverse effects of *scatter PRP* include decreased color and night vision, reduced contrast sensitivity, and decreased peripheral vision. A patient can lose one or two lines of visual acuity or see "glares." There are transient adverse effects such as loss of accommodation and corneal sensitivity, as well as photopsias. A PRP procedure can precipitate or worsen macular edema. The use of more peripheral laser placement may be able to stop progression of proliferative diabetic retinopathy and preserve the biggest central visual field. When the horizontal meridians (the pathways of long ciliary vessels and nerves) are spared, accommodation and corneal innervation are protected. When needed, extensive treatment is performed in retinal areas where vision loss is not as noticeable or is related to less morbidity. The nasal and superior retina receive extensive treatment last because they correspond to essential temporal and inferior peripheral vision. Extra care is taken to avoid foveal photocoagulation, especially when image-inverting contact lenses are used.

Prevention

The prevention of diabetic retinopathy is based on controlling BP and blood glucose. Onset of retinopathy is delayed if there is intensive blood glucose control. A newer preventive method is the use of carbonic anhydrase inhibitors such as *dorzolamide* (*Trusopt*) to dilate the retinal capillaries and decrease the amount of capillaries that become occluded. Also, *renin-angiotensin system inhibitors* may electively prevent or delay retinopathy's progression. Topical treatment with anti-VEGF agents may be effective for advanced retinopathy, to reduce the need for laser photocoagulation.

Prognosis

The prognosis of diabetic retinopathy is quite varied due to the expensive of treatments, which may limit patient access to treatment and worsen prognosis. The outlook is based on the *Early Treatment for Diabetic Retinopathy Study*, which found that laser surgery for macular edema reduces incidence of MVL from 30% to 15% over 3 years. The *Diabetic Retinopathy Study* found that panretinal laser photocoagulation reduces risks for severe visual loss by more than 50%.

CLINICAL CASE

1. What is the definition of proliferative retinopathy?
2. What are the differences in the signs and symptoms of nonproliferative and proliferative retinopathy?
3. What does the prevention of diabetic retinopathy require?

A 52-year-old man previously diagnosed with type 2 diabetes mellitus but no diabetic retinopathy went to his ophthalmologist because of vision changes. At that time, he was diagnosed with proliferative retinopathy. The patient lost nearly all the vision in his left eye, and oral hypoglycemic agents were prescribed to prevent further progression of the disease. These were effective, but it was decided to hospitalize the patient and initiate insulin therapy. The patient's right eye also had begun to worsen with regard to visual acuity, but it was nowhere as serious as his left eye. The patient eventually had to retire from his career as a truck driver due to his eyesight, and instead took a job in which he could work from home.

ANSWERS

1. Proliferative retinopathy is a severe form of retinopathy that can lead to vitreous hemorrhage and traction retinal detachment. There is abnormal neovascularization. It can continue into the vitreous cavity, where it causes vitreous hemorrhage. Neovascularization is often present with preretinal fibrous tissue. Along with the vitreous, it can contract and cause traction retinal detachment. Vision loss can be severe.
2. Initial signs of nonproliferative retinopathy include capillary microaneurysms, soft exudates (cotton-wool spots), dot-and-blot hemorrhages of the retina, and hard exudates. Later, signs include macular edema, intraretinal microvascular abnormalities, and venous dilation. The symptoms of proliferative retinopathy include blurred vision, flashing lights in the visual field, and floaters. There can also be painless vision loss that occurs suddenly, which is severe.
3. The prevention of diabetic retinopathy is based on controlling blood pressure and blood glucose. Onset is delayed if there is intensive blood glucose control. A newer preventive method is the use of carbonic anhydrase inhibitors such as dorzolamide (Trusopt) to dilate the retinal capillaries and decrease the amount of capillaries that become occluded. Renin-angiotensin system inhibitors by electively prevent or delay disease progression. For advanced retinopathy, topical treatment with anti-VEGF agents may be effective to reduce the need for laser photocoagulation.

KEY TERMS

- Cystoid fluid
- Floaters
- Fluorescein angiography
- Focal laser photocoagulation
- Funduscopy
- Laser photocoagulation
- Macular edema
- Müller cell
- Optical coherence tomography
- Paracentral scotomata
- Pericytes
- Retinal neuropil
- Stereobiomicroscopy
- Vitrectomy
- Vitreoretinal traction

REFERENCES

Abraham, C., and Mathai, A. (2019). *Diabetic Retinopathy for the Clinician.* Jaypee Brothers Medical Publishers Ltd.

Academia.edu. (2021). *A Case Study of a Patient with Diabetic Retinopathy.* Academia. https://www.academia.edu/Register ToDownload/BulkDownload

American Diabetes Association – Diabetes Care. (1992). *Epidemiology of Proliferative Diabetic Retinopathy*. American Diabetes Association. https://care.diabetesjournals.org/content/15/12/1875

ARVO Journals / Investigative Ophthalmology & Visual Science / Retina. (2016). *The Evaluation of Diabetic Macular Ischemia Using Optical Coherence Tomography Angiography*. The Association for Research in Vision and Ophthalmology. https://iovs.arvojournals.org/article.aspx?articleid=2496245

Baumal, C.R., and Duker, J.S. (2017). *Current Management of Diabetic Retinopathy*. Elsevier.

BMC / Springer Nature / Eye and Vision. (2021). *Prevalence of Diabetic Macular Edema among Diabetic Subjects*. BioMed Central Ltd. https://eandv.biomedcentral.com/articles/10.1186/s40662-015-0026-2/tables/4

BMC / Springer Nature / Ophthalmology. (2021). *Subretinal Leakage of a Retinal Capillary Microaneurysm – A Case Report*. BioMed Central Ltd. https://bmcophthalmol.biomedcentral.com/articles/10.1186/s12886-021-01984-6

Boehringer Ingelheim. (2021). *Advancing a Vision for Pioneering Treatments in Diabetic Macular Ischemia*. Boehringer Ingelheim International GmbH. https://www.boehringer-ingelheim.com/human-health/science-stories/research-in-diabetic-macular-ischemia

Boyer, D.S., and Tabandeh, H. (2014). *Diabetic Retinopathy: From Diagnosis to Treatment*. Addicus Books.

Carter, D., and Montgomery, E. (2014). *Diabetic Retinopathy: Causes, Tests, and Treatment Options*. Carter.

El-Baz, A.S., and Suri, J.S. (2020). *Diabetes and Retinopathy* (Computer-Assisted Diagnosis, Volume 2). Elsevier.

Karger. (2021). *Retinal Diseases Amenable to Pharmacotherapy – Diabetic Retinopathy and Diabetic Macular Edema*. S. Karger AG, Basel. https://www.karger.com/Article/Fulltext/438970

Kayte, S., Kayte, J., and Kayte, C. (2019). *Non-Proliferative Diabetic Retinopathy Detection by Digital R-Images*. Scholars' Press.

Khorram, D., and Liu, A. (2020). *Diabetic Eye Disease: An Easy to Understand Guide to Keeping Your Vision for People with Diabetes*, 2nd Edition. Khorram.

Kychenthal, A.B., and Dorta, P.S. (2017). *Retinopathy of Prematurity: Current Diagnosis and Management*. Springer.

The Lancet. (2009). *Prevention of Diabetic Retinopathy*. Elsevier Inc. https://www.thelancet.com/journals/lancet/article/PIIS0140-6736(09)60750-9/fulltext

Leslie, R.D.G., and Pozzilli, P. (2003). *Diabetic Complications: New Diagnostic Tools and Therapeutic Advances (International Bart's Symposium)*. CRC Press.

Marashi, A. (2017). *Clinical Diabetic Retinopathy: Step by Step for Management and Decision Making*. Lap Lambert Academic Publishing.

Medscape. (2020). *What Is the Prognosis of Diabetic Retinopathy?* WebMD LLC. https://www.medscape.com/answers/1225122-100711/what-is-the-prognosis-of-diabetic-retinopathy

National Library of Medicine – National Center for Biotechnology Information. (2016). *A Case Study of a Patient with Diabetic Retinopathy*. National Library of Medicine. https://pubmed.ncbi.nlm.nih.gov/26907970/

National Library of Medicine – National Center for Biotechnology Information. (2011). *Prevention and Treatment of Diabetic Retinopathy: Evidence from Clinical Trials and Perspectives*. National Library of Medicine. https://pubmed.ncbi.nlm.nih.gov/21438851/

National Library of Medicine – National Center for Biotechnology Information. (2001). *Prognostic Significance of Retinal Microaneurysm Number and Localization in Type-1 Diabetes Mellitus*. National Library of Medicine. https://pubmed.ncbi.nlm.nih.gov/11582732/

NIH / National Library of Medicine / National Center for Biotechnology Information. (2020). *Gender-Related Differences in Patients Treated with Intravitreal Anti-Vascular Endothelial Growth Factor Medication for Diabetic Macular Edema*. National Library of Medicine. https://pubmed.ncbi.nlm.nih.gov/31937122/

Ohji, M. (2019). *Surgical Retina (Retina Atlas)*. Springer.

Ortega, A.L. (2021). *Oxidative Stress in Diabetic Retinopathy*. Mdpi AG.

Review of Ophthalmology. (2018). *Managing Retinal Macro-aneurysms*. Jobson Medical Information LLC. https://www.reviewofophthalmology.com/article/managing-retinal-macroaneurysms

Scanlon, P.H., Sallam, A., and van Wijngaarden, P. (2017). *A Practical Manual of Diabetic Retinopathy Management*, 2nd Edition. Wiley-Blackwell.

Sivaraj, R.R., and Dodson, P. (2020). *Diabetic Retinopathy: Screening to Treatment*, 2nd Edition. Oxford University Press.

Springer Link / Diabetic Retinopathy. (2010). *Diabetic Macular Ischemia*. Springer Nature Switzerland AG. https://link.springer.com/chapter/10.1007/978-0-387-85900-2_8

StatPearls. (2021). *Diabetic Macular Edema*. StatPearls. https://www.statpearls.com/articlelibrary/viewarticle/24631/

Stewart, M.W. (2017). *Diabetic Retinopathy: Current Pharmacologic Treatment and Emerging Strategies*. Adis.

TvAssignmentHelp. (2021). *Mr. Hank Johnson Case Study – Diabetic Retinopathy – Nursing Assignment Help*. TvAssignmentHelp. https://www.tvassignmenthelp.com/questions/mr-hank-jackson-case-study-diabetic-retinopathy-nursing-assignment-help

Wiley Online Library – Clinical & Experimental Ophthalmology. (2015). *Diabetic Retinopathy: Global Prevalence, Major Risk Factors, Screening Practices and Public Health Challenges: A Review*. John Wiley & Sons, Inc. https://www.onlinelibrary.wiley.com/doi/full/10.1111/ceo.12696

World Health Organization. (2009). *Diabetes and Diabetic Retinopathy*. Dr. Silvio Paolo Mariotti. https://www.iapb.org/wp-content/uploads/Diabetes-and-Diabetic-Retinopathy_Silvio-Mariotti_14Sept2013.pdf

CHAPTER 6 Diabetic Nephropathy

Diabetic nephropathy is a primary cause of chronic kidney disease. There is thickening of the glomerular basement membrane, glomerular sclerosis, and mesangial expansion. Diabetic nephropathy is one of the major complications of diabetes mellitus that results in kidney failure and death without treatment. The changes that occur lead to glomerular hypertension and a steady decline in the glomerular filtration rate. If there is systemic hypertension present, the progression of diabetic nephropathy may occur more quickly. It is usually asymptomatic until the development of nephrotic syndrome or renal failure. The detection of urinary albumin prompts the diagnosis of diabetic nephropathy. Once the presence of diabetes is diagnosed, urinary albumin should be monitored regularly, at least once per year, by measuring the albumin: creatinine ratio. Diabetic nephropathy is managed with strict blood glucose and blood pressure control.

GLOMERULAR BASEMENT MEMBRANE NEPHROPATHY

The glomerular basement membrane (GBM) is a thin structure within the nephrons of the kidneys. Each nephron consists of three parts, which include a tiny blood vessel that brings in unfiltered blood, the **glomerulus**, and another tiny blood vessel that returns filtered blood to the body. The earliest change in the kidneys that often occurs because of diabetes is a thickening of the GBM, which separates the blood from the urine. If the membrane is damaged, proteins leak from the blood into the urine. Albumin can be detected in the urine even when kidney disease is in its early stages and is only mild. Damage to the GBM can be seen in electron microscope studies. If the disease progresses chronically, the kidneys eventually cannot function normally, leading to renal failure. GBM nephropathy is also called *thin basement membrane nephropathy.*

Epidemiology

GBM nephropathy is estimated to affect between 1% and 10% of the population, though many experts agree that the percentage is probably closer to 1% or 2%. This type of nephropathy affects a higher percentage of type 1 diabetes patients than type 2 diabetes patients. Aside from its links to diabetes, it is also the most common inherited renal disease. Globally, GBM has been documented in Caucasians, Africans, Chinese, and Indians. Median ages of presentation are 37 years for adults and 7 years for children. Hematuria caused by the disease has been reported in an age range from 1 to 86 years. It is 1.6 times more common in females than in males.

Etiology and Risk Factors

GBM nephropathy is caused by thickening of the glomerular basement membrane. The exact reason that this occurs is not known, but it results in abnormal function and large amounts of protein being lost in the urine. This form of nephropathy may be a primary kidney disease or related to other conditions. Risk factors for GBM nephropathy are increased by lung and colon cancers, exposure to toxins such as gold and mercury, infections, medications, and autoimmune disorders such as **systemic lupus erythematous**, rheumatoid arthritis, and **Graves' disease**. Causative infections include endocarditis, hepatitis B, malaria, and syphilis. Causative medications include penicillamine, creams used for skin lightening, and trimethadione.

Pathophysiology

GBM diabetic nephropathy most often damages the glomeruli of the kidneys. There may be thickening of the capillary basement membrane, diffuse glomerular sclerosis, and nodular lesions in the glomerular capillaries, which impairs blood flow, leading to progressive kidney function loss and renal failure. When the basement membrane changes, plasma proteins escape in the urine. This causes albuminuria, edema, hypoalbuminemia, and various signs of kidney impairment. There are five stages in the pathophysiology of GBM diabetic neuropathy, which include the following:

- **Hyperfiltration** – This increases the glomerular filtration rate (GFR), with increased capillary glomerular pressure. It occurs because of renal hypertrophy and may be partly caused by intrarenal hemodynamic abnormalities from diabetes, contributing to glomerular hypertension.

- **Silent stage** – In this stage, albuminuria is not present. There can be basement membrane thickening, mesangial expansion, and slight increases in BP.

- **Microalbuminuria** – This occurs 5–15 years after the initial diagnosis of type 1 diabetes. There are many glomerular structural changes and increases in BP. With no treatment, microalbuminuria may cause severe nephropathy. In most cases of type 1 diabetes, microalbuminuria resolves by itself.

DOI: 10.1201/9781003226727-8

- **Macroalbuminuria** – In GBM diabetic nephropathy, macroalbuminuria is worsened. Without treatment, renal failure can occur. Urinary albumin excretion is over 300 mg in 24 hours. It may be seen after the patient has had diabetes for 10–15 years. Over 70% of patients have serious systemic hypertension.

- **Uremia** – This develops in about 40% of patients with type 1 diabetes. Dialysis of kidneys may be needed. However, a kidney transplant is the ultimate indicated treatment.

Clinical Manifestations

The clinical manifestations include edema of the feet, ankles, and lower legs, due to water retention. The urine may darker due to the presence of blood. Dyspnea and fatigue are often present. Nausea or vomiting are common, and there may also be a metallic taste in the mouth.

Diagnosis

Diabetes is often signified initially by hyperfiltration, kidney enlargement, and nephron hypertrophy. This means that the kidneys must work much hard to reabsorb excessively large amounts of glucose. In diabetic nephropathy, there is often an initial increase of urinary albumin excretion. This means a loss of urine protein that is greater than 30 mg per day. Systolic or diastolic hypertension makes diabetic nephropathy develop more quickly. Risk of chronic kidney disease can be reduced even with moderate lowering of blood pressure. Regular monitoring of the estimated GFR should occur.

Treatment

Treatment of GBM diabetic neuropathy avoiding nonsteroidal anti-inflammatory drugs (NSAIDs) and cyclooxygenase-2 (COX-2) inhibitors. Their use may cause poor BP control, and reduce effects of antihypertensive drugs. Medications and dosing of oral hypoglycemics are critical. The patient at high risk for progressive renal deterioration should be referred to a nephrologist for consultation to manage renal failure. Other options include hemodialysis, peritoneal dialysis, and renal transplantation. Most of the patients prefer hemodialysis over peritoneal dialysis.

Prevention

Smoking cessation, controlling blood pressure, treating hyperlipidemia, and good glycemic control are the keys for preventing or reducing proteinuria. Smoking increases the risks of chronic kidney disease. Type 2 diabetics have a higher risk of increased excretion of urinary albumin.

Prognosis

The prognosis of GBM nephropathy is generally good. Up to 33% of patients go into remission even without treatment within 5 years. With immunosuppressive therapy, most patients go into remission. However, relapse is common and has a worsened prognosis since it may lead to end-stage kidney disease. Better prognostic factors include lower levels of protein in the urine, female gender, and age less than 60 years.

GLOMERULAR SCLEROSIS

Glomerular sclerosis, also known as *glomerulosclerosis*, is hardening of the glomeruli in the kidneys. The term generally describes progressive scarring of the glomeruli, which is linked to diabetes mellitus. Lumpy nodules of scar tissue may form, which is referred to as *nodular diabetic glomerulosclerosis*. Scattered, segmental mesangial sclerosis beginning in some glomeruli that will eventually affect all of the glomeruli is described as *focal segmental glomerulosclerosis*. This is usually an idiopathic condition, but can be secondary to obesity, *atheroembolic disease*, loss of the nephrons, sickle cell disease, use of drugs such as heroin, and HIV infection. The disease is the most common cause of primary **nephrotic syndrome** in adults.

Epidemiology

Diabetic glomerular nephropathy, including sclerosis, is the most common cause of chronic renal failure in adults, and causes 45% of kidney transplants. It is increasing in prevalence, along with type 2 diabetes, obesity, and metabolic syndrome. Between 30% and 40% of type 1 diabetics develop nephropathy after 20 years, and between 15% and 20% of type 2 diabetics develop it within the same length of time. However, type 2 diabetes affects 90% of all diabetic patients; therefore, more patients with diabetic glomerular nephropathy have type 2 diabetes. Men are affected more than women, and more people from African American, Native American, and Pacific Islander ethnic groups are affected.

Etiology and Risk Factors

Aside from diabetes causing glomerular sclerosis and other nephropathies, risk factors include persistent hyperglycemia (glucotoxicity), hyperlipidemia, hypertension, lack of physical activity, smoking, and a diet that is high in fat and protein. Genetics are also linked to the disease, and a family history of any diabetic glomerulopathy increases risks.

Pathophysiology

Diabetic glomerular sclerosis is characterized by thickening of the GBM, and increased permeability. The mesangial space gradually enlarges because of deposits of proteins, which is initially diffuse but then becomes nodular. When diffuse, the deposits appear on the basement membranes of the capillary loops of the glomeruli, as well as the basement membranes of the tubules and arterioles. When nodular, periodic acid-Schiff (PAS)-positive deposits may appear in the mesangial space. They contain collagen, fibrils, and mucopolysaccharides, and may be located at the periphery of the glomerulus, pushing against the capillaries. They are focal lesions – not affecting all of the glomerulus – and are also known as *Kimmelstiel-Wilson lesions*.

The nodular lesions are round or oval in shape. Over time as they expand, the capillaries become compressed and the entire glomerulus can be destroyed. **Hyalinosis** is also present, which affects the afferent and efferent arterioles of the glomerulus. In the capillary loops, they are referred to as *fibrin caps*. In the Bowman capsules, they are called *capsular drops*. Over time, ischemia develops, followed by interstitial fibrosis and atrophy of the tubules. These changes cause the kidney to contract. Therefore, on a clinical basis, glomerular sclerosis is often seen as renal failure begins.

Clinical Manifestations

The most important sign of glomerular sclerosis is proteinuria, which is often discovered during a routine examination. Losing a large amount of protein can cause swelling in the ankles as well as buildup of **ascites**, and "puffy" eyes.

Diagnosis

The diagnosis of glomerular sclerosis is based on the presence of proteinuria. A kidney biopsy is often required. Between 7% and 15% of patients with proteinuria have glomerular sclerosis.

Treatment

Treatments for glomerular sclerosis are based on patient age, medical history, overall health, progression of the disease, toleration of various therapies, how long the condition will likely last, and patient choice. The scarring of the glomeruli cannot be healed. Treatments are focused on prevention of further damage and avoiding dialysis. Choices for treatment include the following:

- Dietary changes
- Antihypertensive medications
- Immunomodulators
- Diuretics
- Dialysis
- Kidney transplantation

Even with adequate treatment, some patients develop complications, leading to lifelong dialysis or a kidney transplant.

Prevention

The prevention of glomerular sclerosis requires adequate health management to stop diabetes mellitus from developing, as well as avoiding causative infections or drugs. If the disease develops idiopathically, there is no method of prevention. It is important to alert a physician as soon as any signs or symptoms of glomerular sclerosis develop.

Prognosis

When glomerular sclerosis progresses and is accompanied by fibrosis, prognosis is worsened. Urinary biomarkers that affect prognosis include **eosinophil-derived neurotoxin** and **haptoglobin**. If these are present, the prognosis is worse than when they are not.

CLINICAL CASE

1. What is the pathology of the GBM in glomerular sclerosis?
2. What are the risk factors for developing glomerular sclerosis?
3. What are the treatment options for diabetic glomerular sclerosis?

A 57-year-old man with type 2 diabetes and hypertension is evaluated because a recent urine test revealed proteinuria to be present. He is clinically obese and does not have any signs of retinopathy, thyromegaly, congestive heart failure, or peripheral vascular disease. However, his eyes appear "puffy" and his ankles are swollen. Further testing revealed proteinuria. The patient is diagnosed with glomerular sclerosis, and his medications for diabetes and hypertension are increased. He was also started on a new exercise regimen in order to lose weight, and was referred to a dietitian to discuss better food options and create a diet plan.

ANSWERS

1. Diabetic glomerular sclerosis is characterized by thickening of the GBM, and increased permeability. The mesangial space gradually enlarges because of deposits of proteins such as collagen IV, which is initially diffuse but then becomes nodular.
2. Aside from diabetes, risk factors for glomerular sclerosis include persistent hyperglycemia, hyperlipidemia, hypertension, lack of physical activity, smoking, and a high-fat, high-protein diet.
3. The treatment options for glomerular sclerosis are antihypertensive medications, immunomodulators, diuretics, dialysis, and kidney transplantation.

GLOMERULAR HYPERTENSION

In many diabetic patients, systematic hypertension causes changes in the **hemodynamics** of the glomeruli, and progressive damage. The glomerular perfusion pressure increases in the still-functioning glomeruli to allow for compensatory hyperfiltration to occur. This **glomerular hypertension** involves increased mechanical stress upon the glomerular cells. These include endothelial cells, mesangial cells, and podocytes. The afferent arteriolar resistance determines the fraction of pressure transmitted to the glomerular capillary network. The efferent arteriolar resistance determines the outgoing pressure. The glomerular capillary pressure is determined by the relationship between these two resistances, the renal plasma flow, and the ultrafiltration coefficient. The glomerular capillary pressure usually increases because the reduction in the afferent arteriolar resistance is higher than the reduction in the efferent resistance. A reduction in systemic hypertension may or may not reduce the glomerular capillary pressure. Other terms used to describe glomerular hypertension include *renal hypertension* and *renovascular hypertension*. Systematic hypertension will be discussed in detail in Chapter 7.

Epidemiology

Glomerular hypertension affects about 70% of type 1 diabetics and 30% of type 2 diabetics, often early in the disease course. Younger type 1 diabetics are often affected. However, the majority of people diagnosed with glomerular hypertension are older than age 67. In various studies, there have been no significant differences in prevalence or incidence between men and women. However, certain ethnic groups have glomerular hypertension more than others, including Native Americans, African Americans, Asian Americans, and Pacific Islanders. While global statistics are not well-documented, more than 72 million Americans have systemic hypertension, and less than 2% of these also have glomerular hypertension.

Etiology and Risk Factors

Glomerular hypertension is caused by the complications of diabetes mellitus, chronic glomerulonephritis (including focal segmental glomerular sclerosis), and *IgA nephropathy. Renal artery stenosis* is a narrowing of the arteries that deliver blood to the kidneys. Causative factors include altered tubuloglomerular feedback changes and activation of vasoactive mediators (nitric oxide, the renin-angiotensin system, protein kinase C, and endothelins), which increase glomerular capillary pressure and secondary GFR. With chronic glomerulonephritis, glomerular hypertension is mostly dependent upon blood volume, and not related to deteriorated kidney function. Renal parenchymal hypertension develops along with diabetic nephropathy, acute or chronic glomerulonephritis, hypertensive nephrosclerosis, polycystic kidney disease, and renal microvascular disorders. Glomerular hypertension has also been linked to sickle cell disease, **hyperaldosteronism**, pregnancy, obesity, and metabolic syndrome.

Pathophysiology

Glomerular hypertension speeds up the progression of chronic renal disease. Exactly how the condition develops is still not fully understood. The pathophysiological mechanisms of action need more study. The condition is known to be caused, in diabetic patients, by afferent arteriolar vasodilation. It also develops after high-protein meals, as well as by efferent arteriolar vasoconstriction, due to activation of the renin-angiotensin-aldosterone system. Glomerular hypertrophy and increased pressure may be a cause of kidney injury, but also a complication of it. To prevent further damage, it is important to understand how the kidneys adapt to injury.

Clinical Manifestations

When the kidneys receive less blood flow than is needed, they respond as if the body is dehydrated and release aldosterone that stimulates

63

the retention of sodium and water. The blood vessels fill with extra fluid and pressure increases. Usually, there are no symptoms, but when there is also severely elevated systemic blood pressure, there may be headache, blurry or double vision, bloody urine, confusion, and nosebleeds. The eventual outcome is chronic kidney disease. Often, systemic hypertension is more difficult to control with multiple medications when glomerular hypertension is also present. Some patients have stable systemic hypertension that suddenly worsens. Kidney abnormalities may develop suddenly, and there can sometimes be a fast development of pulmonary edema.

Diagnosis

It is important to have regular hypertension monitoring to assess whether glomerular hypertension may also be present. Narrowed renal arteries may be found via stethoscope examination, if a **bruit** is heard. Imaging studies such as CT may be ordered to see narrowed renal arteries. These include Duplex ultrasound, computerized tomographic angiography (CTA), magnetic resonance angiogram (MRA), and catheter angiogram.

Treatment

The most important blood pressure medications used for glomerular hypertension include the ACE inhibitors and ARBs. Examples of ACE

inhibitors include benazepril, captopril, lisinopril, and ramipril. Examples of ARBs include candesartan, losartan, olmesartan, and valsartan. Procedures that may be helpful include percutaneous transluminal angioplasty, to flatten plaques against the artery walls and insert a stent, allowing blood to flow more freely through the renal arteries. Renal bypass surgery is another surgical option for some patients. When renal artery stenosis can be reversed, the hypertension usually resolves.

Prevention

The best methods to prevent glomerular hypertension involve controlling diabetes mellitus and prevention of systemic hypertension. These include a healthy diet, regular exercise, weight control, avoiding or quitting smoking, reducing alcohol intake, limiting caffeine intake, limiting dietary sodium, and stress reduction.

Prognosis

Generally, the prognosis for glomerular hypertension is good with adequate treatment. However, complications that can occur because of this condition along with systemic hypertension that give a worsened prognosis include renal failure, myocardial infarction, pulmonary edema, stroke, left ventricular hypertrophy, retinopathy, aneurysm, congestive heart failure, and vascular dementia.

CLINICAL CASE

1. How common is glomerular hypertension in people with diabetes?
2. What is the pathophysiological process involved with glomerular hypertension?
3. How does percutaneous transluminal angioplasty work in the treatment of glomerular hypertension?

A 21-year-old woman with type 1 diabetes developed shortness of breath and was taken by her boyfriend to the hospital. She was hypertensive, and tests revealed that she also had glomerular hypertension. An abdominal CT scan revealed bilateral renal artery stenosis. Percutaneous transluminal angioplasty was performed, and stents were placed successfully. Her blood pressure normalized.

ANSWERS

1. Glomerular hypertension affects about 70% of type 1 diabetes and 30% of type 2 diabetes, often early in the disease course. Younger type 1 diabetics are often affected.
2. Glomerular hypertension speeds up the progression of chronic renal disease, but more study is needed about its progression. In diabetic patients, it is caused by afferent arteriolar vasodilation. It also develops after high-protein meals, as well as by efferent arteriolar vasoconstriction due to activation of the renin-angiotensin-aldosterone system. Glomerular hypertrophy and increased pressure may be a cause of kidney injury, but also a complication of it.
3. Percutaneous transluminal angioplasty flattens plaques against the artery walls so that a stent can be inserted, to allow blood to flow more freely through the renal arteries.

NEPHROTIC SYNDROME

Nephrotic syndrome is urinary excretion of more than 3 g of protein per day, because of a glomerular disorder accompanied by edema and hypoalbuminemia. It is more common in children and may be primary or secondary. In adult cases, secondary nephrotic syndrome may occur along with diabetic nephropathy. The disease is diagnosed by determining the urine protein:creatinine ratio, via a random urine sample, or a 24-hour urine collection. Nephrotic syndrome is also defined as nephrotic urine sediment, with edema and hypoalbuminemia. Usually, hypercholesterolemia and hypertriglyceridemia are also present. With nephrotic urine sediment, there are fatty casts, oval fat bodies, and small amounts of cells or cellular casts present.

Epidemiology

Nephrotic syndrome is most prevalent in children between the ages of 18 months and 4 years, and there are congenital nephrotic syndromes that appear in the first year of life. In children under 8 years of age, boys are affected more often than girls. In older-aged patients, the male:female predilection is nearly even.

Etiology and Risk Factors

Nephrotic syndrome is of different causes based on patient age. The most common primary causes include **minimal change disease**, focal segmental glomerulosclerosis, and **membranous nephropathy**. Minimal change disease causes a fast onset of edema and heavy proteinuria, and usually affects children, with renal function remaining normal in most cases. Secondary causes only make up fewer than 10% of childhood cases. However, secondary causes make up more than 50% of adult cases, and include diabetic nephropathy and **preeclampsia**. Amyloidosis causes 4% of all cases. HIV-associated nephropathy occurs in patients with AIDS, and is a form of focal segmental glomerulosclerosis.

Pathophysiology

The pathophysiology of nephrotic syndrome involves proteinuria caused by alterations of the capillary endothelial cells, GBM, or podocytes. Normally, serum protein is selectively filtered based on size and electrical charge. Exactly how these structures are damaged in primary and secondary glomerular diseases is not fully understood. It may be that T cells upregulate circulating *permeability factors* or downregulate their inhibitors to respond to unknown cytokines or immunogens. There may also be inherited protein defects that are required to the glomerular slit diaphragms. Also, activation of complement may damage the glomerular epithelial cells, or there could be a loss of negative groups that are attached to proteins of the basement membrane and epithelial cells. Over time, there is a loss of macromolecular proteins in the urine. These are mostly albumin, immunoglobulins, **erythropoietin**, thyroid-binding globulin, and transferrin. Protein deficiencies can increase complications of the disease.

Clinical Manifestations

The primary symptoms of nephrotic syndrome include anorexia, frothy urine because of high protein concentrations, and malaise. Fluid retention may result in abdominal pain, arthralgia, and dyspnea. The abdominal pain may be due to ascites, or in children, due to mesenteric edema. Arthralgia is due to *hydroarthrosis*, an accumulation of watery fluid in joint cavities. Dyspnea is caused by laryngeal edema or pleural effusion. Edema can obscure signs of muscle wasting, and also cause **Muehrcke lines** in the fingernail beds, which appear as parallel white-colored markings. Additional signs and symptoms may exist, due to complications the syndrome. These include infections such as cellulitis, and spontaneous bacterial peritonitis. There can also be anemia, changes in thyroid function test results, hypercoagulability and thromboembolism (most often being renal vein thrombosis and pulmonary embolism, in as many as 40% of adults and 5% of children), pediatric protein undernutrition (sometimes causing alopecia, brittle nails and hair, and growth stunting), and dyslipidemia.

Diagnosis

The diagnosis of nephrotic syndrome is based on edema and proteinuria during urinalysis. It is confirmed by random urine protein and creatinine levels, or via a 24-hour urinary protein measurement. Clinical findings suggestive of a cause include cancer, preeclampsia, and systemic lupus erythematosus. If the cause is not easy to determine, serologic testing and renal biopsy should be done. During urinalysis, nephrotic syndrome can be diagnosed if proteinuria is present at 3 g of protein within a 24-hour collection, since normal excretion is under 150 mg per day. Also, the protein:creatinine ratio in random urine specimens can accurately estimate grams of protein per 1.73 m^2 of body surface area, in a 24-hour collection. A random urine sample with 40 mg/dL of protein and 10 mg/dL is equivalent to a 24-hour collection with 4 g/1.73 m^2.

Random specimens may be less accurate if the creatinine is high or low, such as during athletic activities or cachexia, respectively.

Even so, random specimen calculations are usually preferred over 24-hour collections because of convenience and less likelihood of error, such as not adhering to the collection instructions. Urinalysis may also show casts that are epithelial cell, fatty, granular, hyaline, or waxy in type. A glomerular order is suggested to be the cause of nephrotic syndrome if there is lipiduria, as fatty casts, oval fat bodies in tubular cells, or present as free globules. Plain microscopy can detect urinary cholesterol, showing a **Maltese cross pattern** when crossed polarized light is used. Triglycerides can be revealed by the use of **Sudan staining**.

Adjunctive testing can be done to determine the severity and complications of nephrotic syndrome. Blood urea nitrogen (BUN) and creatinine levels can vary based on the amount of kidney dysfunction. The serum albumin is often below 2.5 g/dL (which is 25 g/L). There are usually increases in total cholesterol and triglycerides. Though not regularly required to be measured, there can also be low levels of alpha-globulins, gamma-globulins, hormone-binding proteins, immunoglobulins, **ceruloplasmin**, complement components, and transferrin.

For secondary causes of nephrotic syndrome, additional tests are needed, including serum glucose, HbA1C, antinuclear antibodies, cryoglobulins, hepatitis B and C antibodies, HIV test, rheumatoid factor, and serum and rapid plasma reaginic serology for syphilis. If nephrotic syndrome is idiopathic, a renal biopsy is needed for adult patients. In children, idiopathic nephrotic syndrome is usually minimal change disease, with biopsy only done if the child does not improve after being given corticosteroids.

Treatment

Treatment of nephrotic syndrome may be based on the cause, including angiotensin inhibition, diuretics, restricted sodium, statins, and in rare cases, nephrectomy. Prompt treatment of infections such as malaria, schistosomiasis, staphylococcal endocarditis, or syphilis must occur. To reduce systemic or intraglomerular pressure as well as proteinuria, angiotensin inhibition is achieved with ACE inhibitors or ARBs.

However, they can cause or worsen hyperkalemia if the patient has renal insufficiency. Protein restriction is not recommended due to insufficient stoppage of disease progression. For edema, sodium is restricted to less than 2 g per day. Loop diuretics are usually needed, though they can exacerbate hypercoagulability, hyperviscosity, hypovolemia, and renal insufficiency. Therefore, they are only used when sodium restriction is not effective or there is an overload of intravascular fluid. When nephrotic syndrome is severe, intravenous albumin is infused, followed by a loop diuretic.

For dyslipidemia, statin drugs are used. Cholesterol and saturated fat are limited in the diet. For thromboembolism, anticoagulants are used, though they have not been proven as a primary preventive treatment measure for the disease. In rare cases, a bilateral nephrectomy is needed for severe disease due to chronic hypoalbuminemia. Sometimes, the renal arteries can be embolized with coils, avoiding surgery for patients at high risk. Dialysis is used when needed.

Prevention

The only preventive measures for nephrotic syndrome involve methods to avoid the development of diabetes mellitus. Dietary restrictions and adequate exercise will help to maintain normal BP, blood glucose, and healthy levels of fats. Avoiding smoking and excessive alcohol use are also potentially preventive.

Prognosis

The prognosis of nephrotic syndrome is varied because of the different causes. Total remission can occur with or without treatment. Prognosis is usually good when the patient responds well to corticosteroids. Worsened prognosis is given if there is hematuria, hypertension, infection, severe **azotemia**, or thromboses of the cerebral, peripheral, pulmonary, or renal veins. Recurrence of nephrotic syndrome is high after a kidney transplant if the patient has focal segmental glomerulosclerosis, IgA nephropathy, or membranoproliferative glomerulonephritis.

CLINICAL CASE

1. What is the definition of nephrotic syndrome?
2. On which factors is the diagnosis of nephrotic syndrome based?
3. What is the likely prognosis for this patient?

A 27-year-old woman with type 1 diabetes had developed hypertension, which was treated with an antihypertensive medication. She also had nonproliferative diabetic retinopathy. Over time, her hypertension increased, and she developed edema in both lower legs. She quickly developed renal insufficiency. Urinalysis revealed proteinuria and hematuria. Hyaline and red blood cell casts were also present. Random urine protein and creatinine levels were assessed, and the patient was diagnosed with nephrotic syndrome. A renal biopsy showed proliferative and focal membranous glomerulonephritis. There were also changes present that suggested early diabetic glomerular sclerosis. The patient was put on a restricted sodium diet, started on a diuretic as well as a statin, and monitored closely for additional changes.

ANSWERS

1. Nephrotic syndrome is urinary excretion of more than 3 g of protein per day, because of a glomerular disorder accompanied by edema and hypoalbuminemia. In adults, secondary nephrotic syndrome may occur along with diabetic nephropathy.
2. The diagnosis of nephrotic syndrome is based on edema and proteinuria during urinalysis. It is confirmed by random urine protein and creatinine levels, or via a 24-hour urinary protein measurement.
3. The prognosis of nephrotic syndrome in this patient is likely worsened by the presence of hematuria and hypertension.

CHRONIC RENAL FAILURE

Chronic renal failure is also known as *chronic kidney disease* (CKD). It is a long-term and progressive deterioration of kidney function, with slowly developing symptoms. The majority of cases are diagnosed with the disease has reached stage 3 of its development.

Epidemiology

Overall, the prevalence of CKD is estimated to affect 14.8% of adults in the United States. African American, Native American, and Asian American people have higher incidence and prevalence of CKD than other groups. Global prevalence is estimated as being between 11% and 15% of the population, with most cases being stage 3 at diagnosis. Patients with end-stage kidney disease that require kidney transplants number between 4.9 and 7.1 million worldwide. Areas of the world with the highest amount of cases include Europe, the United States, Canada, Australia, Japan, South Korea, and the Oceanic countries. Most people that are affected are older than 40 years, since the kidneys naturally begin to lose filtration by about 1% per year after the age of 40, and conditions that damage them such as diabetes are also more common with aging. Though various studies have given different results, most studies show that chronic renal failure is slightly more common in women than in men.

Etiology and Risk Factors

Chronic renal failure may be caused by anything that results in the kidneys functioning abnormally. The most common causes are diabetic nephropathy, hypertensive nephrosclerosis, and glomerulopathies, which can be primary or secondary. Primary glomerulopathies include focal segmental glomerulosclerosis, idiopathic crescentic glomerulonephritis, IgA nephropathy, membranoproliferative glomerulonephritis, and membranous nephropathy. Systemic diseases that may cause secondary glomerulopathies include amyloidosis, diabetes mellitus, **Goodpasture syndrome**, granulomatosis with polyangiitis, hemolytic-uremic syndrome, mixed cryoglobulinemia, postinfectious glomerulonephritis, and systemic lupus erythematosus. Metabolic syndrome with hypertension and type 2 diabetes mellitus is an increasingly common cause of kidney damage.

Other causes include chronic tubulointerstitial nephropathies, inherited nephropathies, obstructive uropathy, and macrovascular disease of the renal arteries and veins. Inherited nephropathies include autosomal dominant interstitial kidney disease, **Alport syndrome**, polycystic kidney disease, and nail-patella syndrome. Risk factors for CKD include diabetes mellitus, cardiovascular disease, smoking, obesity, family history, older age, and the African American, Native American, and Asian American racial or ethnic groups.

Pathophysiology

Initially, chronic renal failure is distinguished by reduced kidney reserve or insufficiency. This can progress to end-stage renal disease – another term for renal failure. As the tissues lose function, the remaining healthy tissues adapt and increase their function, limiting any obvious signs or symptoms. The kidneys, over time, cannot maintain normal electrolyte and fluid homeostasis. Concentration of the urine is an early change. There are then decreases in the ability to excrete excessive acid, phosphate, and potassium. Once renal failure is advanced, the GFR becomes less than or equal to 15 mL/minute/1.73 m². Then, the kidneys cannot dilute or concentrate the urine effectively. Urine osmolality remains at about 300–320 milliosmoles/kg, which is close to the plasma osmolality (275–295 mOsm/kg). Variations in water intake no longer affect the urinary volume to any large degree. As the GFR is reduced, plasma concentrations of creatinine and urea rise. A normal GFR is more than 90 mL/minute/1.73 m², but once this falls to under 15 mL/minute/1.73 m², the creatinine and urea levels become high, and uremia manifests systemically. The creatinine and urea are markers for substances that cause the uremic symptoms.

The balance of sodium and water is maintained by increased fractional sodium excretion in the urine, plus a normal thirst response. Plasma sodium is usually normal. Hypervolemia usually occurs when dietary intake of sodium or water is restricted or excessive. Heart failure may be caused by an overload of sodium and water. This is more common if the patient has decreased cardiac reserve. Potassium is a substance with secretion mostly controlled via distal nephron secretion. Therefore, renal adaptation usually regulates normal plasma levels of potassium. This cannot occur when renal failure is advanced or the patient consumes too much potassium in the diet. Plasma potassium can be increased when renal failure is not as advanced by the use of ACE inhibitors, potassium-sparing diuretics, beta-blockers, cyclosporine, NSAIDs, tacrolimus, pentamidine, trimethoprim/sulfamethoxazole, or ARBs.

There may be abnormalities of calcium, parathyroid hormone (PTH), phosphate, and vitamin D metabolism. Renal osteodystrophy is also possible. Reduced renal production of the active vitamin D hormone *calcitriol* adds to hypocalcemia. Reduced renal excretion of phosphate causes hyperphosphatemia. Secondary hyperparathyroidism is often seen, developing in kidney failure prior to abnormal calcium or phosphate concentrations manifesting. Therefore, it is important to monitor PTH in patients with moderate CKS prior to hyperphosphatemia occurring. Renal osteodystrophy is abnormal bone mineralization. It occurs because of a deficiency of calcitriol, hyperparathyroidism, excessive serum phosphate, or low to normal serum calcium. There is usually increased bone turnover because of osteitis fibrosa, a hyperparathyroid bone disease. There may be decreased bone turnover, however, caused by an adynamic disease from increased suppression of the parathyroid glands, or osteomalacia. If there is a calcitriol deficiency, this may result in osteomalacia or osteopenia.

Slight metabolic acidosis is usually seen, with a plasma bicarbonate concentration of 15–20 mmol/L. Muscle wasting occurs because acidosis causes protein catabolism. There is bone loss from the bones buffering acid. Kidney disease progression is accelerated. Stage 3 or higher CKD usually involves anemia that is normochromicnormocytic. The hematocrit is at 20%–30%, or with polycystic kidney disease, 35%–40%. The anemia usually results from insufficient erythropoietin production because the function kidney mass is reduced. Other causes include folate, iron, and vitamin B12 deficiencies.

Clinical Manifestations

When the kidney reserve is slightly diminished, the patient is asymptomatic. Mild to moderate renal insufficiency usually only causes elevated blood creatinine and BUN. However, since the kidneys cannot sufficiently concentrate the urine, nocturia is common. The earliest manifestations of uremia include anorexia, decreased mental acuity, fatigue, and lassitude. Once kidney disease worsens, neuromuscular symptoms may develop. These can include coarse muscular twitching, muscle cramps, peripheral motor and sensory neuropathies, hyperreflexia, restless legs syndrome, and seizures. The seizures are usually due to hypertensive or metabolic encephalopathy. Patients usually develop anorexia, an unpleasant taste in the mouth, nausea, vomiting, stomatitis, and weight loss. The skin can become yellowish brown in color. In some individuals, uremic frost forms on the skin due to the crystallization of sweat. Itching may be extreme. Chronic uremia results in prominent undernutrition and generalized tissue wasting. When CKD is advanced, gastrointestinal ulceration with bleeding and pericarditis may occur. Over 80% of patients are hypertensive with advanced CKD – usually because of hypervolemia. Coronary artery disease or hypertension may cause heart failure. Renal retention of sodium and water may cause edema, dyspnea, or both.

Diagnosis

The diagnosis of chronic renal failure involves measurements of BUN, electrolytes, creatinine, calcium, and phosphate. A complete blood count (CBC) is routinely done. Urinalysis includes examination of urinary sediment. Quantitative urine protein is assess in a 24-hour protein collection, or a spot urine protein: creatinine ratio. Ultrasonography is often performed, and sometimes, renal biopsy. When serum creatinine is found to be high, the disease is usually suspected. There must be a determination if kidney failure is acute, chronic, or *acute superimposed on chronic*. This is an acute form of disease that causes more complications of renal function in a person that already has CKD. The cause of kidney failure must be determined. The duration of the disease sometimes reveals the cause, or vice versa.

Specific serologic tests are sometimes needed. A history of the patient's elevated creatinine or abnormal urinalyses helps distinguish CKD from acute kidney injury. Broad casts, more than 3 white blood cell diameters in width, or highly refractile and waxy casts are often obvious with advanced kidney failure, regardless of its cause. Ultrasonography of the kidneys helps evaluate obstructive uropathy. Based on kidney size, it also helps distinguish CKD from acute kidney injury. In most cases, CKD causes the kidneys to shrink to less than 10 cm in length. They have a thin, hyperechoic cortex. As kidney function nears values of end-stage disease, an accurate diagnosis is hard to make. Renal biopsy is the best diagnostic tool, but is not suggested if the kidneys are already small and fibrotic due to dangerous risks. The different stages of chronic renal failure are follows:

- Stage 1 – Normal GFR + persistent albuminuria or identified hereditary or structural kidney disease

- Stage 2 – GFR 60–89 mL/minute/1.73 m^2

- Stage 3a – GFR 45–59 mL/minute/1.73 m^2

- Stage 3b – GFR 30–44 mL/minute/1.73 m^2

- Stage 4 – GFR 15–29 mL/minute/1.73 m^2

- Stage 5 – GFR less than 15 mL/minute/1.73 m^2

The *Chronic Kidney Disease Epidemiology Collaboration* (CKD-EPI) creatinine equation is used to estimate the GFR in chronic renal failure. It is as follows:

$$141 \times (\text{serum creatinine})^{-1.209} \times 0.993^{\text{age}}$$

The result is then multiplied by 1.018 (for females) or by 1.159 (for African Americans). In the case of female African Americans, the result is multiplied by 1.018 × 1.159, which equals 1.1799. It can also be determined using another method in which the GFR is estimated via a timed urine creatinine clearance (usually over 24 hours, using serum and urine creatinine), though this usually overestimates it by 10%–20%. This is done if assessment of serum creatinine is likely to be less accurate, such as in patients that are very thin, very obese, or physically inactive. Another endogenous GFR marker is serum cystatin C. It is used for confirmation in individuals with nonrenal factors that affect levels of serum creatinine. These include amputations, neuromuscular diseases, very high or low muscle mass, exogenous intake of creatine, or diets that are high in proteins or only plant-based. Other formulas used to calculate GFR are less accurate than the CKD-EPI equation. They include the *Modification of Diet in Renal Disease* (MDRD) *formula* and the *Cockcroft-Gault formula*. The CKD-EPI method of calculation has less false-positive results and also predicts the outcome more accurately.

Treatment

Treatment begins with a focus on any underlying causative disorders or factors that contribute to renal failure. For those with diabetic nephropathy, it is important to control hyperglycemia. For all patients, control of hypertension is crucial. Guidelines for BP control are of some controversy between various experts, between 110/80 and 140/90 mm Hg. The rate of decline in GFR is controlled by ACE inhibitors and ARBs, for most causes but especially with proteinuria. Combined use of these types of drugs reduces proteinuria better, but also increases incidence of complications. There is no need to restrict physical activity, though most patients are unable to exercise enough.

To prevent ketosis, adequate carbohydrate and fat should be consumed. A dietitian should be involved if a patient has been prescribed a protein-restricted diet of less than 0.8 g/kg/day. For symptomatic heart failure, loop diuretics such as furosemide may be needed, often in large doses. They are usually effective even with greatly reduced kidney function. If there is depressed left ventricular function, the ACE inhibitors, ARBs, and beta-blockers are indicated. For advanced stages of heart failure, the aldosterone receptor antagonists are recommended. Digoxin may be added, but renal function determines dosages. Moderate to severe hypertension must be treated. If the patient does not respond to sodium restriction, diuretics are used. Loop and thiazide diuretics may be combined if edema or hypertension are not controlled. These combinations are used with great care to avoid excessive diuresis. Sometimes, dialysis is needed to control heart failure. When the extracellular fluid volume is reduced but BP is not controlled, conventional antihypertensives are indicated. Azotemia can be increased, but this may be necessary in order to adequately control heart failure, hypertension, or both.

With renal failure, renal excretion of drugs is often poor. Revised doses are required for common drugs that include cephalosporins, penicillins, aminoglycosides, fluoroquinolones, digoxin, and vancomycin. Serum concentrations of drugs can be reduced by hemodialysis, so they should be supplemented when the procedure is done. The NSAIDs are usually avoided with CKD since they can reduce kidney function, worsen hypertension, and cause electrolyte disturbances. Drugs that should never be used with CKD include nitrofurantoin and phenazopyridine. Gadolinium, used as an MRI contrast agent, has caused nephrogenic systemic fibrosis in some CKD patients. Since risks are very high with a GFR of less than 30 mL/min/1.73 m^2, gadolinium must be avoided whenever this is possible in CKD patients.

Dialysis is usually needed once uremic symptoms develop, there is difficulty in controlling fluid overload, hyperkalemia manifests, or there is acidosis even with use of drugs and lifestyle changes. All of these changes usually happen after the GFR reaches 10 mL/min or less (if the patient does not have diabetes) or 15 mL/min or less (if diabetes is present). Patients must be carefully monitored so that these signs and symptoms are caught early. When dialysis is planned for, preparations can be done and the emergency use of a hemodialysis catheter will not be needed. The patient can be educated about dialysis and choose the type that is preferred.

When there is a live kidney donor, transplantation earlier rather than later provides a better long-term result.

Prevention

Prevention of CKD and its complications involves the management of risk factors. Treatments can slow disease progression and reduce complication risks. At-risk patients should be tested for CKD regularly. Both the blood and urine can be tested. Patients with diabetes must be tested every year. Tips to prevent CKD include losing weight, having regular physical activity, stopping smoking, asking for a kidney examination during a standard physical examination, following medication regimens, keeping blood pressure below 140/90, managing blood glucose closely if diabetes is present, staying in the targeted cholesterol range, reducing dietary salt, and eating more fruits and vegetables. Patients with diabetes should take antihypertensives if their BP is too high.

Prognosis

The progression of CKD is usually predicted by the amount of proteinuria present. A worsened prognosis exists for those with nephrotic-range proteinuria, which is more than 3 g per day or a urine protein:creatinine ratio higher than 3. These patients usually reach renal failure more quickly than those with less proteinuria. Even when the underlying causative disorder is not active, progression can still occur. Patients with urine protein of less than 1.5 g per day usually have slow progression, or no progression. Faster disease progression is also linked to acidosis, hyperparathyroidism, and hypertension.

CLINICAL CASE

1. What are the most common causes of chronic renal failure?
2. What neuromuscular symptoms may develop with further progression of chronic renal failure?
3. Will this patient require dialysis?

A 47-year-old man has a history of poorly controlled type 2 diabetes and hypertension. He had recently been diagnosed with stage 3 chronic renal failure. His efforts to lose weight, reduce dietary sugar, and increase exercise have not been successful, and the patient explains that his job as a restaurant manager involves working long hours. When he gets home, he is too tired to cook healthy meals or do much exercise. He has bone pain in his arms and legs, reduced urine output, and describes that his urine is darker in color than before and has bubbles in it. The patient has itchy skin, peripheral edema of the feet and ankles, and a foul breath odor. Further testing reveals that his disease has progressed to stage 4, and is likely to reach stage 5 soon.

ANSWERS

1. The most common causes of chronic renal failure are diabetic nephropathy, hypertensive nephrosclerosis, and glomerulopathies, which can be primary or secondary. Primary glomerulopathies include focal segmental glomerulosclerosis, idiopathic crescentic glomerulonephritis, IgA nephropathy, membranoproliferative glomerulonephritis, and membranous nephropathy. However, this patient's diabetes and hypertension indicate that his condition is secondary.
2. Later neuromuscular symptoms include coarse muscular twitching, muscle cramps, peripheral motor and sensory neuropathies, hyperreflexia, restless legs syndrome, and seizures.
3. Yes, this patient must be prepared for and educated about dialysis so that the type can be chosen, and an arteriovenous fistula can be created or a peritoneal dialysis catheter can be placed. There should also be counseling about kidney transplantation.

KEY TERMS

- Alport syndrome
- Ascites
- Azotemia
- Bruit
- Ceruloplasmin
- Eosinophil-derived neurotoxin
- Erythropoietin
- Glomerular hypertension
- Glomerular sclerosis
- Glomerulus
- Goodpasture syndrome
- Graves' disease
- Haptoglobin
- Hemodynamics
- Hyalinosis
- Hyperaldosteronism
- Maltese cross pattern
- Membranous nephropathy
- Minimal change disease
- Muehrcke lines
- Nephrotic syndrome
- Preeclampsia
- Sudan staining

REFERENCES

American Diabetes Association – Clinical Diabetes. (2001). *Case Study: Renal Disease in Type 1 Diabetes*. American Diabetes Association. https://clinical.diabetesjournals.org/content/19/2/74

American Society of Nephrology – Clinical Journal. (2015). *A Systematic Review of Glomerular Hyperfiltration Assessment and Definition in the Medical Literature*. American Society of Nephrology. https://cjasn.asnjournals.org/content/10/3/382

Aronoff, G.R., Bennett, W.M., Berns, J.S., Brier, M.E., Kasbekar, N., Mueller, B.A., Pasko, D.A., and Smoyer, W.E. (2007). *Drug Prescribing in Renal Failure: Dosing Guidelines for Adults and Children*, 5th Edition. American College of Physicians.

Atlas of Pathology. (2021). *Kidney Pathology – Diabetic glomerulosclerosis*, 4th Edition. Atlas of Pathology. https://pathologyatlas.ro/diabetic-glomerulosclerosis.php

Avner, E.D., Harmon, W.E., Niaudet, P., Yoshikawa, N., Emma, F., and Goldstein, S.L. (2016). *Pediatric Nephrology Volume 1*, 7th Edition. IPNA / SpringerReference.

Baer, P.C., Koch, B., and Geiger, H. (2020). *Kidney Inflammation, Injury and Regeneration*. MDPI Ag.

Blaine, J. (2016). *Proteinuria: Basic Mechanisms, Pathophysiology and Clinical Relevance*. Springer.

Boston University School of Medicine – Pathology & Laboratory Medicine. (2021). *Glomerular Hypertension*. Boston University. https://www.bumc.bu.edu/busm-pathology/research/glomerular-hypertension-research/

Centers for Disease Control and Prevention – Chronic Kidney Disease Initiative. (2021). *Prevention & Risk Management (CKD)*. U.S. Department of Health & Human Services / USA.gov / CDC. https://www.cdc.gov/kidneydisease/prevention-risk.html

Cleveland Clinic. (2021). *Renal Hypertension*. Cleveland Clinic. https://my.clevelandclinic.org/health/diseases/16459-renal-hypertension

Clinical Diabetes. (2000). *Case Study: A 57-Year-Old Man with Type 2 Diabetes, Hypertension, and Microalbuminuria*. American Diabetes Association. http://journal.diabetes.org/clinicaldiabetes/V18N32000/pg132.htm

Daugirdas, J.T., Blake, P.G., and Ing, T.S. (2014). *Handbook of Dialysis*, 5th Edition. Wolters Kluwer.

DeFronzo, R.A., Ferrannini, E., Zimmet, P., and Alberti, G. (2015). *International Textbook of Diabetes Mellitus*, 2 Volume Set, 4th Edition. Wiley Blackwell.

Feehally, J., Floege, J., Tonelli, M., and Johnson, R.J. (2018). *Comprehensive Clinical Nephrology*, 6th Edition. Elsevier.

Fogo, A.B., Alpers, C.E., Cohen, A.H., Colvin, R.B., and Jennette, C. (2014). *Fundamentals of Renal Pathology*, 2nd Edition. Springer.

Geary, D.F., and Schaefer, F. (2017). *Pediatric Kidney Disease*, 2nd Edition. Springer.

Gilbert, S.F., Weiner, D.E., Bomback, A.S., Perazella, M.A., and Tonelli, M. (2017). *National Kidney Foundation's Primer on Kidney Diseases*, 7th Edition. Elsevier / National Kidney Foundation.

Greenberg, A. (2009). *Primer on Kidney Diseases*, 5th Edition. Saunders / National Kidney Foundation.

Hellman, P. (2014). *Primary Aldosteronism: Molecular Genetics, Endocrinology, and Translational Medicine*. Springer.

Hewitt, J., and Gabata, M. (2011). *Childhood Nephrotic Syndrome: Causes, Tests and Treatments*. Hewitt.

Johns Hopkins Medicine. (2021). *Health – Glomerulosclerosis*. The Johns Hopkins University, The Johns Hopkins Hospital, and Johns Hopkins Health System. https://www.hopkinsmedicine.org/health/conditions-and-diseases/glomerulosclerosis

Kaneko, K. (2015). *Molecular Mechanisms in the Pathogenesis of Idiopathic Nephrotic Syndrome*. Springer.

Kidney International / ISN. (2000). *Glomerular Hypertension, Abnormal Glomerular Growth, and Progression of Renal Diseases*. Elsevier Inc. https://www.kidney-international.org/article/S0085-2538(15)47058-9/fulltext

King Strasinger, S., and Schaub Di Lorenzo, M. (2020). *Urinalysis and Body Fluids*, 7th Edition. F.A. Davis.

Korkula, A. (2018). *Renal Biopsy Interpretation*. Jaypee Brothers Medical Publishers Ltd.

Kowsar – Nephro-Urology Monthly. (2014). *Urinary Prognostic Biomarkers in Patients with Focal Segmental Glomerulosclerosis*. Kowsar. https://sites.kowsarpub.com/num/articles/17114.html

Koyner, J.L., Topf, J.M., and Lerma, E.V. (2021). *Handbook of Critical Care Nephrology*. Lippincott, Williams, and Wilkins.

Lager, D.J., and Abrahams, N. (2012). *Practical Renal Pathology, A Diagnostic Approach: A Volume in the Pattern Recognition Series*. Elsevier/Saunders.

Lecturio. (2020). *Diabetic Glomerulopathy – Pathogenesis and Management*. Lecturio GmbH. https://www.lecturio.com/magazine/diabetic-glomerulopathy/

Lerma, E.V., and Rosner, M. (2013). *Clinical Decisions in Nephrology, Hypertension and Kidney Transplantation*. Springer.

Lerma, E.V., Rosner, M., and Perazella, M. (2018). *Current Diagnosis & Treatment – Nephrology & Hypertension*, 2nd Edition. McGraw-Hill / Medical.

Mastenbjork, M., Meloni, S., and Andersson, D. (2018). *Fluids and Electrolytes: A Thorough Guide covering Fluids, Electrolytes and Acid-Base Balance of the Human Body*. Medical Creations.

Mayo Clinic. (2021). *Chronic Kidney Disease*. Mayo Foundation for Medical Education and Research (MFMER). https://www.mayoclinic.org/diseases-conditions/chronic-kidney-disease/symptoms-causes/syc-20354521

Miligui, J. (2019). *Nutrition during Nephrotic Syndrome: E012 (Diet recommendations)*, 2nd Edition. Books on Demand.

Murray, P.T., Brady, H.R., and Hall, J.B. (2005). *Intensive Care in Nephrology*. Taylor & Francis Group.

Naseri, M. (2011). *Focal Segmental Glomerulosclerosis: FSGS: Clinical Manifestation, Diagnosis, Treatment and Outcome*. Lap Lambert Academic Publishing.

National Kidney Foundation. (2021). *Understanding Glomerular Diseases – What Is Glomerular Disease?* National Kidney Foundation. https://www.kidney.org/atoz/content/understanding-glomerular-diseases

NIH / National Library of Medicine / National Center for Biotechnology Information. (1991, updated 2021). *Glomerular Capillary Pressure and Hypertension*. National Library of Medicine. https://pubmed.ncbi.nlm.nih.gov/1927890/

NIH / National Library of Medicine / National Center for Biotechnology Information. (2012). *Glomerular Hyperfiltration: Definitions, Mechanisms and Clinical Implications*. National Library of Medicine. https://pubmed.ncbi.nlm.nih.gov/22349487/

NIH / U.S. National Library of Medicine / MedlinePlus. (2021). *Membranous Nephropathy*. U.S. National Library of Medicine – U.S. Department of Health and Human Services – National Institutes of Health. https://medlineplus.gov/ency/article/000472.htm

NURS 2534 Chronic Kidney Disease Blog, The. (2021). *7) Case Study & Answers*. My Chronic Kidney Disease. https://mychronickidneydisease.wordpress.com/7-case-study-answers/

Oblouk Darovic, G. (2002). *Hemodynamic Monitoring: Invasive and Noninvasive Clinical Application*, 3rd Edition. Saunders.

Orlando, G., Remuzzi, G., and Williams, D.F. (2017). *Kidney Transplantation, Bioengineering, and Regeneration: Kidney Transplantation in the Regenerative Medicine Era*. Academic Press.

Oxford Academic – Nephrology Dialysis Transplantation. (2012). *Glomerular Hyperfiltration: A Marker of Early Renal Damage in Pre-Diabetes and Pre-Hypertension*. Oxford University Press. https://academic.oup.com/ndt/article/27/5/1708/1843853

PMC - US National Library of Medicine – National Institutes of Health – Electrolytes & Blood Pressure. (2015). *Hypertension in Chronic Glomerulonephritis*. National Center for Biotechnology Information, U.S. National Library of Medicine. https://www.ncbi.nlm.nih.gov/pmc/articles/PMC4737660/

Ragosta, M. (2017). *Textbook of Clinical Hemodynamics*, 2nd Edition. Elsevier.

Reddi, A.S. (2016). *Absolute Nephrology Review: An Essential Q&A Study Guide*. Springer.

Ronco, C., Bellomo, R., Kellum, J.A., and Ricci, Z. (2017). *Critical Care Nephrology*, 3rd Edition. Elsevier.

Schrier, R.W. (2014). *Manual of Nephrology*, 8th Edition. Lippincott, Williams, and Wilkins.

ScienceDirect. (2008). *Glomerulosclerosis*. Elsevier B.V. https://www.sciencedirect.com/topics/pharmacology-toxicology-and-pharmaceutical-science/glomerulosclerosis

Turner, N., Lameire, N., Goldsmith, D.J., Winearls, C.G., Himmelfarb, J., and Remuzzi, G. (2015). *Oxford Textbook of Clinical Nephrology*, Volume 1–3, 4th Edition. Oxford University Press.

UNC School of Medicine / UNC Kidney Center. (2021a). *Kidney Health Library – Diabetes*. UNC School of Medicine / UNC Kidney Center. https://unckidneycenter.org/kidneyhealthlibrary/glomerular-disease/diabetes/

UNC School of Medicine / UNC Kidney Center. (2021b). *Membranous Nephropathy – What Is Membranous Nephropathy?* UNC School of Medicine / UNC Kidney Center. https://unckidneycenter.org/kidneyhealthlibrary/glomerular-disease/membranous-nephropathy/

WebMD. (2020). *What Is Renal Hypertension?* WebMD LLC. https://www.webmd.com/hypertension-high-blood-pressure/guide/what-is-renal-hypertension

Welcome Cure. (2021). *Nephrotic Syndrome Preventions*. Welcome Cure Pvt. Ltd. https://www.welcomecure.com/diseases/nephrotic-syndrome/prevention

Wilcox, C.S., Berl, T., Himmelfarb, J., Mitch, W.E., Murphy, B., Salant, D.J., and Yu, A.S.L. (2008). *Therapy in Nephrology & Hypertension – A Companion to Brenner & Rector's The Kidney*, 3rd Edition. Saunders.

Yevzlin, A., Asif, A., and Salman, L. (2014). *Interventional Nephrology: Principles and Practice*. Springer.

Yu, A.S.L., Chertow, G.M., Luyckx, V., Marsden, P.A., Skorecki, K., and Taal, M.W. (2019). *Brenner & Rector's The Kidney*, 2-Volume Set, 11th Edition. Elsevier.

PART III

MACROVASCULAR COMPLICATIONS OF DIABETES

CHAPTER 7 Hypertension

Hypertension is defined as chronic elevation of blood pressure, and it may result in macrovascular complications of diabetes and hyperglycemia. Hypertension is signified as a resting systolic blood pressure of 130 mm Hg or higher, a resting diastolic blood pressure of 80 mm Hg or higher, or both of these. The most common type of hypertension is primary hypertension (90%–95% of cases), which is of unknown cause, and was previously called *essential hypertension*. Secondary hypertension has an identified cause such as diabetes mellitus, obesity, chronic kidney disease, sleep apnea, or primary aldosteronism. In fact, hypertension is two times more likely in diabetic patients than in nondiabetics. A person with diabetes and hypertension is four times more likely to develop heart disease than others that do not have either of these conditions.

PRIMARY HYPERTENSION

Primary hypertension is of no identifiable cause and has been described as "essential" hypertension. In most cases, it develops slowly over many years. Prevalence usually increases with age in most populations. However, in recent years, younger people have increasingly developed primary hypertension. Another name for primary hypertension is *idiopathic hypertension*. The disease often causes no symptoms until is become advanced and damaged various organs. Since it is a "silent killer," people should have their blood pressure checked at least once every year. Warning signs for primary hypertension include many things that can also be attributed to other diseases, including blurred vision, dizziness, elevated blood pressure, headaches, nosebleeds, palpitations, and tinnitus.

Epidemiology

Of the people with hypertension, approximately 81% are aware that they have the condition, and only three of every four are being treated. Just over 51% of people have blood pressure that is sufficiently controlled. Blood pressure increases with age, and approximately 66% of people older than 65 have the condition. Adults with normal BP at the age of 55 have a 90% lifetime risk for hypertension. Higher BP increases the likelihood of complications and deaths. Over 75 million people having hypertension in the United States. An estimated 1.13 billion people have hypertension throughout the world, mostly in low- and middle-income countries. Hypertension occurs more often in African Americans (41%) than in other races, with Caucasians and Mexican

Americans each having a 28% prevalence (see Figure 7.1). Complications and deaths from hypertension also occur more often in African Americans.

Etiology and Risk Factors

Primary hypertension is probably caused by multiple factors, since hemodynamics and physiological factors may be very different. These factors include activity of the renin-angiotensin system and plasma volume. If one factor is the first cause, many factors are likely involved in keep BP high. Chronic increase of vascular tone may develop in afferent systemic arterioles, as abnormal function of the ion pumps affects the sarcolemmal membranes of smooth muscle cells. Though not fully understood, heredity is implicated in this. In older patients, over age 65, hypertension is usually linked to high sodium intake. However, environmental factors such as stress and dietary sodium seem to affect just younger people that are genetically susceptible.

Pathophysiology

Blood pressure is determined by multiplying cardiac output (CO) by the total peripheral vascular resistance (TPR). Pathogenesis of hypertension involves an increase in one or both of these. Most hypertensive patients have a normal or slightly increased CO, but the TPR is increased. This signifies primary hypertension, or hypertension caused by **pheochromocytoma**, primary aldosteronism, renal parenchymal disease, and renovascular disease.

Many times, a hypertensive patient has abnormal sodium transport across cell wells. This is because of a defect or inhibition of the sodium-potassium

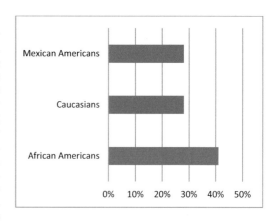

Figure 7.1 Racial/ethnic groups with the highest prevalence of primary hypertension.

DOI: 10.1201/9781003226727-10

pump known as *Na+, K+-ATPase*, or due to increased sodium ion permeability. Intracellular sodium increases, making the cells more easily stimulated by the sympathetic nervous system. Since calcium follows sodium, this increased sensitivity may be caused by increasing intracellular calcium. Since Na+, K+-ATPase can pump norepinephrine back to the sympathetic neurons, this neurotransmitter is inactivated. If this process is inhibited, the effects of norepinephrine may be enhanced, and BP rises. Sodium transport defects have been seen in children with normal BP that have hypertensive parents.

Blood pressure is increased by sympathetic stimulation. This is usually greater in individuals with elevated BP and hypertension than in those that are not hypertensive. It is not known if this hyperresponsiveness is within the sympathetic nervous system, or in the vascular smooth muscle and myocardium. A high resting pulse rate predicts hypertension. It may be caused by increased sympathetic nervous activity. Some hypertensive people have higher than normal plasma **catecholamine** levels while they are resting.

The renin-angiotensin-aldosterone system works in the regulation of blood volume and BP. In the juxtaglomerular apparatus, the enzyme known as *renin* is formed. It catalyzes the conversion of **angiotensinogen** into angiotensin I, which is inactive. Angiotensin I is cleaved by angiotensin-converting enzyme (ACE) – mostly in the lungs, but additionally in the brain and kidneys – into angiotensin II. This product is a strong vasoconstrictor. It stimulates the brain's autonomic centers to increase sympathetic discharges, while stimulating release of vasopressin and aldosterone. These cause retention of sodium and water, and the BP elevates. **Aldosterone** additionally increases potassium excretion. Vasoconstriction is increased by closure of potassium channels due to low plasma potassium of less than 3.5 mEq/L. In the blood circulation, angiotensin III stimulates release of aldosterone as much as is stimulated by angiotensin I. However, angiotensin III has much lower **pressor activity**. Chymase enzymes also convert angiotensin I into angiotensin II. Therefore, drugs that inhibit ACE are not able to completely suppress the production of angiotensin II. There are at least four mechanisms of renin secretion, which may interact. They are summarized as follows:

- Changes in tension in the afferent arteriolar wall cause a renal vascular receptor to respond.

- Changes in the delivery rate of sodium chloride, or concentration of this in the distal tubule, are detected by a macula densa receptor.

- There is a negative feedback effect upon renin secretion by circulating angiotensin.

- Renin secretion is stimulated by the sympathetic nervous system, and mediated by beta-receptors because of the renal nerve.

Angiotensin causes renovascular hypertension in the early phase or possible other phases. It is not understood how the renin-angiotensin-aldosterone system is implicated in primary hypertension. Renin levels are usually low in African American and older hypertensive patients. Older patients also usually have low angiotensin II.

Early in the development of hypertension, there are no pathologic changes, but when it is severe or prolonged, target organs are damaged. These are usually the cardiovascular system, brain, and kidneys. Damage increases risks for coronary artery disease (CAD), heart failure, myocardial infarction (MI), hemorrhagic and other types of stroke, renal failure, and death. Pathological damage occurs with general arteriolosclerosis, plus increased progression of atherogenesis. Arteriolosclerosis involves medial hypertrophy, hyalinization, and hyperplasia. It is obvious in small arterioles such as those of the eyes and kidneys. As the renal arteriolar lumen narrows, TPR increases.

The left ventricle slowly hypertrophies due to increased afterload, and diastolic dysfunction develops. Eventually, the ventricle dilates, resulting in dilated cardiomyopathy and heart failure from systolic dysfunction. This is often made worse by arteriosclerotic CAD. Hypertension often causes thoracic aortic dissection. Nearly all patients with abdominal aortic aneurysms have hypertension.

Clinical Manifestations

Note that patients having systolic and diastolic BP in different categories must be classified in the higher BP category. As clinical manifestations of hypertension develop, the often include dizziness, facial flushing, fatigue, headache, epistaxis, and nervousness. These do not occur when hypertension is uncomplicated. Severe hypertensive emergencies can result in extreme cardiovascular, retinal, renal, and neurologic symptoms. These include symptomatic coronary atherosclerosis, heart failure, renal failure, and **hypertensive encephalopathy**. A very early sign of hypertensive heart disease is a fourth heart sound. In the retinas, there may be arteriolar narrowing, exudates, hemorrhages, and if encephalopathy is also present, papilledema – known as *hypertensive retinopathy*.

Diagnosis

In adults, blood pressure is classified as normal, elevated, and stage 1 or 2 hypertension. The categories of BP are explained in Table 7.1.

Hypertension is diagnosed and confirmed by multiple BP measurements. The patient should be seated in a chair for more than 5 minutes with the back supported and feet on the floor. Measurement of BP should not be done while the patient is sitting on the examination table. The arm being used for the procedure should be supported at heart level. For at least 30 minutes before, the patient should not exercise, smoke, or drink any caffeinated beverage. During the first examination, the BP is measured in both arms. Follow-up procedures should use the arm that had the higher BP reading.

Blood pressure is measured in both arms since BP 15 mm Hg higher or more in one arm than the other means that the upper vasculature must be evaluated. When BP is measured in a thigh, using a larger cuff, this can rule out **coarctation of the aorta** – mostly in patients with reduced or delayed femoral pulses. The BP is much lower in the legs if coarctation of the aorta exists. This likely accounts for **white coat syndrome**, with BP high while the patient is in the physician's office, but normal at home or when ambulatory BP monitoring is used. It should be noted that extreme elevation of BP that alternates with normal readings is not common. This may suggest pheochromocytoma, drug use, or sleep apnea and other sleep disorders.

Patient history must include how long hypertension has been known to be present, and history of CAD, heart failure, loud snoring, or sleep apnea. There should also be discussion of coexisting disorders such as diabetes mellitus, renal dysfunction, stroke, dyslipidemia, peripheral arterial disease, and gout. Family history of any of these disorders must be taken into account. Social history should include use of alcohol, stimulants – whether prescribed or illegal – and tobacco products. Dietary history includes the amount of salt intake, coffee, tea, energy drinks, and sodas that contain caffeine.

Evaluations are more detailed for severe hypertension and younger patient age. For a new diagnosis of hypertension, routine testing can detect target-organ damage and identify risk factors for cardiovascular disease. Tests include urinalysis, spot urine albumin:creatinine ratio, blood tests for creatinine, potassium, fasting blood glucose, sodium, lipid profile, and thyroid-stimulating hormone. If there is hypokalemia that is not related to use of diuretics, the patient is evaluated for high salt intake and primary aldosteronism.

On electrocardiogram (ECG), a broad and notched P-wave means that atrial hypertrophy is present. It is a nonspecific sign, but can indicate early hypertensive heart disease. Left ventricular hypertrophy is shown by a sustained apical thrust, with elevated QRS voltage, with or without any indication of ischemia. This is a later development of hypertension. If these findings exist, echocardiography is often indicated. With an abnormal lipid profile, or CAD symptoms, CRP testing may be needed. All possible cardiovascular risk factors must be assessed. For suspected coarctation of the aorta, diagnosis may be aided by chest X-ray, CT, echocardiography, or MRI. If a patient is labile, with highly elevated BP, headache, palpitations, excessive perspiration, tachycardia, tremor, and pallor – there must be screening for pheochromocytoma. This can be done by measuring plasma free metanephrines. Symptoms must be evaluated if they suggest **Cushing syndrome**, connective tissue disorders, **eclampsia**, hyperthyroidism, acute **porphyria**, or **acromegaly**.

Treatment

Primary hypertension is not curable. Even though treatments can be effective, BP is only lowered to target levels in 33% of hypertensive patients. For most patients, including those with diabetes mellitus or kidney disorders, target BP is below 130/80 mm Hg – regardless of patient age, up to the age of 80 years. Achieving this target level reduces risks for vascular complications. Even so, it increases risks for adverse drug effects. This means that benefits for lowering BP to close to 120 mm Hg systolic must

Table 7.1: Categories of Blood Pressure

Category	Blood Pressure Levels
Normal	Systolic less than 120 mm Hg and diastolic less than 80
Elevated	Systolic 120–129 and diastolic less than 80
Hypertension Stage 1	Systolic 130–139 or diastolic 80 to 89
Hypertension Stage 2	Systolic 140 or higher, or diastolic 90 or higher
Hypertension crisis	Systolic higher than 180 and/or diastolic higher than 120

be evaluated in comparison to increased risks for light-headedness and dizziness as well as potentially worsened kidney functioning. This is a huge concern for patients with diabetes. In this group, a BP lower than 120 mm Hg systolic or a diastolic BP close to 60 mm Hg causes these adverse effects more often.

Older patients, even if frail, can usually tolerate a diastolic BP of 60–65 mm Hg with no increase in cardiovascular events. With proper training, patients or their family members can perform BP measurements at home. There must be close monitoring and regular calibration of the sphygmomanometer. During pregnancy, treatment of hypertension must be done carefully since some antihypertensives are harmful to fetuses.

Lifestyle changes are important for any elevations of BP. There should be more physical activity, in a structured program of exercise. Weight loss must occur in obese or overweight people. The diet must contain fruits, vegetables, low-fat dairy products, whole grains, and reduced saturated fat as well as total fat. Dietary sodium must be less than 1,500 mg/day, which is less than 3.75 g of sodium chloride, or if this is not possible, at least a 1,000 mg/day reduction. Alcohol intake must be no more than 2 drinks per day for men and no more than 1 drink per day for women. Per serving, this means 12 ounces of beer, 5 ounces of wine, and 1.5 ounces of distilled spirits. Smoking must be stopped. Dietary changes help manage diabetes mellitus, dyslipidemia, and obesity. If uncomplicated hypertension is present, activities do not need to be restricted as long as BP is under control.

Medications are indicated because of BP level and whether atherosclerotic cardiovascular disease (ASCVD) or its risk factors exist. Diabetes mellitus and kidney disease are part of the ASCVD risk assessment. The patient must be continually reassessed. If still not at target BP, patient adherence must be improved before any drug is added, or another drug replaces a previous one. Initial medications often are ACE inhibitors, angiotensin II receptor blockers (ARBs), calcium channel blockers, or thiazide-type diuretics such as chlorthalidone or indapamide. However, for African American patients, with or without diabetes mellitus, calcium channel blockers or thiazide-type diuretics are first recommended, unless there is stage 3 or higher chronic kidney disease. If this is present, the ACE inhibitors or ARBs are used first. If two drugs are given initially, there are single-pill combinations with an ACE inhibitor or ARB, plus a diuretic or calcium channel blocker.

Hypertensive emergencies require immediate BP reduction, using parenteral antihypertensives. Not all antihypertensives are used for specific disorders. For example, beta-blockers are contraindicated with asthma. Other drugs are especially indicated for hypertension coexistent with specific disorders. Examples include ACE inhibitors and ARBs for diabetes accompanied by proteinuria, and calcium channel blockers for angina pectoris. When the targeted blood pressure cannot be reached within 1 month, it should be ascertained whether the patient was taking the medication or medications correctly. He or she must be educated about the importance of following the chosen medication regimen. If the patient has been adherent, the doses can be increased or another drug can be added. It is important to realize that ACE inhibitors and ARBs should not be used at the same time, and therapy is often titrated. If the target BP is not achieved with two different drugs, a third one may be needed. If there is no third drug available because of a contraindication in a specific patient population, or a third drug is likely not to be tolerated, drugs from other classes may be chosen. These classes include aldosterone antagonists or beta-blockers. A hypertension specialist may be need to be brought in for BP that is difficult to control.

When the initial systolic BP is higher than 160 mm Hg, regardless of lifestyle factors, two drugs are indicated in the proper dose and combination. There are many single-tablet combination drugs, which are preferred because they make it easier for patients to adhere. Often, four or more drugs are required for **resistant hypertension** that is not reduced with three different antihypertensives. Several changes in medications are often needed to achieve enough BP control. Since lifelong treatment is often needed, insufficient patient adherence can interfere with treatment success. It is important to offer patients empathy about their conditions, and support their needs while educating them. Table 7.2 summaries medications that are used for the initial management of hypertension.

Outside of the United States in places such as Australia and Europe, percutaneous catheter-based radiofrequency ablation is performed (on an experimental level only) for the sympathetic renal artery nerves, to treat resistant hypertension. The procedure is controversial in its effectiveness, and is only done by specialists with widespread experience. Another option is stimulation of the carotid baroreceptor with a surgically implanted device. It is placed around the carotid body, and an attached battery stimulates the baroreceptor. In a dose-dependent method, BP is lowered. Studies have shown that **baroreflex** activation therapy is effective for persistent

Table 7.2: Initial Choices of Antihypertensive Medications

Medications	Indications
Angiotensin-converting enzyme (ACE) inhibitors	Younger patients Left ventricular failure caused by systolic dysfunction Severe proteinuria in chronic kidney disorders or diabetic glomerulosclerosis Erectile dysfunction because of other drugs Nonpregnant patients
Angiotensin II receptor blockers (ARBs)	Younger patients Conditions that could be treated by ACE inhibitors, but when patients cannot tolerate them due to coughing Type 2 diabetes with nephropathy Left ventricular failure and systolic dysfunction Secondary stroke Nonpregnant patients
Long-acting calcium channel blockers	Older patients African American patients Angina pectoris Arrhythmias, including atrial fibrillation and paroxysmal supraventricular tachycardia Isolated systolic hypertension in older patients (the drugs called *dihydropyridines*) Patients with high risk of coronary artery disease (the *nondihydropyridines*)
Thiazide-type diuretics such as chlorthalidone or indapamide	Older patients African American patients Heart failure

reduction in office-measured BP for those with resistant hypertension. There are no major safety issues that have been seen. However, the American Heart Association and American College of Cardiology have not approved the procedure for the management of resistant hypertension as of 2021.

Prevention

Since primary hypertension is of unknown cause, there is no proven method of prevention. Therefore, overall lifestyle changes are recommended, including weight loss, increased physical activity, avoiding smoking, moderate alcohol intake, and a diet high in fruits, vegetables, and low-fat dairy products that is also low in sodium content.

Prognosis

Prognosis is worsened with higher BP and severe retinal changes, as well as additional evidence of target-organ damage. Systolic BP is more predictive of cardiovascular events than diastolic BP. Outlook for 1-year survival is less than 10% of patients with cotton-wool exudates, retinal sclerosis, arteriolar narrowing, and hemorrhage – known as grade 3 retinopathy. Outlook for 1-year survival is less than 5% of patients that also have papilledema – known as grade 4 retinopathy. The most common cause of death in patients treated for hypertension is CAD. When treatment is insufficient, an ischemic or hemorrhagic stroke often occurs. Prognosis is improved with effective control of hypertension, preventing many complications and extending life.

CLINICAL CASE

1. What are the warning signs for primary hypertension?
2. How common is primary hypertension in the African American race?
3. How does left ventricle hypertrophy worsen and lead to a cardiovascular event?

A 45-year-old African American man went for a regular medical checkup, during which his blood pressure was found to be 180/120 mm Hg. He had no prior history of hypertension. Family history revealed that his father died from a stroke at only age 60, and that his mother currently has hypertension. The patient says his health is good and he has no abnormal signs or symptoms. However, he admits to smoking one pack of cigarettes every day and drinking about 12 bottles of beer per week. He also states that he has heard that antihypertensive medications can interfere with his libido. Laboratory studies and tests reveal that the patient has retinopathy, left ventricular hypertrophy, proteinuria, and a high serum creatinine level. He is started on hydrochlorothiazide and a low-sodium diet, and counseled about quitting smoking and reducing his alcohol consumption.

ANSWERS

1. Warning signs for primary hypertension include many factors that can also be attributed to other diseases, including blurred vision, dizziness, elevated blood pressure, headaches, nosebleeds, palpitations, and tinnitus.
2. Hypertension occurs more often in African Americans (41%) than in other races. Complications and deaths from hypertension also occur more often in African Americans.
3. The left ventricle slowly hypertrophies due to increased afterload, and diastolic dysfunction develops. Eventually, the ventricle dilates, resulting in dilated cardiomyopathy and heart failure from systolic dysfunction. This is often made worse by arteriosclerotic CAD.

SECONDARY HYPERTENSION

Secondary hypertension is high blood pressure caused by a medical condition that affects the kidneys, arteries, heart, or endocrine system. Diabetes mellitus is among these conditions. Secondary hypertension can also occur during pregnancy. Proper treatment often is able to control the underlying condition and the hypertension itself, reducing risks of serious complications such as heart disease, kidney failure, and stroke. Resistant hypertension exists when BP remains higher than desired even when three different antihypertensive agents are being used. This type of hypertension causes more complications and deaths than other types. The hypertension that develops before or during pregnancy has its own factors that must be addressed.

Epidemiology

The prevalence of secondary hypertension varies with age. It is more common in children and younger people. Prevalence is approximately 30% in hypertensive patients between 18 and 40 years of age. Between 70% and 85% have an underlying cause, and 17% of adults are 65 and older. The highest prevalence of secondary hypertension is in Africa, while the lowest prevalence is in North, Central, and South America (18% of the population). Overall, secondary hypertension is of similar prevalence in men and women.

Etiology and Risk Factors

Common causes of secondary hypertension include diabetes mellitus, obesity, renovascular disease, primary aldosteronism, obstructive sleep apnea, and renal parenchymal diseases. Examples of renal parenchymal diseases include chronic glomerulonephritis, connective tissue disorders, obstructive uropathy, and polycystic renal disease. There are other causes of secondary hypertension that are much less common. These include Cushing syndrome, pheochromocytoma, congenital adrenal hyperplasia, hyperthyroidism, myxedema, acromegaly, primary hyperparathyroidism, coarctation of the aorta, and excessive mineralocorticoids as part of syndromes that are different from primary aldosteronism. Curable hypertension is often caused by excessive use of alcohol or oral contraceptives. Blood pressure is also increased by NSAIDs, sympathomimetics, cocaine, corticosteroids, and licorice. Risk factors for secondary hypertension include the cardiovascular, endocrine, neurologic, and kidney abnormalities. Table 7.3 lists the cardiovascular, endocrine, neurologic, and renal causes of secondary hypertension.

Pathophysiology

Some patients have increased CO, while the TPR is oddly normal for the degree of the increased CO. The cause of the increase in CO may be large vein vasoconstriction. As the disorder progresses, the TPR increases as the CO normalizes. This is likely because of autoregulation. *Isolated systolic hypertension* is caused by disorders that increase CO – especially as stroke volume is increased. Such disorders include **aortic regurgitation**, arteriovenous fistula, and thyrotoxicosis. In older patients, some develop isolated systolic hypertension, while the CO is normal or low. This is linked to the aorta and its major branches losing elasticity. There is often a decreased CO if a patient has continually elevated diastolic pressure.

Plasma volume usually decreases as BP increases. In rare cases, the plasma volume stays at normal levels or increases. It is usually high in a hypertensive person because of primary aldosteronism or renal parenchymal disease. Plasma volume can be very low as well, because of pheochromocytoma. As the diastolic BP increases and arteriolar sclerosis

Table 7.3: Causes of Secondary Hypertension

Cardiovascular causes	Coarctation of the aorta Increased cardiac output Increased intravascular volume Polyarteritis nodosa Rigidity of the aorta
Endocrine causes	Acromegaly Adrenocortical hyperfunction (congenital adrenal hyperplasia, Cushing's syndrome, ingestion of licorice, primary aldosteronism) Exogenous hormones (estrogen – including oral contraceptives and those due to pregnancy, glucocorticoids, monoamine oxidase inhibitors, sympathomimetics, and tyramine-containing foods) Hyperthyroidism (thyrotoxicosis) Hypothyroidism (myxedema) Pheochromocytoma Pregnancy
Neurologic causes	Acute stress, including from surgery Increased intracranial pressure Psychogenic causes Sleep apnea
Renal causes	Acute glomerulonephritis Chronic renal disease Polycystic disease Renal artery stenosis Renin-producing tumors Renal vasculitis

develops, blood flow through the kidneys gradually decreases. Until much later, the glomerular filtration rate (GFR) remains normal. The filtration fraction increases because of this. Blood flow in the cerebral, coronary, and muscle blood vessels is normal unless severe atherosclerosis is present.

Hypertension caused by chronic renal parenchymal disease is known as **renoprival hypertension**. It develops from the combined effects of mechanisms that depend on renin as well as blood volume. Usually, the peripheral blood shows no evidence of increased renin activity. Hypertension is usually only moderate, and is affected by sodium and water balance. If there is deficiency of a vasodilator such as **bradykinin** or nitric oxide, instead of excessive amounts of vasodilators such as angiotensin or norepinephrine, hypertension may result. If nitric oxide is reduced because of lack of arterial elasticity, this is related to salt-sensitive hypertension. There is an increase of more than 10–20 mm Hg systolic BP after a large amount of sodium is consumed – such as in Chinese food. When the kidneys cannot produce enough vasodilators, BP can also increase. Factors causing insufficient vasodilator production by the kidneys include bilateral nephrectomy and renal parenchymal disease. Endothelin and other vasodilators or vasoconstrictors are also produced by the endothelial cells, so endothelial dysfunction has a large impact upon BP.

Clinical Manifestations

There are no specific signs or symptoms for secondary hypertension, often even when BP has become extremely high. After a diagnosis of hypertension, the following signs may be indicative of secondary hypertension, requiring BP monitoring more often than once per year:

- Hypertension that does not respond to blood pressure medications

- BP that is over 180/120 mm Hg

- Hypertension that previously responded to medications, but no longer does respond to them

- Sudden-onset hypertension before the age of 30 or after 55

- No family history of hypertension

- The patient is not always obese

Diagnosis

Diagnosis of secondary hypertension is based on BP measurements, often 3–6 of these during separate appointments. Home BP monitoring and ambulatory BP monitoring can also be used. During ambulatory BP monitoring, measurements are taken by an automatic device at certain times throughout each day. Other tests that are done to determine the cause of secondary hypertension include the following:

- *Blood tests* – Potassium, creatinine, sodium, blood glucose, total cholesterol, and triglycerides
- *Urinalysis* – For markers of hypertension caused by other conditions
- Kidney ultrasound
- *Electrocardiogram* – If a heart abnormality is suspected to be causative of secondary hypertension

Treatment

Some causes of secondary hypertension are correctable. Control of BP can greatly reduce complications. Medications include thiazide diuretics, beta-blockers, ACE inhibitors, ARBs, calcium channel blockers, and direct renin inhibitors. Lifestyle changes include an improved diet, decreased sodium, maintaining a healthy weight, increased physical activity, limited alcohol, quitting smoking, and stress management.

Prevention

While causes of secondary hypertension such as tumors or blood vessel abnormalities are not preventable, prevention can be achieved by changing medications, weight loss, and other changeable factors. If medication-related, the situation must be discussed with a physician, and the patient should never stop any medication without first consulting a physician.

Prognosis

With treatment, secondary hypertension has a good prognosis. If detected and treated early, results are often extremely successful. Often, patients must still be treated for secondary hypertension even after the underlying condition has been successfully treated.

CLINICAL CASE

1. What happens in secondary hypertension as the disorder progresses with regard to peripheral vascular resistance and CO?
2. What signs may indicate secondary hypertension?
3. What types of medications are used to treat secondary hypertension?

A 49-year-old woman had a history of type 2 diabetes, hypertension, obesity, and migraines. Her diabetes diagnosis was at age 40, accompanied by polyuria and polydipsia. She was initially treated with an oral sulfonylurea, to which metformin was soon added. Her diabetes was fairly well controlled. The secondary hypertension was diagnosed when she was 45, with consistent elevation in the range of 160/90 mm Hg over three different appointments. The patient was started on lisinopril, but her BP has fluctuated. At age 48, microalbuminuria was found in urinalysis. The patient is currently still obese and her BP is 154/86. Her medication doses are increased, and the physician discusses the options of adding a diuretic and a beta-blocker to her regimen.

ANSWERS

1. As secondary hypertension progresses, the TPR increases as the CO normalizes. This is likely because of autoregulation.
2. Signs that may indicate secondary hypertension include the condition not responding to BP medications, or longer responding to them; BP above 180/120 mm Hg; sudden-onset before age 30 or after age 55; no family history of hypertension; and sometimes, not being obese.
3. Medications used for secondary hypertension include thiazide diuretics, beta-blockers, ACE inhibitors, ARBs, calcium channel blockers, and direct renin inhibitors.

MALIGNANT HYPERTENSION

Malignant hypertension is also known as a *hypertensive emergency* or a *hypertensive crisis*. There is severe hypertension and signs of damage to target organs such as the brain, cardiovascular system, and kidneys. The patient is diagnosed by measuring the blood pressure, serum blood urea nitrogen (BUN), and creatinine. Also performed are ECG and urinalysis. There is an urgent need to reduce the BP with intravenous medications. There is no direct link between diabetes mellitus and malignant hypertension, but organ damage from diabetes is likely involved.

Epidemiology

Malignant hypertension develops in only about 1%–2% of hypertensive individuals. However, global cases of the disease are between 1 and 7.3 cases per 100,000 population. Malignant hypertension is most common in older individuals since a history of hypertension is involved, males, and in African Americans as well as African-Caribbeans.

Etiology and Risk Factors

Malignant hypertension mostly occurs in people with a history of hypertension. Smoking is a proven risk factor – especially if the BP has already been above 140/90 mm Hg. Additional risk factors include kidney failure, renal stenosis, amphetamines, cocaine, birth control pills, monoamine oxidase inhibitors (MAOIs), preeclampsia, pregnancy, autoimmune diseases, spinal cord injuries, narrowing of the aorta, and patients that do not follow their antihypertensive drug regimens. Diabetes mellitus may be a risk factor as well, based on the disease damaging target organs.

Pathophysiology

In a normal patient, BP increases and the cerebral vessels constrict, keeping the cerebral perfusion constant. When the mean arterial pressure is 160 mm Hg or higher, the cerebral vessels dilate instead of staying constricted. Therefore, the extremely high BP is directly transmitted to the capillary beds. There is **transudation** and **exudation** of plasma into the brain. Cerebral edema and papilledema result. While many stroke or intracranial hemorrhage patients have elevated BP, the elevation is often an outcome of their conditions, and not a cause. Rapidly lowering the BP for these conditions may be harmful instead of helpful – it is not fully understood. There is also a condition called *hypertensive urgency*, in which diastolic pressure is more than 120–130 mm Hg. There is no target-organ damage except for grade 1–3 retinopathy. Though potentially problematic, acute complications from hypertensive urgency are not likely to occur, and immediate BP reduction is not needed.

Clinical Manifestations

In malignant hypertension, BP is highly elevated, with a diastolic pressure above 120 mm Hg. Neurologic abnormalities include confusion, hemiparesis, hemisensory defects, transient cortical blindness, and seizures. Chest pain and dyspnea are common. Though the kidneys are affected but not causing symptoms, severe azotemia can occur because of advanced renal failure, leading to lethargy, nausea, and vomiting. There may be numbness or weakness in the face, arms, or legs. Shortness of breath, headache, and reduced urine output are common.

Malignant hypertension damages target organs and can cause a variety of complications. These include hypertensive encephalopathy, acute left ventricular failure with pulmonary edema, preeclampsia and eclampsia, acute aortic dissection, myocardial ischemia, and renal failure. The damage progresses quickly and is often fatal. Hypertensive encephalopathy may develop from a failure of the blood flow being autoregulated by the cerebrum. With this condition, there are usually manifestations such as cotton-wool spots, sclerosis, arteriolar narrowing, hemorrhage, and papilledema. Some amount of retinopathy is present in many other types of hypertensive emergencies. Cerebral deficits such as confusion, obtundation, or coma – regardless of the presence of focal deficits – are suggestive of encephalopathy. If there is a normal mental status with focal deficits, this suggests a stroke. Pulmonary edema is suggested by basilar lung crackles, jugular venous distention, and a third heart sound. Aortic dissection is suggested by asymmetry of pulses between the arms.

Diagnosis

Physical examination is focused on target organs and includes cardiovascular examination, funduscopy, and neurologic examination. Testing usually includes ECG, serum BUN and creatinine, and urinalysis. If there are neurologic findings, a CT scan of the head is needed to diagnose intracranial bleeding, edema, or infarction. A chest X-ray is required if the patient has chest pain or dyspnea. Signs of left ventricular hypertrophy or ischemia found on ECG suggest target-organ damage. In urinalysis, abnormalities often include the presence of red blood cells, RBC casts, and proteinuria. Diagnosis, therefore, is based on very high BP and target-organ damage.

Treatment

Malignant hypertension must be treated in an intensive care unit (ICU). The BP is slowly and continually reduced by using a short-acting titratable intravenous medication. Based on the involved target organ, drug choice and the method of BP reduction are varied. Usually, the goal is a 20%–25% reduction in mean arterial pressure over about 1 hour. Additional titration is used based on the patient's symptoms. It is not necessary to achieve a normal BP quickly. First-line agents usually include fenoldopam, nitroprusside, labetalol, and nicardipine. Methyldopa, an aromatic-amino-acid decarboxylase inhibitor, is also used. Nitroglycerin used on its own is not as potent as these drugs. Oral drugs have varied onset and are difficult to titrate. Though short-acting nifedipine reduces BP quickly, it can cause potentially fatal cardiovascular and cerebrovascular events. Thiazide diuretics such as hydrochlorothiazide are also used. Cardiac glycosides include drugs such as digoxin.

Clevidipine is an ultra-short-acting third-generation calcium channel blocker. Within 1–2 minutes, it reduces peripheral resistance while not affecting cardiac filling or venous vascular tone pressures. The drug is quickly hydrolyzed by blood esterases. Its metabolism is therefore not affected by the function of the kidneys or liver. Clevidipine safely and effectively controls perioperative hypertension and hypertensive emergencies. It is implicated in less deaths than nitroprusside. The starting dose is doubled every 90 seconds until the target BP is approached. Then, the dose is increased by less than double every 5–10 minutes. The drug is preferred over nitroprusside for the majority of hypertensive emergencies. While used cautiously for acute heart failure with reduced ejection fraction, there are still negative inotropic effects. Good alternatives if clevidipine is not available include fenoldopam, nicardipine, and nitroglycerin.

Nitroprusside dilates veins and arteries to reduce preload and afterload, so it is very useful for heart failure in hypertensive patients. It is also indicated for hypertensive encephalopathy. With beta-blockers, nitroprusside is used for aortic dissection. Starting doses are titrated in small increments, and the maximum dose is given for 10 minutes or less, reducing risks of cyanide toxicity. Nitroprusside is quickly broken down into cyanide and its active moiety, nitric oxide. Then, the cyanide is detoxified into thiocyanate. Careful administration is required to avoid toxicity to the heart and CNS, signified by agitation, cardiac instability, seizures, and an anion gap metabolic acidosis. However, when given for more than 1 week or more than 3–6 days in renal-insufficient patients, thiocyanate accumulates. This causes abdominal pain, lethargy, tremor, and vomiting. If BP is reduced too quickly, there can be a transitory elevation of the hair follicles known as *cutis anserina*. After three consecutive days of treatment, thiocyanate levels are monitored. The drug is stopped if serum thiocyanate is higher than 12 mg/dL (2 mmol/L). The drug's IV bag and tubing are wrapped in an opaque covering since nitroprusside is degraded by ultraviolet light.

Fenoldopam is a peripheral dopamine-1 agonist. It causes natriuresis, and systemic and renal vasodilation. The drug has a quick onset and a short half-life, so it is a good alternative to nitroprusside. Fenoldopam also does not cross the blood-brain barrier. Via IV infusion, the drug is titrated upward every 15 minutes to reach its maximum dose. Nitroglycerin affects the veins mostly, but also the arterioles. It can manage hypertension during and following acute MI, coronary artery bypass graft surgery, acute pulmonary edema, and unstable angina pectoris. If given IV, nitroglycerin is preferred over nitroprusside for severe CAD since nitroglycerin increases coronary flow. Doses are titrated upward every 5 minutes to achieve a maximal antihypertensive effect. Nitroglycerine must be used with other drugs to achieve long-term BP control. In about 2% of patients, a headache is the most common adverse effects. Other effects include nausea, vomiting, tachycardia, apprehension, muscular twitching, palpitations, and restlessness.

Nicardipine is a dihydropyridine calcium channel blocker that mostly acts as a vasodilator. It has fewer negative inotropic effects than nifedipine. Its primary use is for postoperative hypertension and during pregnancy. Dosages are increased every 15 minutes to the maximum dose, and the drug can cause flushing, headache, and tachycardia. It may decrease the GFR if the patient is renal-insufficient.

Labetalol is a beta-blocker that also has some alpha-1-blocking effects. It causes vasodilation without reflex tachycardia. Labetalol is given as a constant infusion or as regular bolus doses, and the boluses do not cause significant hypotension. Other uses include during pregnancy, after MI, and for intracranial disorders that need control of BP. Constant infusion and boluses are titrated upward to their maximum dosages. There are only slight adverse effects. However, since labetalol has beta-blocking effects, it is not used for asthmatic patients in hypertensive emergencies. If nitroglycerin is given at the same time, low doses of labetalol are used for left ventricular failure.

For *hypertensive urgency*, a 2-drug oral antihypertensive combination is administered and the patient is closely evaluated for a response. This continues on an outpatient basis. Hypertensive urgency often occurs in patients that have not slept well for a few weeks, or in those that are extremely anxious.

Prevention

To prevent malignant hypertension, it is important to monitor preexisting hypertension regularly. All prescribed medications must be taken on schedule. Lifestyle improvements may also be preventative, including the DASH diet, sodium reduction, regular exercise, weight loss, stress management, quitting smoking, and limiting alcohol use. Concurrent health conditions must be treated as well. Early assessment and treatment of any changes in symptoms can help to reduce organ damage from malignant hypertension.

Prognosis

The prognosis for malignant hypertension is poorest in African Americans, with most patients experiencing significant brain damage, heart involvement including systolic dysfunction, and kidney damage. Though in the past malignant hypertension was nearly always fatal, but today, it is successful treated in most patients. About one in five patients will require long-term dialysis.

CLINICAL CASE

1. In which people is malignant hypertension most likely to occur?
2. What neurologic abnormalities may develop as a result of malignant hypertension?
3. Is there any prevention for malignant hypertension?

A 61-year-old woman had experienced her first diagnosis of having hypertension when she was 20, during pregnancy. The hypertension was severe, at 215/130 mm Hg, with proteinuria also present. The hypertension caused harm to the fetus, which spontaneously aborted. After the patient recovered, her hypertension persisted, but at 190/135 mm Hg. She was treated with medications, but by the age of 30, the patient developed symptoms of headache, dyspnea, palpitations, and blurred vision. Chest X-ray confirmed cardiomegaly and pulmonary edema. Electrocardiogram revealed left ventricular hypertrophy. Over the years, her condition was treated with varying degrees of success with multiple hospitalizations in ICU units, but she eventually was able to deliver a healthy baby, after several more spontaneous abortions. By the age of 40, the patient had developed congestive heart failure. Once her medication regimen evolved to include methyldopa, hydrochlorothiazide, and digoxin, she became asymptomatic at age 61, with an average blood pressure of 118/82 mm Hg.

ANSWERS

1. Malignant hypertension mostly occurs in people with a history of hypertension, as in the patient in this case study, who was first diagnosed with hypertension at age 20, but became malignant later in her life.
2. Neurologic abnormalities that may develop as a result of malignant hypertension include confusion, hemiparesis, hemisensory defects, transient cortical blindness, and seizures.
3. To prevent malignant hypertension, it is important to monitor preexisting hypertension regularly. All prescribed medications must be taken on schedule. Lifestyle improvements include diet, sodium restriction, regular exercise, weight loss, stress management, quitting smoking, and limiting alcohol use. Concurrent health conditions must also be treated.

KEY TERMS

- Acromegaly
- Aldosterone
- Angiotensinogen
- Aortic regurgitation
- Baroreflex
- Bradykinin
- Catecholamine
- Coarctation of the aorta
- Cushing syndrome
- Eclampsia
- Exudation
- Hypertensive encephalopathy
- Pheochromocytoma
- Porphyria
- Pressor activity
- Renoprival hypertension
- Resistant hypertension
- Transudation
- White coat syndrome

REFERENCES

American Diabetes Association – Clinical Diabetes. (2004). *Case Study: Treating Hypertension in Patients with Diabetes.* American Diabetes Association. https://clinical.diabetes-journals.org/content/22/3/137

American Family Physician. (2017). *Secondary Hypertension: Discovering the Underlying Cause.* The American Academy of Family Physicians. https://www.aafp.org/afp/2017/1001/p453.html

Bakris, G.L., and Sorrentino, M.J. (2017). *Hypertension: A Companion to Braunwald's Heart Disease*, 3rd Edition. Elsevier.

Berbari, A.E., and Mancia, G. (2018). *Disorders of Blood Pressure Regulation – Phenotypes, Mechanisms, Therapeutic Options – Updates in Hypertension and Cardiovascular Protection.* Springer.

Biessels, G.J., and Luchsinger, J.A. (2009). *Diabetes and the Brain (Contemporary Diabetes)*. Humana Press.

Bogoeva Kostovska, K. (2020). *The Homocysteine and Type 2 Diabetes Mellitus: Homocysteine and Its Correlation with Microvascular and Macrovascular Complications in Patients*. Lap Lambert Academic Publishing.

Byrom, F.B. (2013). *The Hypertensive Vascular Crisis: An Experimental Study*. Butterworth-Heinemann.

Caplan, L.R., Biller, J., Leary, M.C., Lo, E.H., Thomas, A.J., Yenari, M., and Zhang, J.H. (2017). *Primer on Cerebrovascular Diseases*, 2nd Edition. Academic Press.

Chawla, R. (2018). *Recent Advances in Diabetes*. Jaypee Brothers Medical Publishers Ltd.

Chawla, R., and Jaggi, S. (2018). *RSSDI Diabetes Update*. Jaypee Brothers Medical Publishers Ltd.

Cleveland Clinic. (2021). *Can Secondary Hypertension Be Prevented? What Is the Outlook for Those with Secondary Hypertension?* Cleveland Clinic. https://my.clevelandclinic.org/health/diseases/21128-secondary-hypertension#prevention

Cortes, P., and Mogensen, C.E. (2007). *The Diabetic Kidney (Contemporary Retinopathy)*. Humana Press.

DeFronzo, R.A., Ferrannini, E., Zimmet, P., and Alberti, G. (2015). *International Textbook of Diabetes Mellitus*, 2 Volume Set, 4th Edition. Wiley-Blackwell.

Duh, E. (2008). *Diabetic Retinopathy (Contemporary Diabetes)*. Humana Press.

Earlstein, F. (2017). *Hypertension or High Blood Pressure Explained – The Ultimate Information Guide for Hypertension: High Blood Pressure Facts, Diagnosis, Symptoms, Treatment, Causes, Effects, Unconventional Treatments, and More!* Pack & Post Plus, LLC.

Edren.org – from Edinburgh Renal Unit. (2018). *Malignant Hypertension*. The Renal Unit at the Royal Infirmary of Edinburgh and the University of Edinburgh. https://edren.org/ren/edren-info/malignant-hypertension/

Ford, H.J., Heresi, G.A., and Risbano, M.G. (2020). *Pulmonary Hypertension – Controversial and Emerging Topics (Respiratory Medicine)*. Humana Press.

Healthline. (2021). *What Are the Symptoms of a Hypertensive Emergency?* Healthline Media. https://www.healthline.com/health/malignant-hypertension#prevention

Hypertension Center, The. (2021). *Primary Hypertension – Essential Hypertension*. The Hypertension Center. https://www.hypertension-bloodpressure-center.com/primary-hypertension.html

Jenkins, A.J., Toth, P.P., and Lyons, T.J. (2014). *Lipoproteins in Diabetes Mellitus (Contemporary Diabetes)*. Humana Press.

Jenkins, M., and Moore, T.J. (2011). *The DASH Diet for Hypertension*. Gallery Books.

Johns Hopkins Medicine – Health. (2021). *Diabetes and High Blood Pressure*. The Johns Hopkins University, The Johns Hopkins Hospital, and Johns Hopkins Health System. https://www.hopkinsmedicine.org/health/conditions-and-diseases/diabetes/diabetes-and-high-blood-pressure

Johnstone, M.T., and Veves, A. (2005). *Diabetes and Cardiovascular Disease*, 2nd Edition. Humana Press.

Loriaux, L., and Vanek, C. (2021). *Endocrine Emergencies: Recognition and Treatment (Contemporary Endocrinology)*, 2nd Edition. Springer.

Kaplan, N.M., and Victor, G.R. (2014). *Kaplan's Clinical Hypertension*, 11th Edition. Lippincott, Williams, and Wilkins.

Kaufmann, W., Bonner, G., Lang, R., and Meurer, K.A. (2012). *Primary Hypertension – Basic Mechanisms and Therapeutic Implications*. Springer-Verlag.

Lerma, E.V., Rosner, M., and Perazella, M. (2018). *Current Diagnosis & Treatment – Nephrology & Hypertension*, 2nd Edition. McGraw-Hill Education/Medical.

Li, N. (2019). *Secondary Hypertension – Screening, Diagnosis and Treatment*. Springer.

Mann, S.J. (2012). *Hypertension and You: Old Drugs, New Drugs, and the Right Drugs for Your High Blood Pressure*. Rowman & Littlefield Publishers.

Mansoor, G.A. (2004). *Secondary Hypertension – Clinical Presentation, Diagnosis, and Treatment*. Humana Press.

Mayo Clinic. (2021a). *High Blood Pressure (Hypertension)*. Mayo Foundation for Medical Education and Research (MFMER). https://www.mayoclinic.org/diseases-conditions/high-blood-pressure/symptoms-causes/syc-20373410

Mayo Clinic. (2021b). *Secondary Hypertension*. Mayo Foundation for Medical Education and Research (MFMER). https://www.mayoclinic.org/diseases-conditions/secondary-hypertension/symptoms-causes/syc-20350679

McFarlane, S.I., and Bakris, G.L. (2012). *Diabetes and Hypertension: Evaluation and Management (Contemporary Diabetes)*. Humana Press.

Morganti, A., Agabiti Rosei, E., and Mantero, F. (2020). *Secondary Hypertension – Updates in Hypertension and Cardiovascular Protection*. Springer.

NIH – National Library of Medicine – National Center for Biotechnology Information. (2019). *Malignant Hypertension: Diagnosis, Treatment and Prognosis with Experience from the Bordeaux Cohort*. National Library of Medicine. https://pubmed.ncbi.nlm.nih.gov/30160657/

NIH – National Library of Medicine – National Center for Biotechnology Information. (2004). *Primary Prevention of Essential Hypertension*. National Library of Medicine. https://pubmed.ncbi.nlm.nih.gov/14871061/

Oxford Academic – American Journal of Hypertension. (2017). *Malignant Hypertension Revisited – Does This Still Exist?* Oxford University Press. https://academic.oup.com/ajh/article/30/6/543/2990207

Oxford Academic – The Journal of Clinical Endocrinology & Metabolism. (1999). *Hypertension in Men*. Oxford University Press. https://academic.oup.com/jcem/article/84/10/3451/2660462

Pham, P.C.T., and Pham, P.T.T. (2021). *Nephrology and Hypertension Board Review*, 2nd Edition. Lippincott, Williams, and Wilkins.

PMC – US National Library of Medicine – National Institutes of Health – British Journal of Clinical Pharmacology – British Pharmacological Society. (1982). *Malignant Hypertension – A Case Report*. National Center for Biotechnology Information, US National Library of Medicine. https://www.ncbi.nlm.nih.gov/pmc/articles/PMC1401768/?page=1

Prezi. (2014). *Case Study: Primary Hypertension*. Prezi Inc. https://prezi.com/kbd63ri1696m/case-study-primary-hypertension/

Ram, C.V.S. (2014). *Hypertension: A Clinical Guide*. CRC Press.

Regensteiner, J.G., Reusch, J.E.B., Stewart, K.J., and Veves, A. (2009). *Diabetes and Exercise (Contemporary Diabetes)*. Humana Press.

Reusch, J.E.B., Regensteiner, J.G., Stewart, K.J., and Veves, A. (2015). *Diabetes and Exercise – From Pathophysiology to Clinical Implementation*, 2nd Edition (*Contemporary Diabetes*).

Shrikhande, G.V., and McKinsey, J.F. (2012). *Diabetes and Peripheral Vascular Disease – Diagnosis and Management (Contemporary Diabetes)*. Humana Press.

Sima, A.A.F. (2011). *Diabetes & C-Peptide: Scientific and Clinical Aspects (Contemporary Diabetes)*. Humana Press.

Sobel, B.E., and Schneider, D.J. (2002). *Medical Management of Diabetes and Heart Disease*. CRC Press.

Tsatsoulis, A., Wyckoff, J., and Brown, F.M. (2009). *Diabetes in Women: Pathophysiology and Therapy (Contemporary Diabetes)*. Humana Press.

Tsioufis, C., Schmieder, R.E., and Mancia, G. (2016). *Interventional Therapies for Secondary and Essential Hypertension – wwUpdates in Hypertension and Cardiovascular Protection*. Springer.

Vojacek, J., Zacek, P., and Dominik, J. (2018). *Aortic Regurgitation*. Springer.

Walberg Rankin, J. (2015). *Curable Hypertension: Primary Aldosteronism*. Rankin.

Warren, A. (2020). *Type 1 Diabetes for the Newly Diagnosed: What to Expect, What to Do, How to Thrive*. Rockridge Press.

Waxman, A.B., and Singh, I. (2021). *Pulmonary Hypertension, Clinics in Chest Medicine (Volume 42-1)*. Elsevier.

WebMD. (2019). *Malignant Hypertension*. WebMD LLC. https://www.webmd.com/hypertension-high-blood-pressure/guide/what-is-malignant-hypertension#1-3

Wheeler, G. (2020). *Hypertension: A Clinical Guide*. Hayle Medical.

CHAPTER 8 Dyslipidemia

Dyslipidemia is the elevation of total cholesterol, low-density lipoproteins, triglycerides, and lipoprotein-alpha, combined with reduced levels of high-density lipoproteins or apolipoproteins. Dyslipidemia along with hypertension is a significant risk factor for cardiovascular disease. Dyslipidemia is an important modifiable risk factor for atherosclerosis as well. With diabetes mellitus, dyslipidemia often takes on a characteristic pattern that combines low levels of HDL, increased triglycerides, and postprandial lipemia. This is a common occurrence especially with type 2 diabetes mellitus. Adults with diabetes have a composition of lipoproteins that is more atherogenic and influenced by glycemic control than adults that are not diabetic. Diabetic dyslipidemia is often worsened by increased caloric intake and lack of physical activity that is relatively common in the lifestyles of diabetic patients. Women with diabetes may be at a significantly higher risk for cardiovascular disease as a result of diabetic dyslipidemia.

PLASMA CHOLESTEROL

Cholesterol is one of the steroid family of lipids that are waxy, resembling fat. It is present mostly in the cells of humans and animals, where it is also the primary **sterol**. However, cholesterol is present in all body fluids in varying amounts, either in a free form or in a storage form. In the blood plasma, cholesterol levels are measured in mg of cholesterol per dL of blood. Cholesterol is not soluble in the plasma. This is because plasma is water-based, and cholesterol is oil-based. This explains why cholesterol, after entering the bloodstream, solidifies into lumps called *plaques*. Cholesterol is obtained from plants and animals, dairy products, and eggs. Many foods that contain cholesterol are unhealthy. Low-fat dairy products, egg whites, and fresh fruits do not contain cholesterol. Nuts and vegetables are considered excellent sources of soluble fibers, which can reduce cholesterol.

Total cholesterol is the total amount of cholesterol in the bloodstream. Cholesterol, while required in cell membrane formation, healthy skin, normal digestion, and steroid hormones production, can also be extremely harmful. The "good" form is also called high-density lipoprotein (HDL), and high levels of HDL protects against cardiovascular disorders such as myocardial infarction (MI) and stroke. The HDL type carries cholesterol back to the liver. Ranges of HDL should be 40 mg/dL or higher. The "bad" form is also called low-density lipoprotein, and is related to increased risks for coronary heart disease, peripheral artery disease,

and stroke. Excessive LDL in the plasma slowly forms plaques that may block blood flow and form clots. If this occurs in the blood vessels near the heart, it may result in an MI. Ideally, the level of LDL should be 100 mg/dL or lower. Control of LDL in the blood cells is mostly by the liver and intestines.

Factors that influence plasma cholesterol levels include age, gender, weight, genetics, diseases, and lifestyle factors. High cholesterol is mostly caused by diet, but heredity is also implicated. A lack of sufficient exercise can result in heart disease since LDL cholesterol levels are increased. Measuring the plasma cholesterol is a very important component of the clinical management of **dyslipidemia** and **atherosclerosis**. High plasma LDL cholesterol worsens left ventricular function in people with type 2 diabetes mellitus.

PLASMA TRIGLYCERIDES

Triglycerides are the most common form of fat in the bloodstream. A triglyceride is made up of three **fatty acid** chains that are linked together by a molecule of **glycerol**. As we consume food, gastrointestinal enzymes break down fats into component fatty acids. These are reassembled to create particles of triglycerides, which cannot easily move through the bloodstream. Therefore, triglycerides combine with cholesterol and protein, forming *lipoproteins*.

Triglycerides provide energy for the body, and extra triglycerides are deposited in fat tissue. After eating a heavy meal high in fats, the bloodstream may contain excessive triglyceride particles, causing the blood to appear milky. The triglycerides are removed within several hours. When energy is required between meals, hormones release stored triglycerides into the bloodstream. In the liver, carbohydrates are converted into triglycerides. More triglycerides are created when foods rich in carbohydrates are consumed. Triglyceride levels are also raised by being obese or overweight, smoking, and heavy alcohol consumption. High triglycerides are also caused by poorly controlled type 2 diabetes mellitus and diseases of the liver, kidneys, or thyroid.

In healthy adults, normal triglyceride levels are below 150 mg/dL. *Borderline-high* triglyceride levels are between 151 and 200 mg/dL. *High* triglyceride levels are between 201 and 499 mg/dL, and *very high* triglyceride levels are 500 mg/dL or more. Very high triglycerides increase risks of pancreatitis. Abnormally high triglycerides may increases risks for CVD, regardless of the patient's cholesterol levels. The same measures needed for lowering LDL cholesterol are used to lower triglyceride levels – regular exercise, heart-healthy diet, stopping smoking, limiting alcohol consumption, and treating underlying conditions.

LIPOPROTEIN

Lipoprotein is a term describing a complex particle that has a central hydrophobic core of nonpolar lipids. Mostly, these are cholesterol esters and triglycerides. The hydrophobic core is surrounded by a hydrophilic membrane of **apolipoproteins**, free cholesterol, and phospholipids. The plasma lipoproteins actually consist of seven classes. These are based on size, composition of lipid, and the apolipoproteins. Classes of lipoproteins include the following:

- *Chylomicrons* – Density is less than 0.93 g/mL; size is 75–1,200 nanometers (nm); major lipids are triglycerides; and major apolipoproteins are Apo B-48, Apo C, Apo E, Apo A-I, Apo A-II, and Apo A-IV.

- *Chylomicron remnants* – Density is 0.930–1.006 g/mL; size is 30–80 nm; major lipids are triglycerides, and then cholesterol; and major apolipoproteins are Apo B-48 and Apo E.

- *VLDL (very low-density lipoprotein)* – Density is 0.920–1.006 g/mL; size is 30–80 nm; major lipids are triglycerides; and major apolipoproteins are Apo B-100, Apo E, and Apo C.

- *IDL (intermediate-density lipoprotein)* – Density is 1.006–1.019 g/mL; size is 25–35 nm; major lipids are triglycerides, and then cholesterol; and major apolipoproteins are Apo B-100, Apo E, and Apo C.

- *LDL* – Density is 1.019–1.063 g/mL; size is 18–25 nm; major lipid is cholesterol; and major apolipoprotein is Apo B-100.

- *HDL* – Density is 1.063–1.210 g/mL; size is 5–12 nm; major lipids are cholesterol, and then phospholipids; and major apolipoproteins are Apo A-I, Apo A-II, Apo C, and Apo E.

- *Lipoprotein(a) [Lp(α)]* – Density is 1.055–1.085 g/mL; size is approximately 30 nm; major lipid is cholesterol, and major apolipoproteins are Apo B-100 and Apo (α).

Chylomicrons are large triglyceride-rich particles. They are manufactured in the intestines, and involved in transport of dietary triglycerides and cholesterol to the liver. Their size varies based on the amount of fat ingested. After a high-fat meal, large chylomicron particles form because of the higher amounts of triglyceride being carried. During fasting, chylomicron particles are small because less triglyceride is being carried. *Chylomicron remnants* are smaller particles resulting from the removal of triglyceride from the chylomicrons by the peripheral tissues. The remnants are high in cholesterol, and different from chylomicrons, are pro-atherogenic.

Very low-density lipoproteins (VLDL) are rich in triglycerides, and are produced by the liver. They are similar to chylomicrons in size, also varying based on the amount of triglyceride being carried. With increased triglyceride production in the liver, the secreted VLDL particles are larger. The IDL are VLDL remnants. Removal of triglycerides from VLDL is done by the adipose tissue and muscle tissue. Lipoprotein (α) is an LDL particle with apolipoprotein (α) attached to Apo B-100 with a *disulfide bond*. The apolipoproteins play a structural role, serve as ligands for lipoprotein receptors, regulate formation of lipoproteins, and are important activators or inhibitors of enzymes involved in lipoprotein metabolism. Insulin resistance and type 2 diabetes mellitus are related to plasma lipid and lipoprotein abnormalities, increasing the risk for cardiovascular disease.

HYPERLIPIDEMIA

Hyperlipidemia is a condition that involves a variety of factors. It is also called *dyslipidemia*. There can be elevated plasma cholesterol, triglycerides, or both – or there can be a low HDL level, which contributes to atherosclerosis. Dyslipidemia can be primary (genetic) or secondary in cause. Cholesterol, triglycerides, and lipoproteins are all measured to aid in diagnosis. The disorder is treated with changes to diet and exercise, as well as with lipid-lowering drugs. Lipid measurements are continual, so there is no preexisting separation level between the normal and abnormal levels of lipids. With a direct link between lipid levels and cardiovascular risks, even normal levels of cholesterol should be lowered to reduce these risks. Dyslipidemia is difficult to accurately define. The best benefits occur when the LDL levels are lowered. There is less evidence for lowering triglycerides or increasing HDL levels. High HDL levels from genetic disorders may not be protective against cardiovascular disease, and low HDL levels from genetic disorders may not increase risks for CVD. Increased risks may be due to other factors, including hypertriglyceridemia or concurrent lipid and metabolic abnormalities. The dyslipidemia of type 2 diabetes is characterized by high triglyceride levels and decreased HDL.

Epidemiology

In various global studies, dyslipidemia has shown varying levels of abnormal levels in different populations. In the United States alone, more than 18% of adults aged 20 or older have HDL levels that are too low, and more than 12% have total cholesterol that is too high. The Centers for Disease Control and Prevention estimate that 71 million American adults have high levels of LDL cholesterol. Slightly over 50% of U.S. adults that could benefit from cholesterol medications are currently taking them. Even about 7% of children and adolescents in the United States have high total cholesterol. There are gender and racial/ethnic differences in high cholesterol, signified as being 240 mg/dL or higher. In a survey of U.S. adults aged 20 or older from 2015 to 2016, the following statistics were found:

- 14.8% of non-Hispanic Caucasian women had high cholesterol

- 13.1% of Hispanic men

- 11.3% of non-Hispanic Asian men

- 10.9% of non-Hispanic Caucasian men

- 10.6% of non-Hispanic African American men

- 10.3% of non-Hispanic African American women

- 10.3% of non-Hispanic Asian women

- 9% of Hispanic women

These percentages are also shown in Figure 8.1.

Globally, hypercholesterolemia is the most common form of dyslipidemia, with elevated LDL levels being the eighth leading risk factor for death. The global burden of dyslipidemias has increased over the past three decades or more. According to the *Disease Analysis: Dyslipidemia* report, in 2018 there were about 1.5 billion prevalent cases of dyslipidemia in adults aged 20 or higher. This number is likely to reach 1.7 billion prevalent cases by the year 2027.

Etiology and Risk Factors

Primary and secondary causes of dyslipidemia may influence the disease in different amounts. *Familial combined hyperlipidemia* may only develop, for example, when there are strong secondary causes present. Primary causes of dyslipidemia involve single or multiple gene mutations that cause overproduction or poor clearance of LDL and triglycerides. There can also be underproduction or extreme clearance of HDL. Previously, lipoproteins were described by how the separated into alpha (HDL) or beta (LDL) bands on electrophoretic gels.

Secondary causes of dyslipidemia are common in adults. In developed countries, a sedentary lifestyle with excessive intake of total calories, cholesterol, saturated fat, and *trans fats* is the main cause. Trans fats are monounsaturated or polyunsaturated fatty acids with hydrogen atoms added. Trans fats were previously used in a variety of processed foods, and caused as much atherogenesis as saturated fats. The first country to ban trans fats was Denmark (in 2003). Other countries followed, including Norway, Iceland, Hungary, Austria, and Switzerland. In

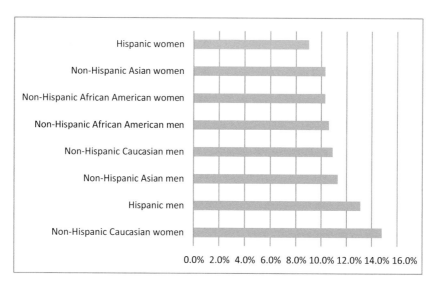

Figure 8.1 Percentages of various individuals with high cholesterol in the United States.

2015, the U.S. Food and Drug Administration began steps to remove artificial trans fats in processed foods. As of January 1, 2020, full compliance had to be met. Manufacturers can no longer legally add *partially hydrogenated fats* (PHOs) to foods – they are the major source of artificial trans fats. The World Health Organization estimates that trans fats will be banned worldwide by 2023. Additional secondary causes of dyslipidemia include diabetes mellitus, alcohol overuse, chronic kidney disease, hypothyroidism, and cholestatic liver diseases such as primary biliary cirrhosis. Also, many drugs can cause dyslipidemia. These include beta-blockers, thiazides, highly active antiretroviral agents, retinoids, cyclosporine, estrogen, progestins, tacrolimus, and glucocorticoids. Low HDL cholesterol can be caused by anabolic steroids, cigarette smoking, HIV infection, and nephrotic syndrome.

Diabetes mellitus is an important secondary cause of dyslipidemia. Affected individuals usually have a combination of the following in relation to atherogenesis: High triglycerides, high small and dense LDL fractions, and low HDL. The combination may be referred to as *diabetic dyslipidemia*. This condition is most prevalent in patients with type 2 diabetes, and is a result of poor diabetic control, obesity, or both. Circulating free fatty acids (FFAs) may increase, causing more VLDL production in the liver. Triglyceride-rich VLDL transfers triglycerides and cholesterol to LDL as well as HDL. This encourages formation of triglyceride-rich small and dense LDL, plus the clearance of triglyceride-rich HDL. Diabetic dyslipidemia is often worsened by higher caloric intake and lack of exercise – which are prime components of a large amount of patients with type 2 diabetes. Because of this type of dyslipidemia, females with diabetes may be at a much higher risk of cardiac disease.

Pathophysiology

Dyslipidemias were first classified by different elevations of lipids and lipoproteins. Today, they are classified as primary or secondary, and via the following considerations:

- Increased cholesterol – *Pure or isolated hypercholesterolemia*

- Increased triglycerides – *Pure or isolated hypertriglyceridemia*

- Increased cholesterol *and* triglycerides – *Mixed or combined hyperlipidemias*

However, there can also be certain abnormalities of HDL and LDL that add to the disease state, while cholesterol and triglyceride levels remain normal.

Clinical Manifestations

Dyslipidemia is usually asymptomatic. However, it leads to vascular disease that does have symptoms, including coronary artery disease, peripheral artery disease, and stroke. Acute pancreatitis can be caused by high levels of triglycerides (more than 500 mg/dL, equivalent to over 5.65 mmol/L). These high levels also cause confusion, dyspnea, hepatosplenomegaly, and paresthesias. High LDL levels may cause **arcus corneae** as well as tendinous **xanthomas** of the Achilles, elbow, and knee tendons, and above the metacarpophalangeal joints (see Figure 8.2). Xanthomas are yellowish in color with surrounding erythematous borders, resulting from increased local extravasation of lipids through the vascular wall to the interstitial spaces of connective tissues. High LDL, as with familial hypercholesterolemia, also causes **xanthelasma**, which may also develop along with primary biliary cirrhosis even when lipid levels are normal. Xanthelasma usually develops on or around the eyelids in a bilateral and symmetric distribution. The lesions are soft, yellow in color, nontender, and nonpruritic.

If the homozygous form of familial hypercholesterolemia is present, the patient may develop arcus corneae, tendinous xanthomas and xanthelasma, along with tuberous or planar xanthomas. **Tuberous xanthomas** are firm, painless nodules usually located above extensor joint surfaces. Planar xanthomas are yellow in color and either flat or slightly raised. Severely elevated triglycerides may cause eruptive xanthomas,

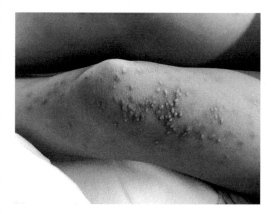

Figure 8.2 Tendinous xanthomas near the knee tendons. (From Sun Yong Lee and Chirag A. Sheth, 2019, Eruptive xanthoma associated with severe hypertriglyceridemia and poorly controlled type 1 diabetes mellitus, *Journal of Community Hospital Internal Medicine Perspectives*, 9:4, 344-346, DOI: 10.1080/20009666.2019.1650591. Used with permission.)

appearing on the back, trunk, elbows, hands, buttocks, knees, and feet. The rare condition called dysbetalipoproteinemia causes palmar and tuberous xanthomas. Severe hypertriglyceridemia exists if triglycerides are above 2,000 mg/dL (22.6 mmol/L). This condition may cause the retinal veins and arteries to have a "creamy" white appearance, known as **lipemia retinalis**. Very high lipid levels cause a milky appearance of the blood plasma.

Diagnosis

Dyslipidemia is suspected because of physical factors or complications such as atherosclerotic disease. Primary lipid disorders are signified by physical manifestations, atherosclerotic disease before 60 years of age, family history of atherosclerotic disease, and serum cholesterol higher than 240 mg/dL (6.2 mmol/L). The serum lipids are measured. A routine lipid profile includes direct measurement of total cholesterol, triglycerides, HDL, and LDL. The total cholesterol and total triglycerides values reveal cholesterol and total triglycerides in all circulating lipoproteins. These include chylomicrons, HDL, intermediate-density lipoprotein (IDL), LDL, and VLDL. Even when no disorder can be diagnosed, total triglycerides can value by up to 25% on a day-to-day basis, and total cholesterol values can vary by 10%. Most patients should have all lipids measured while fasting – usually for 12 hours – to provide the best accuracy and consistency. However, total cholesterol and HDL can be measured when not fasting.

Testing should not be done until any acute illness has resolved, because inflammatory states involve increased total triglycerides and lipoprotein levels, along with decreased cholesterol levels. After an acute MI, lipid profiles can be varied for about 1 month. Even so, the results obtained within 1 day after a MI are usually accurate enough to influence lipid-lowering therapy. LDL values are usually calculated as how much cholesterol is not contained in the HDL and VLDL. The VLDL is estimated by triglycerides divided by 5, since cholesterol in VLDL particles is usually 1/5 of the total amount of lipid in the particles. To calculate this:

- After dividing the triglycerides by 5, they are added to the HDL level.

- This result is then subtracted from the total cholesterol.

- The answer determines the amount of LDL.

However, this is only valid if the triglycerides are below 400 mg/dL (4.5 mmol/L) and the patient is fasting, since eating increases triglycerides.

The LDL value includes measures of all non-HDL, non-chylomicron cholesterol. The LDL can also be directly measured, via plasma ultracentrifugation. This separates the chylomicrons and VLDL fractions from HDL and LDL. Also, an **immunoassay** method can be used to measure LDL. Direct measurement may be sometimes accurate for elevated total triglycerides, but this is not usually needed. Today, apo B testing is being studied. In this, values reveal all non-HDL cholesterol in the VLDL and its remnants, IDL, and LDL. This may have a more accurate predictive rate of risks for coronary artery disease than LDL. Additionally, non-HDL cholesterol may be more predictive of risks for CAD than LDL. This is especially true if hypertriglyceridemia is present. The non-HDL cholesterol is calculated by subtracting HDL from total cholesterol.

Premature atherosclerotic cardiovascular disease, CVD with normal or nearly normal lipid levels, or high HDL refractory to medication therapy requires that the lipoprotein-alpha [Lp(α)] levels be measured. The Lp(α) levels can be measured directly when there are borderline-high LDL levels. This helps determine if drug therapy is likely to be effective. In the same disease states, CRP can also be measured. For patients with increased total triglycerides and metabolic syndrome, it may be good to measure LDL particle numbers or apoprotein B-100 (apo B). Similar information to LDL particle number is provided by measuring apo B, since there is one apo B molecule for each particle of LDL. Measurement of apo B includes every type of atherogenic particle. These include Lp(α) and remnants.

For newly diagnosed dyslipidemia, or when something in the lipid profile has unexpectedly worsened, tests for secondary causes should be done. These include measurements of creatinine, fasting glucose, liver enzymes, thyroid-stimulating hormone (TSH), and urinary protein. A fasting lipid profile is used for screening, taking into account total cholesterol, TGs, HDL, and calculated LDL. Measurement of lipids should include assessment for CVD risk factors such as cigarette smoking, diabetes mellitus, family history of CAD (in a male first-degree relative below age 55, or a female first-degree relative below age 65), and hypertension. For pediatric patients, screening is based on whether there are risk factors present or not, as follows:

- With risk factors (including diabetes, family history of premature CAD or severe hyperlipidemia, or hypertension) – a fasting lipid profile at ages 2 and 8; if the risk factor persists, every 1–3 years after that based on seriousness of the risks

- Without risk factors – a nonfasting or fasting lipid profile one time before puberty, usually at ages 9–11, and one more at ages 17–21

Adults must be screened at the age of 20, and every 5 years after that. Though no certain age has been established to stop screening, studies show that screening past the age of 80 is advised, especially with atherosclerotic cardiovascular disease. Anyone with a significant family history of heart disease should receive additional Lp(α) screening.

Treatment

Treatment is focused on preventing atherosclerotic cardiovascular disease (ASCVD) from developing. This includes atherosclerosis-related acute coronary syndromes, peripheral artery disease, stroke, and transient ischemic attack. Treatment is required as secondary prevention for ASCVD and as primary prevention for some patients without ASCVD. There is controversy about treating children, since diet changes can be difficult, and adult heart disease is not proven to be effectively prevented by previous treatment during childhood. For some children with elevated LDL, the American Academy of Pediatrics does recommend treatment. If a child has heterozygous familial hypercholesterolemia, he or she should be treated initially at ages 8–10. For those with homozygous familial hypercholesterolemia, premature death must be prevented by diet changes, medications, and often, LDL apheresis. Treatments start as soon as the diagnosis is made.

For some patients with hyperlipidemia, just one lipid abnormality may require several types of therapy. For others, just one treatment may be sufficient for several lipid abnormalities. Any present diabetes or hypertension must be treated, and smoking cessation is essential. Low-dose daily aspirin is advised in individuals aged between 40 and 79 years that have a low risk of bleeding and have a risk of MI or death due to CAD.

To prevent ASCVD, a heart-healthy diet and exercise regimen is essential. The lowering of LDL for all age groups also includes medications, dietary supplements, various procedures, and experimental treatments. Regarding diet, there must be less intake of cholesterol and saturated fats, and an increased proportion of complex carbohydrates and dietary fiber. An ideal body weight is the goal. Many people – primarily older patients – benefit from referral to a dietitian. Exercise reduces LDL in most patients and helps maintain an ideal body weight. Medications are indicated for some patients after risks and benefits of *statin therapy* have been discussed.

To reduce LDL, the statins are the treatment of choice. They greatly reduce cardiovascular disease and deaths. The statins inhibit *hydroxymethylglutaryl CoA reductase*. This is an important enzyme in the synthesis of cholesterol. The statins lead to LDL receptor up-regulation and more clearance of LDL. They reduce LDL by as much as 60% while causing small increases in HDL and moderate decreases in total triglycerides. The statins may decrease systemic inflammation, intra-arterial inflammation, or both. They do this by stimulating endothelial nitric oxide production. Other types of lipid-lowering drugs are not as effective as the statins for decreasing ASCVD. There are high, moderate, and low intensity statin regimens, based on the patient's age and conditions. Statins are chosen based on comorbidities, other drugs being taken, intolerance to statins, risk factors for adverse outcomes, cost, and the preference of the patient.

Though adverse effects are not common, statins may cause elevations of liver enzymes, myositis, or **rhabdomyolysis**. Serious liver toxicity is exceedingly rare. About 10% of patient complain of muscle problems, which may be dependent upon dose. Even without enzyme elevation, muscle symptoms can develop. Adverse effects mostly affect older patients, those with multiple conditions, and those on a multiple drug regimen. The fibrate that interacts worst with statins is gemfibrozil. Statins are contraindicated in pregnancy and lactation.

The bile acid sequestrants block reabsorption of intestinal bile acid. This forces the up-regulation of liver LDL receptors to recruit the circulating cholesterol and synthesize bile. These sequestrants reduce cardiovascular-related deaths. They are usually used along with statins or nicotinic acid. The sequestrants are the medications of choice for women planning to become pregnant, or who are already pregnant. Though safe, the sequestrants cause bloating, constipation, cramping, and nausea. They can also increase triglycerides, so they cannot be used if hypertriglyceridemia is present. The drugs called cholestyramine and colestipol interfere with absorption of thiazides, beta-blockers, digoxin, thyroxine, and warfarin. Colesevelam also interferes with these, but not as much. The interference between the drugs can be reduced by administration that is 4 or more hours before or 1 hour after. Bile acid sequestrants are more effective if they are taken during a meal.

PCSK9 monoclonal antibodies are formulated for subcutaneous injection, once to twice per month. They stop proprotein convertase subtilisin/kexin type 9 from attaching to LDL receptors, improving their function. The LDL is lowered by 40%–70%. Trials with alirocumab and evolocumab revealed less cardiovascular events when previous atherosclerotic cardiovascular disease was present. The *cholesterol absorption inhibitors*, including ezetimibe, inhibit absorption of cholesterol and phytosterol in the intestines. The LDL is usually lowered by ezetimibe by 15%–20%, with small increases in HDL and a slight decrease in total triglycerides. Ezetimibe can be used alone if the patient cannot tolerate statins, or it can be added to statins if the patient is on maximum statin dosage, with LDL remaining chronically elevated. Adverse effects of cholesterol absorption inhibitors are rare.

There are dietary supplements that lower LDL, including fiber, margarines, and other products that contain the plant sterols called campesterol and sitosterol, or that contain stanols. Fiber supplements reduce cholesterol by decreasing its absorption and increasing its excretion. The fiber supplements based on oats can provide up to 18% total cholesterol decrease. The plant sterols and stanols displace cholesterol from the **intestinal micelles**, and may reduce LDL by up to 10%, with no effect upon HDL or total triglycerides. For homozygous familial hypercholesterolemia, medications include lomitapide and mipomersen. Lomitapide inhibitors the microsomal triglyceride transfer protein that interfere with secretion of total triglycerides rich lipoproteins in the intestine and liver. Doses start low and are titrated gradually, every 2 weeks. The patient must eat a diet with fewer than 20% of calories from fat. Adverse effects of lomitapide include diarrhea, elevated liver enzymes, and increased fat in the liver. Mipomersen is an apo B antisense oligonucleotide. It decreases apo B synthesis in the liver, while decreasing levels of LDL, apo B, and Lp(α). Mipomersen is injected subcutaneously. Adverse effects include injection site reactions, increased fat in the liver, enzyme elevations, and flu-like symptoms.

For elevated LDL in children, risk factors include family history and diabetes, along with early smoking, hypertension, HDL below 35 mg/dL (0.9 mmol/L), obesity, and physical inactivity. Dietary treatment is recommended if the LDL is above 110 mg/dL (2.8 mmol/L). For children 8 years of older, drug therapy is recommended if either of the following is present:

- LDL at 160 mg/dL (4.13 mmol/L) or higher, plus family history of premature CVD
- Poor response to dietary therapy, LDL at 190 mg/dL (4.9 mmol/L) or higher, and no family history of premature CVD

Elevated triglycerides may or may not independently add to CVD, but they are linked to many metabolic conditions that contribute to CAD. These include diabetes mellitus and metabolic syndrome. Lowering the elevated total triglycerides is likely beneficial. Levels lower than 150 mg/dL (1.7 mmol/L) are the goal, but no pediatric guidelines specially focus on treatment of elevated total triglycerides. Generally, more exercise, weight loss, and avoidance of concentrated dietary sugar are initiated. If a teenager has started drinking alcohol, this must be stopped. Two to four servings of fish high in omega-3 fatty acids should be consumed per week, and omega-3 supplements may be helpful. If the child has diabetes, glucose levels must be rigidly controlled. When these measures fail, lipid-lowering drugs are considered. Those with total triglycerides levels higher than 1,000 mg/dL may need drug therapy immediately, in order to reduce risks for acute pancreatitis.

Fibrates can reduce total triglycerides by approximately 50%. They likely stimulate endothelial lipoprotein lipase (LPL). This results in increased fatty oxidation, within the liver and muscles, and lower hepatic VLDL synthesis. Fibrates also increase HDL by as much as 20%. They may cause abdominal pain, dyspepsia, and elevated liver enzymes. Rarely, they cause **cholelithiasis**. The fibrates may potentiate muscle toxicity if used with statins. They also potentiate the effects of warfarin. Statins can be used if the total triglycerides are below 500 mg/dL (5.65 mmol/L) when elevations of LDL are present. The statins can reduce LDL and total triglycerides by reducing VLDL. When only the total triglycerides are high, the fibrates should be used instead.

To reduce triglycerides, omega-3 fatty acids can be effective in high doses – 1–6 g per day of docosahexaenoic acid (DHA) and eicosapentaenoic acid (EPA). These fatty acids are active ingredients in both ocean fish oil and omega-3 supplements. Adverse effects include diarrhea and **eructation**, but these can be reduced if the supplements not all taken during one meal. Prescription omega-3 fatty acids are used for triglyceride levels above 500 mg/dL (5.65 mmol/L). In some countries, the apo CIII inhibitor called *volanesorsen* is available, and lowers severely elevated triglyceride levels, such as in people with lipoprotein lipase deficiency. The drug is given as a once-weekly injection.

Lifestyle changes and statins are always involved in the reduction of LDL to treat diabetic dyslipidemia. Fibrates can decrease TGs and reduce risks for pancreatitis. Metformin reduces total triglycerides and may be preferred over other oral antihyperglycemic for diabetes. Certain thiazolidinediones (TZDs) increase HDL as well as LDL, and some also decrease total triglycerides – meaning they are not preferred for lipid abnormalities in diabetic patients but can be useful adjunctive medications. Those with very high total triglycerides and poorly controlled diabetes may respond better to insulin than oral antihyperglycemics.

With dyslipidemia, underlying disorder such as chronic kidney disease, hypothyroidism, or liver disease must be treated first. In patients with low to normal thyroid function, hormone replacement may improve abnormal lipid levels. If any drugs are causing lipid abnormalities, they should be reduced or stopped.

Lipid levels are periodically monitored, generally every 2–3 months after starting or changing treatments, and once or twice per year after they are stabilized. Liver and muscle enzyme levels should be measured at the start of treatment. Muscle enzyme levels are only checked regularly if myalgia or other muscle symptoms develop. If it is believed that a statin is damaging the muscles, the drug is stopped and creatine kinase may be measured. Once symptoms subside, a different statin or a lower dose of the same statin is tried. If symptoms continue 1–2 weeks after stopping a statin, another cause is assessed, such as polymyalgia rheumatica.

Prevention

The best methods for preventing development of dyslipidemia include a better diet that includes fiber and antioxidants, along with more exercise. Diets should include vegetables, fruits, whole grains, lean protein, and low-fat dairy products. Alcohol, red meat, and sugary foods and drinks should be limited to the lowest amounts possible. The DASH and Mediterranean diets are known to lower cholesterol levels. As little as 40 minutes of exercise, 3–4 times per week, and regulate cholesterol levels, and simple activities such as walking, dancing, and low-impact aerobics are even safe for older adults. Soluble fiber can lower total cholesterol and LDL, and combined with a low-fat diet, this can balance sugar control, reduce weight, and even prevent certain cancers. Antioxidants such as vitamins C, E, and beta-carotene have properties that can prevent or slow development of atherosclerosis.

Prognosis

Hyperlipidemia usually has a good prognosis if a healthy lifestyle is combined with statins or fibrates. Patients should be instructed about continuing these medications if they effectively manage the condition and there are no significant adverse effects. Some people, without education, reach target cholesterol levels and then mistakenly stop taking their medications. Prognosis is worsened if the patient does not adhere to the drug regimen, or treatment is started late in the disease process when complications have already started to develop.

CLINICAL CASE

1. What is the causative link between diabetes mellitus and dyslipidemia?
2. What type of skin lesions were likely present in this case?
3. Can dyslipidemia actually be prevented?

A 35-year-old man went to his physician because of skin lesions that had developed on his elbows and knees. His blood pressure was 130/80 mm Hg, and laboratory values were very poor. His total cholesterol and triglyceride levels were well beyond the high range of "normal" for their values. There were also some heart changes discovered on electrocardiogram. The physician explained to the patient that his skin lesions were related to dyslipidemia, and there was an urgent need to get his cholesterol and triglycerides under control in order to avoid expected complications such as accelerated atherosclerosis and pancreatitis.

ANSWERS

1. Diabetes mellitus is an important secondary cause of dyslipidemia. Affected individuals usually have a combination of the following in relation to atherogenesis: High triglycerides, high small and dense LDL fractions, and low LDL. The combination may be referred to as diabetic dyslipidemia. This is most prevalent in patients with type 2 diabetes. It is the result of poor diabetic control, obesity, or both. Diabetic dyslipidemia is often worsened by higher caloric intake and lack of exercise.
2. The skin lesions described in this case were likely tendinous xanthomas of the elbow and knee tendons. High LDL levels cause them, and they can also develop over the Achilles tendons and above the metacarpophalangeal joints.
3. The best methods for preventing development of dyslipidemia include a better diet that includes fiber and antioxidants, along with more exercise. Diets should include vegetables, fruits, whole grains, lean protein, and low-fat dairy products. Alcohol, red meat, and sugary foods and drinks should be limited to the lowest amounts possible.

ATHEROSCLEROSIS

Atherosclerosis is defined as the development of **atheromas**, which are intimal plaques collecting in the lumens of medium- and large-sized arteries such as the coronary, carotid, and cerebral arteries. The aorta and its branches as well as the major arteries in the extremities can be affected. The patchy plaques are made up of lipids, inflammatory and smooth muscle cells, and connective tissue. Atherosclerosis is related to dyslipidemia, diabetes mellitus, cigarette smoking, family history, hypertension, obesity, and a sedentary lifestyle. Once the plaques grow or rupture, blood flow can be reduced or obstructed. Atherosclerosis is the most common form of **arteriosclerosis**, which describes disorders that thicken arterial walls and cause them to lose elasticity. Atherosclerosis is very serious, since it results in coronary artery disease (CAD) and cerebrovascular disease (CVD). There are also nonatheromatous forms, which are called *arteriolosclerosis* and *Mönckeberg arteriosclerosis*.

Epidemiology

Atherosclerosis is the primary cause of disease and death in most developed countries worldwide, including the United States. Over recent years, age-related death has been decreasing. However, in 2019, CVD – mostly coronary and cerebrovascular atherosclerosis – caused about 18 million deaths in 2019, making up 32% of all global deaths. About 85% of these were due to heart attack and stroke. Over 75% of CVD deaths occur in low- and middle-income countries. Out of the 17 million deaths under the age of 70 from noncommunicable diseases, 38% were due to CVD. Most people begin to develop a buildup of cholesterol, fat, calcium, and fibrous tissue in their blood vessels while they are in their 20s, and changes can be seen in imaging studies once they reach their 30s. By age 40, about 50% of the population has arterial cholesterol deposits. After age 45, men have significant plaque buildup, and women have this after age 55. According to the Multiethnic Study of Atherosclerosis (MESA), non-Hispanic Caucasian adults have higher levels of atherosclerosis and related CAD than non-Hispanic African, Hispanic, and Asian adults. The top ten countries with the highest rates of atherosclerosis include Slovakia, Hungary, Ireland, Czech Republic, Finland, New Zealand, United Kingdom, Iceland, Norway, and Australia – updated statistics for each of these are not well documented. Slightly different statistics are available for deaths from atherosclerosis-related CAD and CVD. Countries with the most deaths from these conditions include Turkmenistan, Kazakhstan, Mongolia, Uzbekistan, Kyrgyzstan, Guyana, Ukraine, Russia, Afghanistan, Tajikistan, and the Republic of Moldova. All of these have more than 500 deaths per 100,000 population annually. Atherosclerosis is quickly increasing in prevalence in developing countries. Incidence is predicted to increase as people in developed countries live longer.

Etiology and Risk Factors

It is unknown exactly how atherosclerosis starts developing and from what specific cause. Atherosclerosis progresses slowly and may begin as early as childhood. In some patients, it progresses more rapidly. The risk factors for atherosclerosis include diabetes mellitus, dyslipidemia, cigarette smoking, and hypertension. Risk factors are often close to those of metabolic syndrome, which is more prevalent today than in past decades. It combines abdominal obesity, atherogenic dyslipidemia, hypertension, insulin resistance, a prothrombotic state, and in sedentary patients, a proinflammatory state. Insulin resistance may be at the core of the development of metabolic syndrome. Diabetes mellitus causes advanced glycation end products to form, increasing endothelial cell production of proinflammatory cytokines. Oxidative stress and reactive oxygen radicals cause direct injury to the endothelium, promoting atherogenesis. Dyslipidemia results in atherosclerosis by increasing or affecting endothelial dysfunction as well as inflammatory pathways in the vascular endothelium. Oxidation of LDL and subendothelial uptake of LDL increase. The oxidized lipids stimulate adhesion molecule and inflammatory cytokine production. A T cell-mediated immune response and arterial wall inflammation occurs. Today, we know that HDL is not as important in atherogenesis as previously thought. Hypertriglyceridemia has a complex role.

Nicotine and its chemicals are toxic to the vascular endothelium. Smoking increases reactivity of platelets, plasma fibrinogen levels, and hematocrit. Increased platelet reactivity may promote platelet thrombosis, and increased hematocrit results in more blood viscosity. Smoking decreases HDL while increasing LDL. It also results in vasoconstriction – extremely dangerous for atherosclerotic arteries. Proof of the negative effects of smoking can be seen when a patient quits the habit. Within 1 month, the HDL increases by approximately 6–8 mg/dL (0.16–0.21 mmol/L). Hypertension may cause vascular inflammation from angiotensin II-regulated processes. Angiotensin II stimulates endothelial cells, macrophages, and vascular smooth muscle cells. Proatherogenic mediators are produced. These include proinflammatory cytokines, prothrombotic factors, superoxide anions, growth factors, and oxidized LDL receptors that are similar to lectin. Lipoprotein(α) promotes atherogenesis and is an independent CVD risk factor for aortic valve stenosis, MI, and stroke. It also has proinflammatory properties.

Small, dense LDL in high levels is extremely atherogenic and is a common component of diabetes mellitus. This type of LDL may involve higher susceptibility to nonspecific endothelial binding and to oxidation. A high CRP level is able to predict an increased likelihood of an ischemic event. When there are no other inflammatory disorders, increased CRP levels may mean there is a higher risk of rupture of atherosclerotic plaques, increased activity of macrophages and lymphocytes, or chronic thrombosis or ulceration.

Chronic renal disease promotes atherosclerosis because of increasing insulin resistance and hypertension, lower apolipoprotein A-1 levels, and higher C-reactive protein, fibrinogen, homocysteine, and Lp(α) levels. Another factor is heart transplantation. This is often followed by fast-developing coronary atherosclerosis, probably because of endothelial injury that is immune-mediated. Thoracic radiation therapy may also cause accelerated coronary atherosclerosis, which is probably from endothelial injury from the radiation. The likelihood of atherothrombosis is also due to prothrombotic states.

Genetic variants are strongly linked to atherosclerosis and related events. Genetic risk cores add up the total number of small individual risk variants, and are linked to advanced atherosclerosis, plus primary and recurring cardiovascular events. *Hyperhomocysteinemia* is caused by a genetic metabolic defect or a folate deficiency, and is somewhat implicated in atherosclerosis, but is not directly causative. Links between higher **homocysteine** levels and atherosclerosis are not fully understood. It is however well known that atherosclerosis in one vascular area increases the chance for the disease to develop in other vascular areas. Noncoronary atherosclerotic vascular disease carries cardiac event rates similar to those seen in cases of documented CAD. There is definitely a CAD risk equivalence, and treatments should be just as aggressive.

Pathophysiology

The earliest visible lesion of atherosclerosis is called a **fatty streak**, a grouping of foam cells filled with lipid within the intimal arterial layer. The fatty streak evolves into the classic atherosclerotic plaque, which contains lipids, inflammatory cells, smooth muscle cells, and a connective tissue matrix (see Figure 8.3). The matrix may have thrombi that are in different stages of organization. Calcium deposits may also be present. All atherosclerotic pathophysiological stages are inflammatory responses to injury, regulated by cytokines. The first causative factor may be endothelial injury. At branch points within the arterial tree, turbulent or nonlaminar blood flow result in endothelial dysfunction. The endothelial production of nitric oxide is inhibited, and vasodilation and anti-inflammatory effects are reduced. The blood flow stimulates endothelial cells, producing adhesion molecules that recruit and then bind inflammatory cells.

Atherosclerotic plaques are either stable or unstable. *Stable plaques* can grow slowly over several decades until stenosis or occlusion occurs. *Unstable plaques* are weaker and more likely to erode, develop fissures, or rupture. They can cause acute thrombosis, occlusion, and infarction a long time before causing any extreme stenosis. Unstable plaques cause the majority of signs and symptoms. They do not appear to be severe during angiography. Therefore, stabilization of unstable plaques may help reduce disease and death. The rupture of plaques is based on activated macrophages inside that secrete cathepsins, metalloproteinases, and collagenases. After a plaque ruptures, its contents are exposed to the blood circulation, and thrombosis is triggered.

Clinical Manifestations

For decades, atherosclerosis is often asymptomatic until blood flow begins to be affected. When stable plaques enlarge and reduce the arterial lumen by 70% of more, transient ischemic symptoms may appear. These include intermittent claudication, stable exertional angina, and transient ischemic attacks. A lesion that does not limit blood flow can be affected by vasoconstriction so that severe or total stenosis develops. When an unstable plaque ruptures and occludes a major artery along with a superimposition of embolism or thrombosis, symptoms may develop that include unstable angina, MI, ischemic stroke, or limb pain while resting. Unfortunately, atherosclerosis can also cause sudden death without any stable or unstable angina pectoris having ever occurred. If the arterial wall is atherosclerotic, the results can include aneurysms and arterial dissection, causing pain, absent pulses, a pulsatile mass, and sudden death.

Diagnosis

Diagnosis of atherosclerosis is based on whether the patient is symptomatic or asymptomatic. If there are signs and symptoms of ischemia, there must be evaluation for the location and amount of vascular occlusion. Noninvasive and invasive

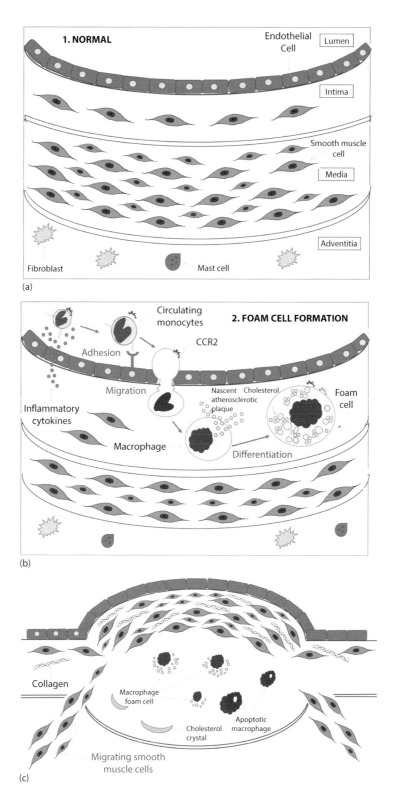

Figure 8.3 (a) Stages in the formation of atherosclerotic plaques. (b) Early atherosclerosis. (c) Plaque progression. (With permission from Boland, J.E., and Muller, David W. M. (2019). *Interventional Cardiology and Cardiac Catheterisation: The Essential Guide,* 2nd Edition. CRC Press/Taylor & Francis.)

tests are available. The patient's history is taken, followed by physical examination, a fasting lipid profile, and plasma glucose as well as glycosylated hemoglobin (HbA1C) levels. If there is disease in one site, the patient is evaluated for disease in other sites. Noninvasive imaging is able to evaluate the morphology and characteristics of atherosclerotic plaques. These methods include CT angiography, MR angiography, and three-dimensional vascular ultrasonography. There are also invasive tests that utilize catheters, such as the following:

- *Angioscopy* – Using fiberoptic catheters to visualize arterial surfaces

- *Elastography* – To identify plaques that are soft and filled with lipids

- *Intravascular ultrasonography* – A transducer on the tip of a catheter produces arterial wall and lumen images

- *Optical coherence tomography* – Using infrared laser light

- *Plaque thermography* – To detect increased temperature in plaques that are actively inflamed

Immunoscintigraphy is an alternative, noninvasive method. It uses radioactive tracers that localize vulnerable plaques. A newer technique uses positron emission tomography (PET) to image the vasculature, and assess vulnerable plaques. For some patients, serum markers of inflammation are also measured, since CRP levels are often accurately predictive of cardiovascular events. For asymptomatic patients, CT imaging for coronary artery calcium, obtaining a *calcium score*, helps to classify risks for cardiovascular events. It also helps to determine which statins may be best to use in patients of intermediate risk or with a family history of early CVD. Lipid profile screening should be performed if the patient fits any of the following:

- Male, 40 years of age or older

- Female, 50 years of age or older, and postmenopausal

- Chronic inflammatory conditions

- Family history of familial hypercholesterolemia, or premature CVD (such as with an age of onset below 55 years in a male first-degree relative, or below 65 years in a female first-degree relative)

- Hypertension

- Metabolic syndrome

- Type 2 diabetes

There is a new recommended method of estimating the 10-year and lifetime risk of atherosclerotic CVD. It is based on age, gender, race, total cholesterol and HDL levels, diabetes mellitus, smoking status, and systolic BP. This method is recommended by the American Heart Association. Also, the European Cardiovascular Society and European Atherosclerosis Society use the Systemic Coronary Risk Estimation (SCORE). This method is based on age, gender, smoking, systolic BP, and total cholesterol. It estimates the 10-year risk for a first atherosclerotic event. If a patient is at intermediate risk, lipoprotein(α) should be measured as well. Urinary albuminuria is a strong marker for cardiovascular and noncardiovascular disease and death as well as for renal disorders. Even so, a direct link between albuminuria and atherosclerosis is not fully understood.

Treatment

Treatment of atherosclerosis includes serious modifications of risk factors, designed to slow down disease progression and cause existing plaques to regress. Today, it is recommended to lower LDL to as much as possible, not only to certain target levels. Lifestyle changes and medications can improve endothelial function, reduce inflammation, and improve the prognosis. Patients must greatly decrease intake of saturated fat, refined or processed carbohydrates, and increase the types of carbohydrates that contain fiber: Fruits and vegetables. These dietary changes are required for all patients. Caloric intake must be limited to keep weight gain in a normal range. Fat intake must be limited to no more than 20 grams per day. This must consist of 6–10 g of polyunsaturated fat with equal proportions of omega-3 and omega-6 fatty acids. There must be 2 g or less of saturate fat, and the remainder must be monounsaturated fat. All sources of trans fats must be avoided.

There must be avoidance of excessive fat and refined sugars – especially if the patient is at risk for diabetes mellitus. Consumption of complex carbohydrates in the form of vegetables and whole grains is encouraged instead. Five daily servings of fruits and vegetable appear to decrease risks for coronary atherosclerosis. Phytochemicals known as **flavonoids** are very protective. They are found in red or purple grapes, black teas, dark beers, and red wine. The high concentrations of flavonoids in red wine help explain the low incidence of coronary atherosclerosis in societies that regularly consume it, such as France. While not preventative of atherosclerosis, flavonoids are somewhat protective.

Increased dietary fiber may affect glucose and insulin levels while decreasing total cholesterol. There should be at least 5–10 g of soluble fiber consumed every day. Good sources include beans, oat bran, psyllium, and soy products. The recommended daily amount of fiber decreases LDL by approximately 5%. Cellulose and lignin are forms of *insoluble fiber* that do not affect cholesterol, but do help reduce risks for colorectal cancer. Excessive fiber should be avoided because it interferes with absorption of some vitamins and minerals. Generally, foods with large amounts of phytochemicals and vitamins also contain large amounts of fiber.

Though alcohol increases HDL and also has some anti-inflammatory, antioxidant, and anti-thrombotic properties, higher doses can cause severe health problems. The "good" effects of alcohol appear to be the same for moderate consumption of beer, wine, and hard liquor. Approximately 30 mL of ethanol is contained in 1 ounce, or 2 average servings of each type of alcoholic beverage. If consumed in this quantity 5–6 times per week, it protects against coronary atherosclerosis. Deaths from atherosclerosis are lowest for men that consume less than 14 alcoholic servings per week, and for women that consume less than 9. Healthcare professionals do not recommend that people that do not drink alcohol should start based only on this slight protective effect.

Except for fish oil supplements, no other vitamin, phytochemical, or trace mineral supplements reduce risks for atherosclerosis. Some alternative medicines and health foods have minor effects upon cholesterol and BP. They are not always safe or effective, and may interact with effective prescription medications. Coenzyme Q10 decreases with aging and may be low if certain heart conditions and other chronic diseases are present. Supplementation with this coenzyme has been recommended, but is still of unproven therapeutic benefit.

Regular physical activity reduces incidence of diabetes mellitus, dyslipidemia, hypertension, CAD, and atherosclerotic-related death. This is true whether there has or has not been any previous ischemic events. It is recommended that patients engage in 30–45 minutes of walking, cycling, swimming, or running for 3–5 days per week. The majority of evidence suggests that there is an inverse, linear relationship between CAD and CVD risk factors and aerobic physical activity. Also, regular walking increases the amount of distance that peripheral vascular disease patients can walk without experiencing pain. Aerobic exercise helps prevent atherosclerosis while promoting weight loss. However, people with CAD or CVD risk factors, and the elderly, should never start an exercise program without approval from a physician. This is based on patient history, physical examination, and risk factors that may be present.

Since most atherosclerotic complications occur from plaque fissure or rupture, followed by platelet activation and thrombosis, oral anti-platelet drugs are extremely important. Aspirin is widely used, and is indicated for secondary prevention. It may be used for primary prevention if the patient is at very high risk (diabetes, those with 20% or higher risk of cardiac events with low risks of bleeding, and those at intermediate risk of atherosclerosis with 10%–20% risks of cardiac events and low risks of bleeding). Use of aspirin is controversial among clinicians, especially in people at low risk. The lowest dose (81 mg per day) is usually recommended to reduce risks of bleeding, especially if other antithrombotic drugs are used. In patients using aspirin for secondary prevention, there is recurrence of ischemic events. The nonsteroidal anti-inflammatory drugs (NSAIDs) must be used carefully since they appear to increase cardiovascular risks.

If ischemic events recur and the patient has been taking aspirin, or if the patient cannot tolerate aspirin, clopidogrel is used instead. It can also be combined with aspirin for acute ST-segment and non-ST-segment elevation MI. This combination may also be given after percutaneous intervention for 9–12 months, to reduce risks of recurring ischemia. There is sometimes resistance to clopidogrel, and newer drugs include prasugrel and ticagrelor. They are more effective than clopidogrel to prevent coronary disease in certain patients. The statin drugs mostly lower LDL, but also enhance endothelial nitric oxide production, reduce arterial wall accumulation of lipid, stabilize atherosclerotic plaques, and assist in plaque regression. They are used for clinical atherosclerotic CVD. Statins can also be used with family history of premature arteriosclerotic CVD, with high-sensitivity C-reactive protein scores, with high coronary artery calcium scores, and with a low ankle:brachial BP index.

The ACE inhibitors, ARBs, ezetimibe, and PCSK9 inhibitors reduce risks of atherosclerosis unrelated to their effects upon BP and levels of lipid and glucose. The PCSK9 inhibitors have been shown to reduce atherosclerosis as well as related cardiovascular events. Rivaroxaban is a factor Xa inhibitor that also decreases risks of cardiovascular events in patients with stable atherosclerotic vascular disease, along with daily aspirin therapy. Though bleeding risks are increased, the chances for cardiovascular death, MI, or stroke are reduced.

Prevention

The prevention of atherosclerosis involves quitting or avoiding smoking, managing hypertension and high cholesterol, becoming more physically active, eating a heart-healthy diet, any other treatment modalities for being obese or overweight, and correctly managing diabetes mellitus. For younger people especially, quitting use of e-cigarettes and vaping devices can be preventive, since both cause inflammation of arteries. Aerobic exercise is of higher benefit than less strenuous forms of exercise. At-risk patients should see their healthcare providers regularly for check-ups, to check BP and cholesterol levels.

Prognosis

The prognosis for atherosclerosis is based on the level of the disease progression. With only the presence of fatty streaks, prognosis is good with proper treatment. Once fibrous plaques develop, prognosis is fair since the likelihood of serious outcomes is much more likely. However, with adequate treatment and lifestyle changes, many patients still are treated effectively. Once fibrous plaques have ruptured, prognosis is poor due to constriction of blood flow. Timely disease management may still save the life of the patient, but many patients do not survive this stage of the disease.

CLINICAL CASE

1. What are atheromas that develop as part of atherosclerosis?
2. How serious is atherosclerosis regarding global mortality?
3. How is diabetes mellitus implicated with atherosclerosis?

A 55-year-old man presents to his local emergency department because of chronic low-grade chest pain that has worsened with exercise. He states that he has to take a lot of breaks while exercising, sitting down for a while, in order to relieve the pain. The patient has been a one pack-per-day smoker for 30 years, and has not seen a physician for at least 5 years. His BP is 160/100 mm Hg, and his heart rate is at 68, which is slightly lower than normal for his age. After patient history, physical examination, and testing, the patient is diagnosed with chronic stable angina due to atherosclerotic plaque buildup in a coronary artery.

ANSWERS

1. Atherosclerosis is defined as the development of atheromas, which are intimal plaques collecting in the lumens of medium- and large-sized arteries such as the coronary, carotid, and cerebral arteries. The patchy plaques are made up of lipids, inflammatory and smooth muscle cells, and connective tissue. Once the plaques grow or rupture, blood flow can be reduced or obstructed.
2. Atherosclerosis is the primary cause of disease and death in most developed countries worldwide. Age-related death has been decreasing over recent years, yet coronary and cerebrovascular atherosclerosis caused most of the 18 billion CVD deaths in 2019, making up 32% of all global deaths. About 85% of these were due to heart attack and stroke.
3. With atherosclerosis, diabetes mellitus causes advanced glycation end products to form, increasing endothelial cell production of proinflammatory cytokines. Small, dense LDL in high levels is extremely atherogenic and is a common component of diabetes mellitus.

KEY TERMS

- Apolipoproteins
- Arcus corneae
- Arteriosclerosis
- Atheromas
- Atherosclerosis
- Cholelithiasis
- Chylomicrons
- Dyslipidemia
- Eructation
- Fatty acid
- Fatty streak
- Flavonoids
- Glycerol
- Homocysteine
- Immunoassay
- Immunoscintigraphy
- Intestinal micelles
- Lipemia retinalis
- Rhabdomyolysis
- Sterol
- Tuberous xanthomas
- Xanthelasma
- Xanthomas

REFERENCES

American Diabetes Association – Diabetes Care. (2005). *Racial / Ethnic Differences in Subclinical Atherosclerosis among Adults with Diabetes – The Multiethnic Study of Atherosclerosis.* American Diabetes Association. https://care.diabetesjournals.org/content/28/11/2768

Baliga, R.R., and Cannon, C.P. (2011). *Dyslipidemia (Oxford American Cardiology Library).* Oxford University Press.

Ballantyne, C.M. (2014). *Clinical Lipidology: A Companion to Braunwald's Heart Disease,* 2nd Edition. Elsevier.

Ballantyne, C.M., O'Keefe, Jr., J.H., Gotto, Jr., A.M. (2009). *Dyslipidemia & Atherosclerosis Essentials,* 4th Edition. Physician's Press.

Banach, M. (2015). *Combination Therapy in Dyslipidemia.* Adis.

Bray, G.A., and Bouchard, C. (2014). *Handbook of Obesity – Volume 2: Clinical Applications*, 4th Edition. CRC Press.

BYJU's Classes. (2021). *What Is Cholesterol?* BYJU's Classes. https://byjus.com/biology/cholesterol/

Centers for Disease Control and Prevention. (2017). *High Cholesterol in the United States*. U.S. Department of Health & Human Services – USA.gov – CDC. https://www.cdc.gov/cholesterol/facts.htm

Cision – PRNewswire – ResearchAndMarkets. (2021). *Global Dyslipidemia Disease Analysis 2020–2027*. Verizon Media, Inc. https://finance.yahoo.com/news/global-dyslipidemia-disease-analysis-2020-190000812.html

Covic, A., Kanbay, M., and Lerma, E.V. (2014). *Dyslipidemias in Kidney Disease*. Springer.

Dullaart, R. (2020). *Novel Aspects of Lipoprotein Metabolism with Focus on Systemic Inflammation (Journal of Clinical Medicine)*. Mdpi AG.

Food and Drug Administration. (2021). *Food Additives & Petitions – Trans Fat*. U.S. Food and Drug Administration. https://www.fda.gov/food/food-additives-petitions/trans-fat

Garg, A. (2015). *Dyslipidemias: Pathophysiology, Evaluation and Management (Contemporary Endocrinology)*. Humana Press.

Harvard Health Publishing – Harvard Medical School. (2020). *Heart Health - Understanding Triglycerides*. The President and Fellows of Harvard College. https://www.health.harvard.edu/heart-health/understanding-triglycerides

Haverich, A., and Boyle, E.C. (2019). *Atherosclerosis Pathogenesis and Microvascular Dysfunction*. Springer.

Healthline. (2021). *Dyslipidemia – Prevention Tips*. Healthline Media. https://www.healthline.com/health/dyslipidemia#outlook

Kwiterovich, M.D. (2009). *The Johns Hopkins University Textbook of Dyslipidemia*. Wolters Kluwer Health / Lippincott, Williams, and Wilkins.

Lee, S.H., and Kyoung Kang, M. (2021). *Stroke Revisited: Dyslipidemia in Stroke*. Springer.

Mosca, L.J. (2009). *Contemporary Diagnosis and Management of Dyslipidemias in Women*, 2nd Edition. Handbooks in Health Care Company.

Myerson, M. (2018). *Dyslipidemia: A Clinical Approach*. Wolters Kluwer Health.

NationMaster – Health. (1998). *Heart Disease Deaths: Countries Compared*. NationMaster.com. https://www.nationmaster.com/country-info/stats/Health/Heart-disease-deaths

NCBI – Endotext. (2021). *Introduction to Lipids and Lipoproteins*. National Center for Biotechnology Information, U.S. National Library of Medicine. https://www.ncbi.nlm.nih.gov/books/NBK305896/

NIH – National Library of Medicine – National Center for Biotechnology Information. (2021). *Global Epidemiology of Dyslipidaemias*. National Library of Medicine. https://pubmed.ncbi.nlm.nih.gov/33833450/

Ojo, O. (2019). *Dietary Intake and Type 2 Diabetes (Nutrients)*. Mdpi AG.

Schaefer, E.J. (2010). *High Density Lipoproteins, Dyslipidemia, and Coronary Heart Disease*. Springer.

SlideShare – a Scribd company. (2012). *Dyslipidemia Case Study*. SlideShare from Scribd. https://www.slideshare.net/gamalbadr54/dyslipidemia-case-study

Sorrentino, M.J. (2011). *Hyperlipidemia in Primary Care: A Practical Guide to Risk Reduction (Current Clinical Practice)*. Humana Press.

Study.com. (2021). *Atherosclerosis: Stages & Prognosis*. Study.com. https://study.com/academy/lesson/atherosclerosis-stages-prognosis.html

Taylor, A.J., and Villines, T.C. (2012). *Atherosclerosis: Clinical Perspectives Through Imaging*. Springer.

Texas Tech University Health Sciences Center – El Paso. (2021). *Clinical Cases: Atherosclerosis*. Texas Tech University. https://anatomy.elpaso.ttuhsc.edu/clinicalcases/atherosclerosis/atherosclerosis2.html

Thompson, D. (2015). *Prevention and Management of Dyslipidemia*. Foster Academics.

University of Rochester Medical Center Health Encyclopedia. (2021). *What You Can Do to Prevent Atherosclerosis*. University of Rochester Medical Center. https://www.urmc.rochester.edu/encyclopedia/content.aspx?ContentTypeID=1&ContentID=1583

WebMD. (2015). *Atherosclerosis: Your Arteries Age by Age*. WebMD LLC. https://www.webmd.com/heart-disease/features/atherosclerosis-your-arteries-age-by-age

World Economic Forum – Industry Agenda. (2015). *Which Countries Have the Most Deaths from Heart Disease?* World Economic Forum. https://www.weforum.org/agenda/2015/10/which-countries-have-the-most-deaths-from-heartdisease/

World Health Organization. (2021). *Cardiovascular Diseases (CVDs)*. World Health Organization. https://www.who.int/news-room/fact-sheets/detail/cardiovascular-diseases-(cvds)

World Health Organization Regional Office for Europe. (2015). *Eliminating Trans Fats in Europe*. WHO Europe. https://www.euro.who.int/en/health-topics/disease-prevention/nutrition/news/news/2015/09/eliminating-trans-fats-in-europe

Yassine, H. (2015). *Lipid Management: From Basics to Clinic*. Springer.

CHAPTER 9 Coronary Artery Disease

Coronary artery disease is the most common cause of death in developed countries. Accurate, early diagnosis and treatment are imperative because of the extreme complications, deaths, and socioeconomic factors related to the disease. In relation to diabetes mellitus, coronary artery disease is a primary factor in determining prognosis. Diabetes mellitus is linked with a 2 to 4 times higher risk for death from heart disease. There is an increased mortality after myocardial infarction in diabetic patients, and a worsened prognosis with coronary artery disease.

STRUCTURE OF THE CORONARY ARTERIES

The right and left coronary arteries arise from the coronary sinuses in the root of the aorta, above the aortic valve orifice. The arteries divide into large and medium-sized arteries running along the heart surface, known as *epicardial coronary arteries*, and then smaller arterioles that extend into the myocardium. The left coronary starts as the left main artery. It soon divides into the left anterior descending (LAD) artery, circumflex artery, and sometimes an intermediate artery called the *ramus intermedius*. The structure of these arteries is not identical in every person. For example, the LAD artery usually follows the anterior interventricular groove. However, in other people, it continues over the heart apex. This artery supplies the anterior septum, which includes the proximal conduction system. It also supplies the anterior free wall of the left ventricle (LV). The circumflex artery is smaller than the LAD artery. It supplies the free wall of the lateral LV. The majority of people have *right dominance* of the coronary arteries. The right coronary artery continues along the atrioventricular (AV) groove and right side of the heart. It supplies the right atrium, right ventricle, and often, the inferior myocardial wall.

CORONARY ARTERY DISEASE

Coronary artery disease (CAD) develops when atheromas or other factors impair blood flow through the coronary arteries. This causes the development of angina pectoris, myocardial infarction (MI), and sudden death. Development of CAD can be reversed by treating hypercholesterolemia, hypertension, obesity, and diabetes mellitus, and by lifestyle changes such as increasing physical activity, healthy diet, and quitting smoking.

CAD is the most common cause of death in developed countries. In relation to diabetes mellitus, coronary artery disease is a primary factor in determining prognosis. Diabetes mellitus is linked with a 2–4 times higher risk for death from heart disease. There is an increased mortality after myocardial infarction in diabetic patients, and a worsened prognosis with coronary artery disease.

Epidemiology

CAD is the leading cause of death in developed countries in both men and women. For postmenopausal women, the death rate from CAD is increased. By the age of 75, it is equal to and sometimes higher than the death rate for men. Globally, CAD, deaths occur in low- and middle-income countries. In the United States, CAD is the most common type of heart disease. It causes over 365,000 deaths annually. Approximately 18.2 million adults aged 20 and older have CAD, and about 20% of deaths from this disease occur in adults younger than age 65. Though data from many countries is not well documented, some studies are very revealing. For example, CAD has increased by 300% in India over the past 30 years. People in India have the highest mortality and morbidity rates from CAD compared to any other ethnic group. It has been projected that more than 60 million Indians have CAD. Of this number, 23 million are less than 40 years of age, and 10 million are less than age 30. The World Health Organization projects that 2.9 million deaths occur in India every year from CAD. Males are affected more than females.

Etiology and Risk Factors

CAD is usually caused by *atherosclerosis*, in which there are subintimal **atheromas** in the large and medium-sized coronary arteries. Vascular endothelial dysfunction promotes atherosclerosis and coronary artery spasm. This dysfunction is a cause of angina when there is no epicardial coronary artery stenosis or spasm – known as **syndrome X**. This syndrome is cardiac microvascular constriction or dysfunction, and causes angina even when the epicardial coronary arteries appear normal during angiography. Rare causes of CAD include coronary artery embolism, aneurysm as seen in **Kawasaki disease**, dissection, and vasculitis as seen in systemic lupus erythematosus or syphilis. Risk factors for CAD are increased LDL cholesterol, low levels of HDL cholesterol in the blood, diabetes mellitus (especially type 2), high levels of apoprotein B, high blood levels of CRP, lack of physical exercise, obesity, and smoking. Risks for CAD are also increased by smoking tobacco products, a diet that is high in calories and fat but has low vegetables, fruits, and fibers,

DOI: 10.1201/9781003226727-12

insufficient dietary vitamins C, D, and E, insufficient omega-3, and stress.

Pathophysiology

Atherosclerosis in CAD often has distribution in different vessels that is highly irregular. It occurs most at vessel bifurcations or other areas of turbulence. With growth of atheromatous plaques, the arterial lumen becomes progressively narrowed, and ischemia develops. This often causes angina pectoris. The amount of stenosis that will cause ischemia is different with varying oxygen demands. Sometimes an atheromatous plaque splits or ruptures, likely due to morphology, calcium content, or plaque softening because of an inflammatory condition. An acute thrombus is formed, interrupting coronary blood flow. *Acute coronary syndromes,* including acute ischemia, are based on the degree of obstruction and its location. A transmural infarction can occur. Additional complications include conduction defects, ventricular arrhythmias, heart failure, and sudden death.

Coronary artery spasm is defined as a transient and focal increase in vascular tone. The lumen is greatly narrowed and blood flow is reduced. If an atheroma is present, it causes local hypercontractility. The vasoconstrictors may be produced in larger quantities near the atheroma which include angiotensin II, endothelin, serotonin, leukotrienes, and thromboxane. When there are recurring spasms, the intima may be damaged, resulting in formation of an atheroma. Coronary spasms are also triggered by emotional stress and the use of vasoconstricting drugs such as cocaine and nicotine.

Clinical Manifestations

Initially, decreased coronary artery blood flow causes no symptoms. With plaque buildup, signs and symptoms include angina pectoris, shortness of breath, and MI. Angina is described as chest pressure or tightness, usually on the middle portion or left side. The pain usually subsides a few minutes after stopping any stressful activity. For some patients – primarily women – the pain can be brief or sharp, in the left arm, neck, or back. With activity, the patient develops shortness of breath or extreme fatigue. If a coronary artery becomes totally blocked, an MI occurs. There is crushing pressure in the chest and pain in the arm or shoulder, often with shortness of breath and sweating. However, an MI can occur without any obvious signs or symptoms. Also, women are more likely than men to have more unusual signs and symptoms, such as jaw or neck pain, sometimes accompanied with nausea, fatigue, and shortness of breath.

Diagnosis

Diagnosis of CAD is based on medical history, physical examination, and routine blood tests. Other diagnostic tests include ECG, echocardiogram, an exercise stress test, a nuclear stress test, cardiac catheterization, and cardiac CT scan. Electrocardiogram can reveal evidence of a previous heart attack or even one that is currently happening. Echocardiogram allows for examination of all parts of the heart wall, revealing signs of CAD. An exercise stress test involves walking on a treadmill or riding a stationary bicycle as an ECG is being performed, and sometimes an echocardiogram is done as well. For some patients, a medication is used to stimulate the heart instead of exercise. A nuclear stress test is similar to an exercise stress test, but provides images as well as ECG recordings, measuring blood flow to the heart muscle during stress and at rest via specialized cameras. In cardiac catheterization, a catheter is inserted into a groin, neck, or arm artery or vein and carefully pushed to the heart, guided by the use of various imaging techniques. Dye may be injected to improve imaging of the blood vessels and any blockages. A cardiac CT helps visualize calcium deposits in the arteries that can narrow them, indicating likely CAD. Also, in a CT coronary angiogram, a contrast dye is injected intravenously to produce detailed images of the coronary arteries (see Figure 9.1).

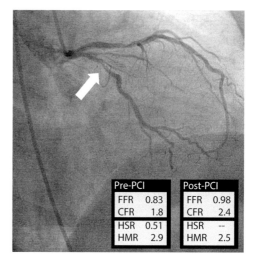

Pre-PCI		Post-PCI	
FFR	0.83	FFR	0.98
CFR	1.8	CFR	2.4
HSR	0.51	HSR	--
HMR	2.9	HMR	2.5

Figure 9.1 Coronary angiography. The white arrow indicates moderate stenosis in the left circumflex artery. (With permission from Grech, E.D. (2017). *Practical Interventional Cardiology,* 3rd Edition. CRC Press/Taylor & Francis.)

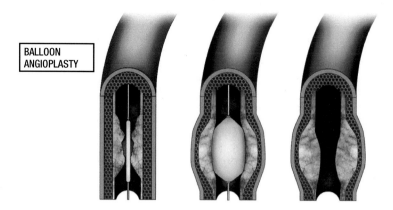

Figure 9.2 Balloon angioplasty. (With permission from Laflamme, D. (2016). *Cardiology: A Practical Handbook*, 1st Edition. CRC Press/Taylor & Francis.)

Treatment

Treatment of CAD is focused on reducing the cardiac workload. This is achieved by decreasing oxygen demand while improving blood flow through the coronary artery. Over time, the goal is to stop and reverse atherosclerosis. *Percutaneous coronary intervention* (PCI) and *coronary artery bypass grafting* (CABG) can improve coronary artery blood flow. Fibrinolytic drugs may be used to dissolve an acute coronary thrombosis, for some patients. The medical treatments for CAD are based on cardiac function, present symptoms, and underlying disorders. Antiplatelet drugs are recommended to stop clot formation. Statins are used to lower LDL cholesterol, improving outcomes in part by stabilizing atheromatous plaques and also by causing better endothelial function. Beta-blockers can reduce angina symptoms by decreasing myocardial oxygen demand and reducing heart rate and contractility. Calcium channel blockers are often effective, especially when used with beta-blockers to manage angina and hypertension. Nitrates slightly dilate the coronary arteries to decrease venous return. For patients with CAD and LV dysfunction, the angiotensin-converting enzyme (ACE) inhibitors and angiotensin II receptor blockers (ARBs) are the preferred medications.

PCI may be used for some patients with acute coronary syndromes as well as those with stable ischemic heart disease when there is angina that persists even with medications, balloon angioplasty may be done (see Figure 9.2). In some cases, CABG is required.

Prevention

CAD can be prevented by quitting smoking, losing weight, exercising regularly, eating a healthy diet, reducing serum lipid levels and salt intake, and controlling diabetes mellitus and hypertension. When serum lipid levels are modified, mostly by using statins, progression of CAD may be slowed or partially reversed. Patients are chosen for treatment based on risks of atherosclerotic cardiovascular disease.

Prognosis

There is no cure for CAD, but treatments often provide a good prognosis. Advances in medications, surgery, and other interventions have improved prognosis for many CAD patients. Morbidity and mortality have been greatly decreased. Cardiac rehabilitation programs can reduce second MI or death in up to 30% of patients. Prognosis is worsened if a patient has had a cardiac event, and becomes poor with multiple events. The worst prognosis is given for people who have diabetes mellitus, hypertension and continue to smoke.

CLINICAL CASE

1. How common is CAD as a cause of death in developed countries?
2. What are the common causes of CAD?
3. Aside from electrocardiogram, what other diagnostic tests are used for CAD?

A 61-year-old man with type 2 diabetes is taken to the emergency room by his wife, because of tightness in his chest. The patient says his discomfort started in the middle of his chest after he was working outside in his yard. He is sweating and says that he feels nauseous. The pain is slightly better when sitting down, but his chest still feels "heavy." The patient smokes two packs of cigarettes per day, drinks alcohol regularly, and has a stressful job. He is also obese. His BP is 145/95 mm Hg. An ECG and other tests are ordered and the patient is diagnosed with CAD.

ANSWERS

1. CAD is the leading cause of death in developed countries, causing approximately 33% of all deaths – in both men and women.
2. CAD is usually caused by atherosclerosis, in which there are subintimal atheromas in the large and medium-sized coronary arteries. Rare causes of CAD include coronary artery embolism, aneurysm as seen in Kawasaki disease, dissection, and vasculitis as seen in systemic lupus erythematosus or syphilis.
3. Other diagnostic tests include echocardiogram, an exercise stress test, a nuclear stress test, cardiac catheterization, and cardiac CT scan.

STABLE ANGINA

Stable angina is defined as a syndrome of uncomfortable, precordial pressure or pain caused by transient myocardial ischemia. It is also called **angina pectoris**, or simply, *angina*. There is no infarction that is part of this syndrome. In most cases, angina pectoris, follows psychologic stress or physical exertion. It is often relieved by rest or by the use of nitroglycerin, administered sublingually. Angina is a common condition – especially in people over age 55. Having type 2 diabetes results in an additional and very significant risk factor for angina pectoris.

Epidemiology

The prevalence of stable angina is difficult to determine since it is diagnosed based on patient history using clinical assessment. It is known to increase in prevalence with age, for both men and women. In older adults between ages 65 and 84, stable angina affects 10%–12% of women, yet is more prevalent in men, affecting 12%–14%. In the United States, almost 10 million people are diagnosed with stable angina every year. There are slight variances in the percentage of people of various racial or ethnic groups affected by angina, as follows – this is also shown in Figure 9.3.

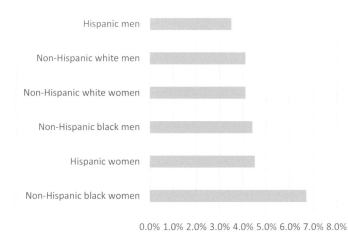

Figure 9.3 Percentages of various individuals with angina in the United States.

- Non-Hispanic black women – 6.7%

- Hispanic women – 4.5%

- Non-Hispanic black men – 4.4%

- Non-Hispanic white women – 4.1%

- Non-Hispanic white men – 4.1%

- Hispanic men – 3.5%

Etiology and Risk Factors

The cause of angina pectoris is from a cardiac workload that requires more myocardial oxygen than the coronary arteries are able to supply via the oxygenated blood in the body. This occurs when the arteries have become narrowed, usually from coronary artery atherosclerosis, but also from coronary artery spasm. A rare cause is coronary artery embolism. Acute coronary thrombosis may cause angina with partial or transient obstruction, but in most cases, it causes acute MI. Myocardial oxygen demand is mostly determined by heart rate, systolic wall tension, and contractility. Therefore, narrowing of a coronary artery usually causes angina during exertion. It is relieved by rest. Cardiac workload can also be increased by aortic stenosis, hypertension, aortic regurgitation, or hypertrophic cardiomyopathy. If these are present, angina may occur with or without any atherosclerosis. Angina can be precipitated or aggravated by a decreased oxygen supply due to severe hypoxia or anemia. Risk factors for stable angina include diabetes mellitus, being overweight or obese, history of heart disease, high cholesterol, hypertension, smoking, and insufficient exercise.

Pathophysiology

With stable angina, it is usually easy to predict the relationship between the cardiac workload and ischemia. Atherosclerotic narrowing of the coronary arteries varies with normal fluctuations in **arterial tone**. When arterial tone is relatively high, such as in the morning, angina is most common. Abnormal endothelial function may aid in varying the arterial tone. This occurs when the endothelium is damaged by atheromas when a stressful surging of catecholamines causes vasoconstriction instead of dilation, which would be the normal response. With an ischemic myocardium, the coronary sinus blood pH decreases. There is a loss of cellular potassium and an accumulation of lactate. On ECG, there are obvious abnormalities. Systolic and diastolic ventricular function deteriorates. The LV diastolic pressure usually increases during an episode of angina. This may cause dyspnea and pulmonary congestion. The discomfort from ischemia may involve nerve stimulation from hypoxic metabolites.

Clinical Manifestations

For some patients, stable angina is only a slight aching sensation. It can quickly become severe and intense, usually described as a crushing sensation, but not usually described as pain. Discomfort is most common under the sternum. It may radiate to the left shoulder and outside portion of the left arm. The discomfort can reach the fingers, move to the back, and jaws. Some patients have described discomfort in the upper abdomen. **Atypical angina** is less common and involves abdominal distress, bloating, and gas. The patient often believes that indigestion is the cause. Ischemic symptoms usually require a minute or longer to resolve, so very brief sensations are usually not from angina.

Nocturnal angina can occur if a dream or nightmare triggers large changes in BP, pulse rate, and respiration. When lying down, venous return is increased, which stretches the myocardium and increases arterial wall stress. Oxygen demand is therefore increased. *Silent ischemia* may occur with CAD – especially in patients with diabetes mellitus. It may appear as transient and asymptomatic ST-T heart abnormalities. These can be seen in stress tests or during 24-hour **Holter monitoring**. In radionuclide studies, there can be proof of asymptomatic myocardial ischemia during mental or physical stress. Silent ischemia and angina pectoris can exist together, and occur a different times.

Diagnosis

When a patient has chest discomfort caused by exertion and relieved by rest, the diagnosis of stable angina is likely. It is more accurate when significant risk factors for CAD are present. Patients are assessed for an acute coronary syndrome if their chest discomfort lasts for more than 20 minutes. It is important to understand that chest discomfort can also be caused by anxiety, panic attacks, costochondritis, GI disorders, and hyperventilation. ECG is performed, and for some cases, stress testing with ECG or myocardial imaging and coronary angiography may order. Myocardial imaging methods include echocardiography, MRI, and radionuclide imaging. The noninvasive tests are performed first.

Stress testing confirms diagnosis and determines the extent of the disease. It helps to identify levels of exercise that should be tolerated by the patient and also predicts prognosis. For men with suspicious chest discomfort, stress ECG testing is 70% specific and 90% sensitive. In women, the specificity is lower while the sensitivity is similar. This is especially true in women under age 55, in which the specific is below 70%. Women with CAD are more likely than men to have an abnormal resting ECG. Coronary angiography is preferred to diagnose CAD, but is not required for confirmation of diagnosis in every case.

Cardiac MRI is an excellent method to evaluate a large amount of abnormalities. It can evaluate CAD in several ways. There can be assessment of blood flow in the coronary arteries, direct views of coronary stenosis, assessment of myocardial metabolism and perfusion, evaluation of a myocardium that is either viable or infarcted, and assessment of wall motion abnormalities. Cardiac MRI is indicated to evaluate cardiac structure and function, and to assess myocardial viability. To diagnose and assess risks for patients with suspected or known CAD, specific forms of cardiac MRI include stress perfusion MRI and quantitative analysis of myocardial blood flow.

Treatment

Sublingual nitroglycerin is the most effective drug to relieve symptoms during an acute angina attack. It is a strong smooth-muscle relaxant and also a vasodilator. It works primarily in the peripheral vascular tree, primarily of the capacitance or venous system, and in the coronary blood vessels. Sublingual nitroglycerin can also be taken before exertion to prevent an attack. Effective relief occurs in 1.5–3 minutes in most cases, completely by 5 minutes, and lasting as long as 30 minutes. Doses can be repeated every 4–5 minutes, up to three times, if the effects are incomplete. The patient must always carry nitroglycerin, regardless of its dosage form, for prompt use when needed. If tablets are used, they must be stored in a light-resistant glass container that is tightly sealed in order to retain their potency. The drug deteriorates very quickly, so small amounts should be frequently purchased.

Ischemia is prevented by antiplatelet drugs, beta-blockers, long-acting nitrates, and calcium channel blockers. Antiplatelet drugs inhibit the aggregation of platelets. Aspirin binds to the platelets irreversibly, inhibiting platelet aggregation and cyclooxygenase. Other antiplatelet drugs include clopidogrel, prasugrel, and ticagrelor. These block platelet aggregation induced by adenosine diphosphate. They are able to reduce risks of MI or sudden death, and are most effective when administered together. If a patient cannot tolerate one of them, he or she should receive one of the drugs that can be tolerated.

Calcium channel blockers are used for persistent symptoms after nitrates are used, or if they cannot be tolerated. These blockers are best used if there is concurrent coronary spasm or hypertension. The dihydropyridines, including amlodipine, felodipine, and nifedipine do not have chronotropic effects, but have widely different negative inotropic effects. The shorter-acting dihydropyridines can cause reflex tachycardia. They are linked to more deaths of patients with CAD, and are not used alone to treat stable angina.

Sodium channel blockers and sinus node inhibitors can also be used for stable angina. Ranolazine is a sodium channel blocker that treats chronic angina. Common adverse effects include constipation, dizziness, headache, and nausea. Ivabradine, a sinus node inhibitor, inhibits the inward sodium/potassium current in the gated channel in sinus node cells. It slows down the heart rate without causing decreased contractility. Ivabradine is used for chronic stable angina pectoris when there is a normal sinus rhythm, and the patient cannot tolerate beta-blockers. It is also used in combination with beta-blockers when the patient's symptoms are not adequately controlled only by a beta-blocker, and the heart rate is more than 60 beats per minute.

If angina continues even with drug therapy and the quality of life is poor, or if anatomic lesions found during angiography may cause death, revascularization can be done. This is either with PCI such as angioplasty or stenting, or CABG. The choice is based on where the anatomic lesions are located and how severe they are, along with experience of the surgical team and patient preference. The PCI procedure is most often used for cases in which one or two vessels are involved. It is also becoming more popular for three vessel disease. However, long lesions or those close to bifurcation points are often not highly treatable with PCI. The process is being used for more complex cases today due to improvements in stent technology. It is being use more often for unprotected left main coronary stenosis, such as with no LAD or circumflex graft being present.

For certain patients, CABG is highly effective. It is better than PCI for diabetic patients and for those with multiple diseased vessels that likely will be responsive to grafting. Ideally, CABG is used for severe angina pectoris that is localized, or for those with diabetes. Approximately 85% of patients have significant or total symptom relief. There is a positive relationship between graft patency and better exercise tolerance, as shown on exercise stress testing. However, exercise tolerance can still remain better even with graft closure. Survival is improved with CABG for patients with left main disease, 3-vessel disease with poor LV function, and for some patients with 2-vessel disease.

Prevention

The best methods of preventing angina include a heart-healthy diet, avoiding smoking, limiting alcohol use, exercising regularly, maintaining a healthy weight, and keeping diabetes mellitus controlled.

Prognosis

The prognosis of stable angina varies because of adverse outcomes that can occur. Stable angina carries a better prognosis than unstable angina. About 1.4% of patients with this form of angina die annually without a history of MI, and with a normal resting ECG and BP. However, MI or arrhythmias worsen prognosis. Women with CAD and stable angina have a worse prognosis also. Death rates are highest with abnormal ECG results (8.4%), when systolic hypertension is present (7.5%), or when both are present (12%). The death rates for each of these are nearly doubled when type 2 diabetes mellitus is present. Prognosis is also worse with older age, anatomic lesions, poor ventricular function, and symptoms that increasingly worsen. An extremely poor prognosis exists if there are lesions within the left main coronary artery or the proximal LAD artery. Also, prognosis is based on how many coronary arteries are diseased, and to what extent. The prognosis is good for stable angina if ventricular function is normal, even if there is disease of 3 vessels.

UNSTABLE ANGINA

Unstable angina involves potentially dangerous and unpredictable changes, such as new-onset angina, rest angina, or increasing angina. These are serious if the chest discomfort is severe. It occurs from an acute obstruction of a coronary artery, with no MI. Rest angina usually lasts for more than 20 minutes, and new-onset angina is at least class 3 in severity. Increasing angina is disease that was previously diagnosed but has become more frequent, severe, of longer duration, or of lower threshold. An example is when class 1 disease increases to at least class 3 in severity. Therefore, unstable angina requires prompt diagnosis and treatment. Diabetic patients with unstable angina usually have more severe disease and poorer outcomes in comparison with nondiabetic patients.

Epidemiology

The most accurate global data on unstable angina is based on the Organization to Assess Strategies for Ischemic Syndromes registry (OASIS-2). Aside from the United States, this registry contains data for Australia, Canada, Brazil, Poland, and Hungary. The mean age at diagnosis is between 62 and 65 years, with men diagnosed more than women in a ratio of slightly more than 1.5:1. One interesting factor is that women diagnosed with unstable angina are approximately 5 years older than men when

CLINICAL CASE

1. Which test may confirm stable angina?
2. Which cardiac disorders can cause stable angina?
3. How much does quitting smoking affect possible MI related to stable angina?

A 59-year-old man previously diagnosed with stable CAD sees his physician after developing chest discomfort every time he exercised. The patient also has hyperlipidemia and chronic obstructive pulmonary disease (COPD). His physician asks him about smoking, and the patient confesses that he has tried to stop many times, but still smokes about 5 cigarettes per day. He has smoked since being in the Army when he was in his 20s. The patient is given a beta-blocker to relieve the stable angina, but he finds that it worsens his COPD symptoms. The patient is then started on nitrates, but due to severe headaches, they also are stopped. A calcium channel blocker is tried, and is successful in relieving the patient's angina.

ANSWERS

1. Stress testing confirms diagnosis and determines the extent of the stable angina. It helps to identify levels of exercise that should be tolerated by the patient and also predicts prognosis. For men with suspicious chest discomfort, stress ECG testing is 70% specific and 90% sensitive.
2. Cardiac disorders that can cause stable angina include aortic dissection, atrial fibrillation, mitral valve prolapse, pericarditis, and supraventricular tachycardia.
3. The risk of MI related to stable angina is reduced in 2 or more years of quitting smoking – to the level of a person that has never smoked.

they are diagnosed. There is no specific racial or ethnic predilection, except that black patients often are diagnosed at younger ages than other groups.

According to the Global Unstable Angina Registry and Treatment Evaluation (GUARANTEE) and the CRUSADE registry of the American College of Cardiology and American Heart Association, every year in the United States there are almost 1 million primary diagnoses of unstable angina in hospitalized patients. There may be as many cases that occur outside of hospitals that are unrecognized or managed on an outpatient basis. Average ages of diagnosed patients are between 62 and 69 years, though 44% of all diagnosed patients are aged 65 or older. Men are affected more than women, in a ratio of 1.5:1. Most patients with unstable angina (60%–73%) are hypertensive, and hypercholesterolemia is present in 43%–50%. Unstable angina affects 66% of patients that previously had angina of any form. There are no specific racial or ethnic differences.

Etiology and Risk Factors

Unstable angina is caused by blood clots that block an artery partially or completely. They can form, partially dissolve, and reform, with unstable angina occurring each time. The condition is related to coronary heart disease from the buildup of atherosclerotic plaques along arterial walls. Risk factors for unstable angina include diabetes mellitus, obesity, family history of heart disease, hypertension, high LDL, low HDL, male gender, use of tobacco products, and having a sedentary lifestyle. Men are at the highest risk after age 45, and women are at the highest risk after age 55.

Pathophysiology

Ruptures at points of high-grade stenosis within the epicardial coronary arteries occur along with thrombi that block vessels while vasoconstriction occurs. This develops into a condition in which the same amount of oxygen consumption occurs, yet the coronary blood flow may be insufficient even while resting. The development of severe ischemia, MI, or sudden cardiac death is therefore possible. Unstable angina worsens over time, and can occur at rest. It may occur more often over time or become more intense each time it happens. The disease progresses to often cause MI or arrhythmias. Less often, sudden death occurs.

Clinical Manifestations

Chest pain or discomfort are the common symptoms of unstable angina. However, these are usually more intense, longer in duration, precipitated by little exertion or occurs while resting. Unstable angina is classified by severity and the clinical situation as follows:

- *Class 1 severity* – New onset of severe angina or increasing angina, but no angina at rest.

- *Class 2 severity* – There is angina at rest over the previous month, but not within the preceding 48 hours; this is designated as subacute angina at rest.

- *Class 3 severity* – There is angina at rest over the preceding 48 hours; this is designated as acute angina at rest; the **troponin** status as negative or positive is evaluated, which affects prognosis.

- *Clinical situation A* – The condition develops secondary to an extracardiac condition that worsens the myocardial ischemia; designated as secondary unstable angina.

- *Clinical situation B* – The condition develops without a contributing extracardiac condition being present; the troponin status as negative or positive is evaluated, which affects prognosis; designated as primary unstable angina.

- *Clinical situation C* – The condition develops within 2 weeks of an acute MI; designated as post-myocardial infarction unstable angina.

The basic classification of the level of unstable angina consists of both a Roman numeral to assess severity and a letter to assess the clinical situation, for example, the least severe would be class IA. There is a consideration of whether the unstable angina occurs during treatment for chronic stable angina, and if transient changes in the ST-T waves occur during the angina attack. If the discomfort has occurred within 48 hours and there is no contributing extracardiac condition present, the troponin levels may be measured to estimate prognosis. Troponin-negative gives a better prognosis than troponin-positive.

Diagnosis

For unstable angina, early stress testing cannot be performed. Diagnosis begins with initial and serial electrocardiograms, plus serial measurements of cardiac biomarkers. This helps determine whether unstable angina is present or an acute MI is imminent. There can be non-ST-segment elevation MI (NSTEMI) or ST-segment elevation MI (STEMI) used for this determination. It is important since fibrinolytics are helpful for patients with STEMI, but can increase risks for patients with NSTEMI and unstable angina. For acute STEMI, urgent cardiac catheterization is required, but not usually for patients with

NSTEMI or unstable angina. An ECG must be done within 10 minutes of the patient arriving to the chosen medical facility. During unstable angina, transient ECG changes may include ST-segment depression or elevation, or T-wave inversion. When unstable angina is suspected, there must be a high-sensitivity assay of cardiac troponin done immediately and then 3 hours later. When a standard troponin assay is used, it is performed at zero and 6 hours. The creatinine kinase will not be elevated. However, cardiac troponin – especially in the high-sensitivity troponin test, may be slightly increased.

After symptoms resolve, most patients undergo coronary angiography in the first 24–48 hours after being hospitalized. This detects lesions requiring treatment. The procedure usually combines diagnosis with PCI to perform angioplasty and/or place a stent. Later, coronary angiography can be used if there are signs of continuing ischemia, based on symptoms or ECG, hemodynamic instability, recurring ventricular tachyarrhythmias, and any abnormality suggesting recurrence of ischemia.

Treatment

Treatment of unstable angina begins with establishing a good intravenous route. Oxygen is given, usually 2 L via nasal cannula. Single-lead ECG monitoring is initiated. Prior to hospitalization, emergency medical personnel can lessen risks for complications and death by monitoring the ECG, using nitrates to manage pain, and giving 325 mg of chewable aspirin. Once the diagnosis is confirmed within the emergency department, drug therapy and the scheduling of revascularization are confirmed. If the patient is clinically unstable, because of continuing symptoms or arrhythmias, or is hypotensive, urgent angiography with revascularization must take place. Morphine must be used carefully, such as when nitroglycerin is contraindicated, or the patient still has symptoms after nitroglycerin has been administered. Unstable angina can be complicated by recurring attacks, infarction, heart failure, or sustained and recurring ventricular arrhythmias.

CABG is preferred over PCI if the patient has *left main* or *left main equivalent* angina, left ventricular dysfunction, or diabetes mellitus that is being treated. Lesions that are long or close to bifurcation points are often not successfully treated with PCI. All unstable angina patients are given anticoagulants, antiplatelet drugs, and when chest pain is present, antianginal drugs. The drug regimen is based on reperfusion strategy. Unless contraindicated, the drugs for unstable angina include unfractionated or low molecular weight heparin (or bivalirudin); aspirin, clopidogrel, or both, with alternatives to clopidogrel being prasugrel or ticagrelor; nitroglycerin or another antianginal drug; beta-blockers; ACE inhibitors; statins; and if PCI is done, a glycoprotein IIb/IIIa inhibitor may be required. Aspirin is not of the enteric-coated type. Chewing the first dose before it is swallowed will speed up absorption, and reduce short- and long-term risks of death. For patients having PCI, a loading dose of clopidogrel, prasugrel, or ticagrelor will improve results, especially when given 24 hours before the procedure. If the patient requires urgent PCI, prasugrel and ticagrelor work more quickly than clopidogrel, so they are often preferred.

Unless contraindicated, such as by active bleeding, a low molecular weight heparin (LMWH), unfractionated heparin, or bivalirudin are usually given. Unfractionated heparin requires dosing every 6 hours in order to achieve the target activated partial thromboplastin time (aPTT). The LMWHs have lower risks for heparin-induced thrombocytopenia, better bioavailability, and are given via simple weight-based doses that do not require monitoring aPTT or dose titration. For patients with known or suspected occurrences of heparin-induced thrombocytopenia, bivalirudin is preferred. A glycoprotein IIb/IIIa inhibitor is considered during PCI if lesions are of high risk, such as when there is no reflow or a high thrombus burden. Drug choice is based on availability, cost, and familiarity, and options with equivalent effectiveness include abciximab, eptifibatide, and tirofiban.

For chest pain, nitroglycerin is usually used, but sometimes morphine is needed. Nitroglycerin is preferred, but morphine is used if the patient has a contraindication to nitroglycerin, or maximal nitroglycerin therapy does not relieve pain. At first, nitroglycerin is given sublingually, which may be followed by a continuous IV drip if required. Morphine is given IV every 15 minutes as needed, but close monitoring is required due to the drug depressing respiration, being a strong venous vasodilator, and reducing myocardial contractility – along with the interference with P2Y12 receptor inhibitors. In a large study, morphine was shown to increase mortality for patients with acute MI. Though bradycardia and hypotension can be secondary to the use of morphine, prompt elevation of the legs usually overcomes these developments. Beta-blockers, ACE inhibitors, and statins are usually used as well. Beta-blockers are recommended, especially for patients at high risk, except if contraindicated because of asthma, bradycardia, heart block, or hypotension. They reduce arterial pressure, contractility, and the heart rate.

This results in reduced oxygen demand and cardiac workload. The ACE inhibitors can improve endothelial function by providing cardioprotection that is long term. It they cannot be tolerated due to coughing or rash, an ARB may be given instead. Statins are used often no matter what the patient's lipid levels are, and continued throughout life. Fibrinolytic drugs are not of benefit for patients with unstable angina. Angiography, performed immediately or within 24–48 hours, is essential. It determines whether CABG or PCI should be done.

For patients that do not have angiography performed, options are based on whether there are high-risk features. These include recurring angina, heart failure, ventricular fibrillation or tachycardia after 24 hours, shock, or new murmurs. Also, if the ejection fraction is higher than 40%, these patients should have stress testing before discharge or shortly afterwards. Because unstable angina is so acute, the patient must be educated about seriously modifying all risk factors. The patient's physical and emotional status must be discussed. Advice about diet, exercise, managing work and family time and stressors, and quitting smoking is crucial. It must be stressed to the patient that prognosis can be improved with aggressive management of risk factors. After discharge, the patient must continue taking prescribed antianginals, antiplatelet drugs, statins, and any other drugs required for underlying conditions.

Prevention

Methods of preventing unstable angina include quitting smoking, avoiding secondhand smoke, exercising regularly, eating a heart-healthy diet to maintain a healthy weight, managing underlying conditions (diabetes mellitus, hypertension, and high cholesterol), and managing stress or depression.

Prognosis

Prognosis of unstable angina is based on the amount of diseased coronary arteries, and the severity. A worse prognosis exists for stenosis of the proximal left main artery, proximal left descending artery, or circumflex artery. Distal stenosis or stenosis of a smaller arterial branch carry a better prognosis. Left ventricular dysfunction that is significant, even with 1- or 2-vessel disease, give less likelihood of revascularization being successful. Approximately 30% of patients will have an MI within 3 months of unstable angina beginning, but sudden death is not as common. Significant ECG changes with chest pain mean there are higher risks of MI or death.

CLINICAL CASE

1. What is the cause of unstable angina, and what are its risk factors?
2. How does the diagnosis of unstable angina begin?
3. Which drugs are often used for the treatment of unstable angina?

A 61-year-old man was hospitalized because of left-sided chest pain that had recurred, with localized pain that continued while resting. The patient's medical history includes diabetes mellitus, hypertension, and ischemic heart disease. He was previously hospitalized for his heart disease, and a right bundle branch block was also found. Tests reveal that the patient has developed low-grade kidney disease. He used to be a chronic smoker but has not smoked for 15 years. The diagnosis is unstable angina, and the patient is given aspirin and clopidogrel, with close monitoring for any signs of bleeding. He is also given a statin and an ACE inhibitor.

ANSWERS

1. Unstable angina is caused by blood clots that block an artery partially or completely. Risk factors include diabetes mellitus, obesity, family history of heart disease, hypertension, high LDL, low HDL, male gender, use of tobacco products, and having a sedentary lifestyle.
2. Diagnosis begins with initial and serial electrocardiograms, plus serial measurements of cardiac biomarkers.
3. Drugs often used for treatment of unstable angina include anticoagulants, antiplatelet drugs, antianginal drugs including nitroglycerin, unfractionated or LMWH or bivalirudin, aspirin, clopidogrel, prasugrel, ticagrelor, beta-blockers, ACE inhibitors, statins, and glycoprotein IIb/IIIa inhibitors.

VARIANT ANGINA

Variant angina is also known as *Prinzmetal angina* or *angina inversa*. The condition is secondary to epicardial coronary artery spasm, signified by angina symptoms occurring at rest, but rarely after exertion. Many patients also have a significant obstruction of one or more major coronary arteries. If there is only mild obstruction or no *fixed obstruction*, the long-term outcome is better than when there are significant fixed obstructions. Having diabetes mellitus and variant angina affects the use of certain medications such as bisoprolol, if there are large fluctuations in blood glucose levels. This is because the drug can mask symptoms of hypoglycemia.

Epidemiology

Variant angina is relatively rare, affecting between 2% and 10% of all angina patients. It usually occurs in younger-aged patients than the other forms of angina – mostly between ages 51 and 57. The condition is not very well documented globally. In the United States, about 4 out of every 100,000 Americans have variant angina. Men are slightly more affected than women. The disease is more common in people of Japanese origin than in any other racial or ethnic group.

Etiology and Risk Factors

Variant angina is usually caused by smoking, hypertension, and high cholesterol. However, it can occur for unknown reasons in people that are otherwise healthy. While diabetes mellitus is not a direct cause of variant angina, it does complicate cardiovascular disease, with variant angina possibly resulting. Risk factors include alcohol withdrawal, exposure to cold temperatures, various medications, stimulants such as cocaine, and stress.

Pathophysiology

The pathophysiology of variant angina involves deficient basal release of nitric oxide because of endothelial dysfunction. There is enhanced vascular smooth-muscle contractility involving the *Rho/Rho-kinase signaling pathway*. Precipitating factors include abnormal autonomic nervous activity, chronic low-grade inflammation, increases in oxidative stress, genetic susceptibility, and magnesium deficiency.

Clinical Manifestations

Variant angina involves discomfort occurring mostly while resting, usually at night. The discomfort only rarely occurs during exertion, and is inconsistent unless there is a significant coronary artery obstruction. Variant angina often occurs regularly at specific times during each day. The pain can be extreme, lasting from several minutes up to 1 half hour. The pain can spread to the left arm, shoulder, neck, or head. Persistent spasms increase risks for serious complications, including life-threatening arrhythmias or MI. Additional manifestations include chest tightness or pressure, heartburn, dizziness, nausea, palpitations, and sweating.

Diagnosis

The diagnosis of variant angina is suspected because of an ST-segment elevation occurring during the time of an attack. In between attacks, the ECG may have a stable yet abnormal pattern, or even be normal. Diagnosis is confirmed by testing with ergonovine or acetylcholine. This may initiate a coronary artery spasm, which is identified by a significant ST-segment elevation on ECG, or when a reversible spasm is seen during cardiac catheterization. Most diagnostic testing for variant angina is done in cardiac catheterization laboratories.

Treatment

Sublingual nitroglycerin is usually able to quickly relieve variant angina. Symptoms can be prevented by using calcium channel blockers. The most commonly used drugs in this class include sustained-release diltiazem, sustained-release verapamil (though doses must be reduced if there is kidney or liver dysfunction), and amlodipine (though doses must be reduced with liver dysfunction or in elderly patients). These drugs do not appear to change the prognosis, however. Though not proven clinically, it is theorized that beta-blockers can worsen spasms by allowing alpha-adrenergic vasoconstriction to occur. For diabetic patients, bisoprolol must be used carefully since it can mask symptoms of hypoglycemia. However, this is not an issue in nondiabetic patients with variant angina.

Prevention

The prevention of variant angina is based on lifestyle changes to remove the known causes and risk factors, or to use medications to stop future attacks from occurring. It is important to quit smoking, manage stress, exercise regularly but not to the point of causing hyperventilation, eating a heart-healthy diet, avoiding extremely cold temperatures, engaging in relaxation therapies, and monitoring your body's circadian rhythms to prepare for the times of day in which the condition may occur regularly.

Prognosis

Variant angina is usually of good prognosis, with average survival over 5 years being 89%–97% of patients. However, risks for death are higher if the disease is accompanied by atherosclerotic coronary artery obstruction. Prognosis is significantly worsened by severe fixed obstructions.

CLINICAL CASE

1. What other names are used to describe variant angina?
2. What are the most common causes and also the risk factors for variant angina?
3. Which factors worsen the prognosis of variant angina?

A 57-year-old former smoker arrived at the emergency department with chest pain. His ST segment was elevated, and in the cardiac catheterization laboratory, angiography revealed moderate disease of the left circumflex artery and first diagonal branch. A bare metal stent was inserted into the proximal left circumflex artery. Once stabilized, the patient was discharged. He returned 2 weeks later with similar chest pain, which had been becoming more severe. Again, there was an ST-segment elevation, but after being started on IV nitroglycerin and bivalirudin, this resolved. The patient was diagnosed with variant angina. He was educated about the need to stay away from secondhand smoke and treated with amlodipine, which was successful.

ANSWERS

1. Variant angina is also known as Prinzmetal angina or angina inversa. The condition is secondary to epicardial coronary artery spasm, with symptoms occurring at rest, but rarely after exertion.
2. Variant angina is usually caused by smoking, hypertension, and high cholesterol. Risk factors include alcohol withdrawal, exposure to cold temperatures, various medications, stimulants such as cocaine, and stress.
3. While variant angina is usually of a good prognosis, risks for death are higher if the disease is accompanied by atherosclerotic coronary artery obstruction. Prognosis is significantly worsened by severe fixed obstructions.

ACUTE CORONARY SYNDROMES

Acute coronary syndromes are outcomes of acute coronary artery obstruction. Severity is based on the location of the obstruction and its degree. Uncontrolled angina can occur, as well as various types of MI, or sudden cardiac death. Diabetes mellitus is a major risk factor. All acute coronary syndromes involve acute coronary ischemia. They are identified by their symptoms, ECG results, and cardiac biomarkers. The uncontrolled angina subtype involves acute coronary insufficiency, preinfarction angina, and is an *intermediate syndrome*. The cardiac biomarkers do not meet the criteria for MI. There is resting angina longer than 20 minutes, new-onset angina of at least class 3 severity, and increasing angina that becomes more regular, severe, longer lasting, or that increases quickly from class 1 to class 3 or higher. With non-ST-segment elevation MI (NSTEMI, also called *subendocardial MI*), there is myocardial necrosis with no acute ST-segment elevation. There may be ST-segment depression, T-wave inversion, or both.

Epidemiology

The global prevalence of acute coronary syndromes is as much as 13.5% of the population. Estimated incidence is 2,149 cases per 1 million population annually. Acute coronary syndromes represent about 1.8 million deaths per year. Ages in which acute coronary syndromes are most likely are over 30 (in men), over 40 (in women), and at younger ages (in diabetic patients). Acute coronary syndromes occur much more often in men under age 60 than in women in the same age range, but most diagnosed patients over 75 years of age are women. There are no significant differences in the predilection of acute coronary syndromes between various racial or ethnic groups.

Etiology and Risk Factors

An acute coronary syndrome is usually caused by an acute thrombus in an atherosclerotic coronary artery. The plaque can become unstable or inflamed, then rupture or split. Thrombogenic material is exposed, activating platelets and the coagulation cascade, resulting in an acute thrombus. Cross-linking and aggregation of platelets occurs. Even with slight obstruction, atheromas can rupture and cause thrombosis. In more than half of all cases, pre-syndrome stenosis is less than 40%. While stenosis severity predicts the symptoms that will occur, it cannot always be predictive of acute thrombotic events. The thrombus quickly slows blood flow to areas of the myocardium. In most cases, spontaneous thrombolysis occurs. However, the obstruction does remain for long enough to cause tissue necrosis.

Rare causes of acute coronary syndromes include coronary artery embolism or dissection, and coronary spasm. Embolism may be due to aortic, mitral valve stenosis, infective endocarditis, atrial fibrillation, or **marantic endocarditis**. Coronary artery dissection may occur in atherosclerotic or nonatherosclerotic coronary arteries. The nonatherosclerotic form is most common in women that are pregnant or have given birth as well as patients with connective tissue disorders such as fibromuscular dysplasia. Diabetic patients with acute coronary syndromes have increased mortality rates compared to non-diabetic patients. Diabetes mellitus is linked to a proinflammatory and prothrombotic state that can lead to plaque rupture. Risk factors for acute coronary syndromes, aside from diabetes, include increased age, hypertension, high cholesterol, smoking, insufficient physical activity, unhealthy diet, being overweight or obese, family history (of angina, heart disease, or stroke), personal history (of hypertension, preeclampsia, or gestational diabetes), and the COVID-19 infection.

Pathophysiology

The pathophysiology of acute coronary syndromes ranges from transient ischemia to infarction. Cell necrosis likely occurs even with milder forms. When tissue is only ischemic, there is impairments of contractility as well as relaxation. **Hypokinetic** or akinetic segments develop, which can bulge or expand during systole. This is known as **paradoxical motion**. The affected area's size determines effects ranging from partial heart failure to cardiogenic shock. Usually, large portions of the myocardium must be ischemic in order to cause severe myocardial dysfunction. In about 66% of hospitalized patients with acute MI, there is some degree of heart failure. When there is low cardiac output and heart failure, the condition is called *ischemic cardiomyopathy*. If ischemia affects the papillary muscle, mitral valve regurgitation may follow. Mural thrombus formation may occur from dysfunctional wall motion.

If a MI occurs, the infarcted tissue becomes permanently unable to function, though there is an area of possible reversible ischemic near to the infarcted tissue. Transmural infarcts involve the entire thickness of the myocardium from epicardium to endocardium. There are usually abnormal Q waves seen on ECG. The nontransmural infarcts do not continue through the ventricular wall. There are only ST-segment and T-wave abnormalities. If there is necrosis of a large area of the interventricular septum or walls of the ventricles, tissue may rupture and cause death.

Clinical Manifestations

Acute coronary syndromes cause a variety of symptoms. Stimuli from the heart and other thoracic organs cause discomfort. This is described as pressure, burning, indigestion, aching, sharp pain, or stabbing pain. It is difficult to assess the amount of ischemia present only by symptoms, unless the infarction is very large. The symptoms often mimic those of angina. Complications of acute coronary syndromes may involve electrical dysfunction, myocardial dysfunction, or valvular dysfunction. Electrical defects include arrhythmias and conduction defects. Myocardial effects include heart failure, free wall rupture, interventricular septum rupture, pseudoaneurysm, ventricular aneurysm, cardiogenic shock, and formation of a mural thrombus. Valvular defects usually involve **mitral regurgitation**. Additional complications of acute coronary syndromes include recurring ischemia and pericarditis. If pericarditis occurs 2–10 weeks after an MI, it is called *post-MI syndrome*, also known as *Dressler syndrome*.

Diagnosis

Acute coronary syndromes are considered for patients with chest pain or discomfort that are over age 30 in male or over age 40 in female – except in diabetic patients, in which these syndromes occur at younger ages. The pain must be differentiated from pain caused by pneumonia, pericarditis, pulmonary embolism, costochondral separation, rib fracture, acute aortic dissection, esophageal spasm, renal calculi, splenic infarction, or abdominal disorders. It is important not to attribute any new symptoms to previous disorders such as hiatal hernia, gallbladder disease, or peptic ulcer.

Initial and serial electrocardiogram plus serial **cardiac biomarker** assessment should be done, distinguishing between the subtypes of acute coronary syndromes. Pulse **oximetry** is indicated. Chest X-rays are important to assess any mediastinal widening, suggesting aortic dissection. An ECG is done within 10 minutes of the patient's arrival, to assess treatments. Urgent cardiac catheterization may be needed. Careful reading of the ECG is required, since there can be only slight ST-segment elevation. It is important not to focus on leads showing ST-segment depression. With the characteristic symptoms, ST-segment elevation on ECG is 90% specific and 45% sensitive to diagnose MI. Diagnosis is usually confirmed when serial tracings are taken, every 8 hours for the first day, then daily, if they show a slow evolution toward a more normal and stable pattern, or the development of abnormal Q waves over several days. Cardiac biomarkers are the serum markers of myocardial cell injury, released into the bloodstream following myocardial cell necrosis. Cardiac biomarkers appear at differing times, with levels decreasing at various rates. The newer testing allows for earlier MI identification and has become the primary cardiac biomarker assay in many locations.

Coronary angiography usually combines diagnosis with PCI. If possible, emergency coronary angiography is done stat after onset of an acute MI. This has greatly lowered complications and deaths and also improved outcomes in the long term. Angiography may be done if there is evidence of continuing ischemia, based on ECG or symptoms, hemodynamic instability, and recurring ventricular tachyarrhythmias, or anything suggesting ischemia.

Treatment

Treatment of acute coronary syndromes is focused on interrupting thrombosis, relieving distress, limiting size of infarctions, reversing ischemia, reducing cardiac workload, and preventing complications. Acute coronary syndromes are medical emergencies. Rapid diagnosis and treatment are essential, which occur simultaneously. There must be aggressive treatment of anemia, heart failure, or any other contributing conditions. Any chest pain remaining after 12–24 hours must be assessed. It may indicate pericarditis, recurring ischemia, pneumonia, pulmonary embolism, gastritis, or an ulcer. A solid IV route is established, oxygen is usually given by nasal cannula, and continual single-lead ECG monitoring begins. Prehospital interventions include ECG, chewable aspirin, and nitrates for pain management. Morphine is only used cautiously.

Before or after discharge, patients often have stress testing based on individual features of their acute coronary syndrome. Physical activity is slowly increased over the first 3–6 weeks after discharge. Moderate physical activities, including sexual intercourse, are encouraged. Most patients can return to full activities after 6 weeks following an acute MI. Regular exercise programs are taught, based on age, cardiac status, and lifestyle. After revascularization, supervised cardiac rehabilitation programs decrease mortality. The patient must be encouraged to modify risk factors and lifestyle, and instructed that doing so can improve the prognosis.

Aspirin and other antiplatelet drugs reduce mortality and reinfarction following an MI. Long-term enteric-coated aspirin every day is recommended. Warfarin, with or without aspirin, also reduces mortality and reinfarction. Beta-blockers are commonly prescribed, including acebutolol, atenolol, metoprolol, propranolol, and timolol. They reduce deaths after MI by approximately 25% for 7 years or more. ACE inhibitors are also standard medications, and are especially indicated after an MI if the ejection fraction is less than 40%. Statins are usually also prescribed and benefit nearly all post-MI patients. Statins are usually continued throughout life barring any extreme adverse effects with doses increased up to a maximally tolerated level.

Prevention

Prevention of acute coronary syndromes requires the same type of lifestyle changes used to prevent CAD: Quitting smoking, a heart-healthy diet, increased physical activity, reducing stress, and taking medications that combat thrombocyte aggregation and reduce the development of atherosclerotic plaques.

Prognosis

High-risk features of acute coronary syndromes that worsen prognosis include heart failure, recurring angina or ischemia at rest or in low-level activities, extreme ECG abnormalities, hypotension during a stress test, complex ventricular arrhythmias, worsening mitral regurgitation, hemodynamic instability, diabetes mellitus, and sustained ventricular tachycardia.

CLINICAL CASE

1. How common are acute coronary syndromes?
2. What are the possible complications of acute coronary syndromes?
3. How serious are acute coronary syndromes?

A 62-year-old man was admitted to the hospital with a diagnosis of an acute coronary syndrome. His cardiac biomarkers and initial electrocardiograms were negative for indications of MI. Six months before, the patient had a PCI for an occlusion of the right coronary artery.

He had recently experienced increasingly severe chest pain, which even occurred at rest. Nitroglycerin was administered, and the patient's chest pain reduced significantly. Another ECG showed ST depression in the inferior leads, and another assessment of the cardiac biomarkers showed that the troponin levels were positive for damage to the myocardium. Morphine was ordered the next time the chest pain increased, and the patient was also started on metoprolol. He was scheduled for a left heart catheterization because it was discovered that he now had an obstruction in the circumflex branch of his left coronary artery.

ANSWERS

1. The global prevalence of acute coronary syndromes is as much as 13.5% of the population. Estimated incidence is 2,149 cases per 1 million population annually. Acute coronary syndromes represent about 1.8 million deaths per year.
2. Complications of acute coronary syndromes may involve electrical dysfunction, myocardial dysfunction, or valvular dysfunction. Electrical defects include arrhythmias and conduction defects. Myocardial effects include heart failure, free wall rupture, interventricular septum rupture, pseudoaneurysm, ventricular aneurysm, cardiogenic shock, and formation of a mural thrombus. Valvular defects usually involve mitral regurgitation. Other complications include recurring ischemia and pericarditis.
3. Acute coronary syndromes are medical emergencies. Rapid diagnosis and treatment is essential, which occur simultaneously. There must be aggressive treatment of anemia, heart failure, or any other contributing conditions. After treatment, the patient must be encouraged to modify risk factors and lifestyle and instructed that doing so can improve the prognosis.

ACUTE MYOCARDIAL INFARCTION

Myocardial ischemia develops when the ability to supply oxygen and nutrients to the myocardium is less than the oxygen and nutrient requirements of the myocardium. The heart is a mostly aerobic organ and has a low threshold for a deficit in oxygen delivery. An acute MI (*heart attack*) involves necrosis of the myocardium because of a coronary artery obstruction. An acute MI causes chest discomfort that is often accompanied by dyspnea, nausea, and sweating. Acute MI is also considered to be one type of acute coronary syndrome. Diabetic patients experience higher mortality rates with acute MI, and also more morbidities in the period following an MI.

Epidemiology

Acute MI is the most common form of coronary heart disease (CHD) throughout the world. It causes more than 15% of all deaths annually. Prevalence is higher in men in all age-specific groups than in women. The prevalence of diabetes mellitus is increasing. A significant proportion of the general population is affected. With metabolic syndrome or diabetes mellitus, there is increased incidence of myocardial ischemia and MI. Incidence is lower in industrialized nations partly due to better healthcare systems, but rates are rapidly increasing in Eastern Europe, Southern Asia, and Latin America. For unknown reasons, the highest prevalence of MI in people younger than age 45 is in the countries for India, Pakistan, Sri Lanka, Bangladesh, and Nepal.

In the United States, there are about 1 million myocardial infarctions per year, and about one American dies from MI every minute of every day. Of these, between 300,000 and 400,000 are fatal. Incidence is declining in the United States, however. According to the American Heart Association, the group with the highest incidence of MI is African American men aged 75–84 (12.9 cases per 100,000 population), followed by African American women of the same age (10.2 cases), Caucasian men (9.1), and Caucasian women (7.8) – see Figure 9.4.

Etiology and Risk Factors

Acute myocardial infarction is caused by narrowing or blockage of the coronary arteries with atherosclerotic plaque. Factors that lead to this include high LDL, and excessive saturated fat and trans fats in the diet. Modifiable risk factors represent over 90% of the risks for acute MI. Risk factors include diabetes mellitus, obesity, smoking, hypertension, high cholesterol, high triglycerides, increased age, and family history of heart disease. Additional risk factors include high stress levels, lack of physical exercise, use of amphetamines or cocaine, and a history of preeclampsia.

116

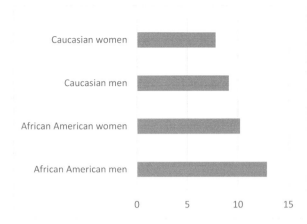

Figure 9.4 Acute MI in various individuals; cases per 100,000 population.

Pathophysiology

Myocardial necrosis as part of acute MI is consistent with myocardial ischemia. Cardiac biomarkers are increased. At least one of the following criteria must also be present:

- Ischemic symptoms
- Development of pathologic Q waves
- Electrocardiogram changes revealing new ischemia, via left bundle branch block or significant ST/T changes
- Imaging studies showing new loss of myocardial tissue, or new regional abnormalities of wall motion
- Angiography evidence of an intracoronary thrombus

An MI mostly affects the LV, but can extend into the right ventricle or atria. *Right ventricular infarction* is usually caused by an obstruction of the right coronary or dominant left circumflex artery. There is high RV filling pressure, and often, severe tricuspid regurgitation with reduced cardiac output. Death is much more likely if there is an RV infarction that complicates an LV infarction. MIs are either transmural or non-transmural, as discussed in acute coronary syndromes.

Clinical Manifestations

The majority of patients experience prodromal symptoms days to weeks before an MI. Symptoms include fatigue, shortness of breath, and crescendo or unstable angina. The first symptom of an infarction is usually deep visceral pain below the sternum that is described as pressure or a severe pain. It often radiates to the back, arms, shoulders, jaw, or all of these locations. The pain is nearly the same as that of angina pectoris, but usually lasts longer and is more severe. There is often sweating, dyspnea, nausea, and vomiting. Relief is usually slight or temporary when the patient rests or takes nitroglycerin. In some patients, the discomfort is mild. Approximately 20% of acute MI cases are *silent*, with these cases more commonly seen in diabetic patients. In silent MI, the patient may not recognize what is happening since the symptoms are so vague. Some patients actually experience no symptoms as the MI occurs. Often, the affected person thinks they are just having indigestion, and relief of the discomfort may be incorrectly believed to be achieved by taking antacids or belching. Syncope is another symptom that may be seen.

Female patients often have atypical chest discomfort, and older patients may have more dyspnea than ischemic-related chest pain. If there is severe ischemia, the pain may be extreme and the patient becomes apprehensive and restless. Nausea and vomiting are more common with *inferior MI*. For some patients, the primary symptoms are dyspnea and weakness (from LV failure), pulmonary edema, significant arrhythmia, and shock. The patient's skin may be moist, pale, and cool, and peripheral or central cyanosis may be seen. Blood pressure can be varied, but many patients first experience early hypertension when the pain manifests. The pulse is often described as **thready**. Heart sounds are often slightly distant, and a fourth heart sound is nearly always present. In some cases, there is a soft systolic *blowing apical murmur*, which indicates dysfunction of the papillary muscle of the heart. Upon first examination, a preexisting heart condition or another type of condition may be suggested by a **friction rub** or more significant murmurs. If a friction rub is found within several hours after MI symptoms begin, acute pericarditis is more likely than MI. Even so, friction rubs described usually as **evanescent**. In about 15% of patients, the chest wall is tender when it is palpated. Signs of RV infarction include distended jugular veins, often with the **Kussmaul sign**, elevated RV filling pressure, lung fields that are clear, and hypotension.

Diagnosis

The diagnosis of acute MI starts with initial and serial ECG. Then, serial measurements of cardiac biomarkers help to identify the subtype of MI that is present, or distinguish between these and unstable angina. Additionally, urgent cardiac catheterization is needed for some patients. An ECG is crucial for diagnosis, and must be done within 10 minutes of the patient's arrival. An initial ECG usually reveals an ST-segment elevation. If possible, emergency coronary angiography and PCI are performed very soon after the onset of an acute MI.

Treatment

For acute MI prior to hospitalization, emergency personnel establish a good IV route, give oxygen by nasal cannula, and begin continuous single-lead ECG monitoring. Medications include antiplatelet drugs, anticoagulants, and antianginal drugs. Antiplatelet drugs include aspirin, clopidogrel, prasugrel, and ticagrelor. Anticoagulants include various types of heparin, and bivalirudin. Nitroglycerin is the predominant antianginal agent, and morphine is used more selectively based on the individual patient. Beta-blockers, ACE inhibitors, and statins are also given.

Fibrinolytics are most effective within a few minutes to 1 hour after onset of acute MI – the earlier the better. Lower-risk patients usually have stress testing before discharge, or soon after. Patients must be educated about closely following all medication regimens and making significant lifestyle changes. Based on any other conditions, all acute MI patients remain taking antiplatelet drugs, statins, antianginals, and any other required medications. By working with physicians to manage risk factors for MI, their prognosis may be improved.

Prevention

Prevention of acute MI, even if it recurs, includes a heart-healthy diet, with plenty of whole grains, fruits, vegetables, and lean protein. There must be large reductions of cholesterol, saturated fat, trans fat, and sugar. This is extremely critical for people with diabetes mellitus, high cholesterol, and hypertension. Exercising regularly, following an approved exercise plan created by a physician, improves cardiovascular health. Any new exercise plan must only be started by consulting a physician. Quitting smoking significantly lowers risks for acute MI and improves heart as well as lung health. Secondhand smoke must also be avoided.

Prognosis

Prognosis is poorer when there are manifestations such as diabetes mellitus, recurring angina or ischemia without significant activity, heart failure, mitral regurgitation, high-risk results of a stress test, hemodynamic instability, continuing ventricular tachycardia. About 10% of hospitalized patients with acute MI die – mostly from cardiogenic shock, but this is varied based on how severe left ventricular failure actually is. Most deaths from cardiogenic shock are due to an infarction or a combined scar and new infarction that affects 50% of more of the LV. Death rates are higher in women and people with diabetes mellitus. After a hospitalization for acute MI, death rates are 8%–10% within the next year. The majority occur within only 3–4 months. Higher risk for death is based on the presence of heart failure, chronic ventricular arrhythmia, poor ventricular function, and recurring ischemia.

CLINICAL CASE

1. What does the pathophysiology of acute MI include?
2. What type of acute MI is more commonly seen in diabetic patients?
3. How is an acute MI diagnosed?

A 48-year-old man went to bed early after feeling unwell. During the night, he awoke, sweating profusely and breathing with difficulty. He then collapsed on the floor, which woke his wife. She called 911, and the emergency personnel arrived within 15 minutes. They performed standard emergency treatments for a suspected acute MI. The man's family history included heart disease, and his father had a heart attack at age 56. The patient was more than 50 pounds overweight, dealt with high levels of stress at his job, and smoked several packs of cigarettes per week. He admitted to not exercising very much at all. At the hospital, tests revealed that the patient had experienced an acute MI. He was admitted to the coronary care unit, and started on beta-blockers, anticoagulants, and aspirin. Angiography was done, revealing several blocked arteries, and angioplasty was scheduled. The patient responded well, and he was discharged within several days, with a strict regimen to follow: Weight reduction and moderate exercise, changing his diet, stopping smoking, and reducing work-related stress.

ANSWERS

1. The pathophysiology of acute MI includes increased cardiac biomarkers. At least one of the following must also be present: Ischemic symptoms, development of pathologic Q waves, electrocardiogram changes revealing new ischemia via left bundle branch block or significant ST/T changes, imaging studies showing new loss of myocardial tissue or new regional abnormalities of wall motion, and angiography evidence of an intracoronary thrombus.
2. Approximately 20% of acute MI cases are silent, with these cases more commonly seen in diabetic patients. In silent MI, the patient may not recognize what is happening since the symptoms are so vague. Some patients actually experience no symptoms as the MI occurs.
3. The diagnosis of acute MI starts with initial and serial ECG. Then, serial measurements of cardiac biomarkers help to identify the subtype that is present, or distinguish between these and unstable angina. Urgent cardiac catheterization is needed for some patients. An ECG is required within 10 minutes of the patient's arrival. Emergency coronary angiography and PCI are performed, if possible, very soon.

KEY TERMS

- Arterial tone
- Atheromas
- Atypical angina
- Cardiac biomarker
- Evanescent
- Friction rub
- Holter monitoring
- Hypokinetic
- Kawasaki disease
- Kussmaul sign
- Marantic endocarditis
- Mitral regurgitation
- Nocturnal angina
- Oximetry
- Paradoxical motion
- Stable angina
- Syndrome X
- Thready
- Troponin
- Unstable angina
- Variant angina

REFERENCES

Aggarwal, N.R., and Wood, M.J. (2021). *Sex Differences in Cardiac Disease: Pathophysiology, Presentation, Diagnosis and Management.* Elsevier.

AHA Journals. (2015). *Acute Myocardial Infarction: Changes in Patient Characteristics, Management, and 6-Month Outcomes over a Period of 20 Years in the FAST-MI Program (French Registry of Acute ST-Elevation or Non-ST-Elevation Myocardial Infarction) 1995 to 2015.* American Heart Association, Inc. www.ahajournals.org/doi/pdf/10.1161/circulationaha.117.030798

American College of Cardiology. (2019). *Current Clinical Implications of Coronary Artery Disease Polygenic Risk Scoring.* American College of Cardiology Foundation. https://www.acc.org/latest-in-cardiology/articles/2019/10/07/06/51/current-clinical-implications-of-coronary-artery-disease-polygenic-risk-scoring

American Heart Association. (2021a). *Unstable Angina.* American Heart Association, Inc. https://www.heart.org/en/health-topics/heart-attack/angina-chest-pain/unstable-angina

American Heart Association (2021b). *Prinzmetal's or Prinzmetal Angina, Variant Angina and Angina Inversa.* American Heart Association, Inc. https://www.heart.org/en/health-topics/heart-attack/angina-chest-pain/prinzmetals-or-prinzmetal-angina-variant-angina-and-angina-inversa

Barsness, G.W., and Holmes, D.R. (2012). *Coronary Artery Disease: New Approaches without Traditional Revascularization.* Springer.

Bel Marra Health. (2021). *Unstable Angina – A Common Cause of Heart Attack: Causes, Symptoms, Treatment, and Prevention.* BelMarraHealth. https://www.belmarrahealth.com/unstable-angina-common-cause-heart-attack-causes-symptoms-treatment-prevention/

BestHeartInfo.com. (2021). *How to Prevent Prinzmetal Angina.* BestHeartInfo.com. https://www.bestheartinfo.com/prevent-prinzmetal-angina/

Bhatt, D.L., and Bavry, A.A. (2009). *Acute Coronary Syndromes in Clinical Practice.* Springer.

Bleifeld, W., Hamm, C.W., and Braunwald, E. (2012). *Unstable Angina.* Springer/Verlag.

British Journal of Cardiology, The. (2020). *Angina Module 1: Epidemiology.* Medinews Cardiology Ltd. https://bjcardio.co.uk/2020/04/angina-module-1-epidemiology-2/

Brubaker, P., Whaley, M., and Kaminsky, L. (2001). *Coronary Artery Disease: Essentials of Prevention and Rehabilitation Programs.* Human Kinetics.

Cardiac Health. (2021). *Your Heart – Your Coronary Arteries – Angina – Prinzmetal's Angina.* Tryzelaar Consulting. https://www.cardiachealth.org/your-heart/your-coronary-arteries/angina/prinzmetals-angina/

Cath Lab Digest. (2012). *Variant Angina: A 53-Year-Old Male with Recurrent ST-Segment Elevation.* HMP Global. https://www.hmpglobellearningnetwork.com/site/cathlab/articles/Variant-Angina-53-Year-Old-Male-Recurrent-ST-Segment-Elevation

Cohn, P.F. (2012). *Diagnosis and Therapy of Coronary Artery Disease,* 2nd Edition. Springer.

Cooper, O. (2020). *Coronary Artery Disease: Causes, Diagnosis and Management.* Hayle Medical.

De Lemos, J., and Omland, T. (2017). *Chronic Coronary Artery Disease: A Companion to Braunwald's Heart Disease.* Elsevier.

Defelice, E. (2005). *Prevention of Cardiovascular Disease: Atherosclerosis, Carotid Artery Disease, Cerebral Artery Disease/ Stroke, Coronary Artery Disease, Peripheral Artery Disease and Hypertension.* iUniverse.

Faergeman, O. (2003). *Coronary Artery Disease: Genes, Drugs and the Agricultural Connection.* Elsevier.

Hanna, E.B. (2017). *Practical Cardiovascular Medicine.* Wiley-Blackwell.

HCPLive – ContagionLive – NeurologyLive – OncLive. (2009). *Angina by the Numbers – Mortality, Incidence, Prevalence, and Other Angina Statistics.* HCPLive. https://www.hcplive.com/view/angina_statistics

Healthline. (2018a). *How Can Acute Myocardial Infarction Be Prevented?* Healthline Media. https://www.healthline.com/health/acute-myocardial-infarction#prevention

Healthline. (2018b). *What Causes Acute Myocardial Infarction?* Healthline Media. https://www.healthline.com/health/acute-myocardial-infarction#causes

iConcept Press. (2017). *Coronary Artery Disease: Research and Practice.* iConcept Press.

IntechOpen. (2018). *Epidemiology of Myocardial Infarction.* IntechOpen Limited. https://www.intechopen.com/chapters/59778

Intermountain Healthcare. (2014). *What Is Angina Pectoris and How Do We Prevent It?* Intermountain Healthcare. https://intermountainhealthcare.org/blogs/topics/heart/2014/03/what-is-angina-pectoris-and-how-do-we-prevent-it/

JAMA Network. (2021). *Diagnosis and Management of Stable Angina – A Review.* JAMA Network / American Medical Association / Silverchair Information/Systems. https://jama-network.com/journals/jama/article-abstract/2779543

Kaski, J.C. (2016). *Essentials in Stable Angina Pectoris.* Springer.

King, M.W., Bambharoliya, T., Ramakrishna, H., and Zhang, F. (2020). *Coronary Artery Disease and The Evolution of Angioplasty Devices (Briefs in Materials).* Springer.

Lyde, W. (2015). *Encyclopedia of Coronary Artery Disease (Physiology and Treatment): Volume III.* Hayle Medical.

Mayo Clinic. (2021). *Coronary artery disease.* Mayo Foundation for Medical Education and Research (MFMER). https://www.mayoclinic.org/diseases-conditions/coronary-artery-disease/symptoms-causes/syc-20350613

McAlpine, W.A. (2012). *Heart and Coronary Arteries: An Anatomical Atlas for Clinical Diagnosis, Radiological Investigation, and Surgical Treatment.* Springer/Verlag.

Medscape. (2020). *What Is the Prognosis of Acute Coronary Syndrome (ACS)?* WebMD LLC. https://www.medscape.com/answers/1910735-178323/what-is-the-prognosis-of-acute-coronary-syndrome-acs

Minatoguchi, S. (2019). *Cardioprotection against Acute Myocardial Infarction.* Springer.

Narayana Health. (2020). *Cardiology – Coronary Artery Disease: Life Expectancy and Prognosis.* Narayana Hrudayalaya Ltd. https://www.narayanahealth.org/blog/coronary-artery-disease-life-expectancy-and-prognosis/

Narila, K. (2021). *Symptoms of Coronary Artery Disease: Chest Pain, Shortness of Breath, Sweating, Palpitations, Tachycardia, Weakness, Dizziness, Nausea, Pedal Edema, Fatigue.* Narila.

NDTV-Food. (2016). *Coronary Artery Disease Up by 300 Per Cent in India: Expert.* NDTV Convergence. https://food.ndtv.com/health/coronary-artery-disease-up-by-300-per-cent-in-india-expert–1427685

NETCE - Continuing Education. (2021). *Acute Coronary Syndrome: An Overview for Nurses.* NetCE. https://www.netce.com/casestudies.php?courseid=1747

NIH – National Center for Advancing Translational Sciences – Genetic and Rare Diseases Information Center. (2021). *Prinzmetal's Variant Angina.* Genetic and Rare Diseases Information Center (GARD). https://rarediseases.info.nih.gov/diseases/7465/prinzmetals-variant-angina

NIH – National Library of Medicine – National Center for Biotechnology Information. (2019). *Acute Coronary Syndrome: Prevention.* National Library of Medicine. https://pubmed.ncbi.nlm.nih.gov/30671595/

NIH – National Library of Medicine – National Center for Biotechnology Information. (2016). *Prevalence and Characteristics of Acute Coronary Syndromes in a Sub-Saharan Africa Population.* National Library of Medicine. https://pubmed.ncbi.nlm.nih.gov/26988750/

NIH – National Library of Medicine – National Center for Biotechnology Information. (2014). *The Incidence and Outcomes of Acute Coronary Syndromes in a Central European Country: Results of the CZECH-2 Registry.* National Library of Medicine. https://pubmed.ncbi.nlm.nih.gov/24602321/

NIH – National Library of Medicine – National Center for Biotechnology Information. (2011). *Variant Angina and Coronary Artery Spasm: The Clinical Spectrum, Pathophysiology, and Management.* National Library of Medicine. https://pubmed.ncbi.nlm.nih.gov/21389642/

NIH – National Library of Medicine – National Center for Biotechnology Information. (1990). *Unstable Angina: Pathophysiology and Drug Therapy.* National Library of Medicine. https://pubmed.ncbi.nlm.nih.gov/1972360/

Ostovar, L., Khadem Vatan, K., and Panahi, O. (2020). *Clinical Outcome of Thrombolytic Therapy in Patients with Acute Myocardial Infarction.* Scholars' Press.

Oxford Medicine Online – European Society of Cardiology. (2018). *Epidemiology of Acute Coronary Syndromes.* Oxford University Press. https://oxfordmedicine.com/view/10.1093/med/9780198784906.001.0001/med-9780198784906-chapter–305

Pharmacy Times. (2013). *Case Studies.* Pharmacy Times. https://www.pharmacytimes.com/view/finerenone-receives-fda-approval-for-treatment-of-chronic-kidney-disease-associated-with-type-2-diabetes

Polimeni, A. (2020). *Coronary Artery Disease (Clinics Review Articles – Cardiology Clinics),* Volume 38-4. Elsevier.

Prescriber.co.uk. (2013). *Stable Angina: Current Guidelines and Advances in Management (Drug Review).* Prescriber co.uk. https://wchh.onlinelibrary.wiley.com/doi/pdf/10.1002/psb.1095

Richardson, R.R. (2020). *Atlas of Pediatric CTA of Coronary Artery Anomalies.* Springer.

Shah, P.K. (2019). *Risk Factors in Coronary Artery Disease.* CRC Press.

Stone, P.H., Underwood, A., Leighton, S., and Linkinhoker, M. (2013). *Diagnosis: Coronary Artery Disease (Special Health Report).* Harvard Health Publications.

Tamburino, C., Di Salvo, M.E., La Manna, A., and Capodanno, D. (2009). *Left Main Coronary Artery Disease: A Practical Guide for the Interventional Cardiologist.* Springer.

Tcheng, J.E. (2009). *Primary Angioplasty in Acute Myocardial Infarction (Contemporary Cardiology),* 2nd Edition. Humana Press.

Thompson Rivers University. (2021). *Coronary Artery Disease: Clinical Case Study.* Thompson Rivers University. https://barabus.tru.ca/hlth2501/cardiovascular/cad/case.html

Tousoulis, D. (2017). *Coronary Artery Disease: From Biology to Clinical Practice.* Academic Press.

UK Essays – Biology. (2017). *Case Study of Unstable Angina.* UKEssays / All Answers Ltd. https://www.ukessays.com/essays/biology/case-study-of-unstable-angina-biology-essay.php

Unstable Angina Blogspot. (2013). *Unstable Angina – Practice Essentials.* Unstable Angina Blogspot. https://unstableangina.blogspot.com/

U.S. Department of Health and Human Services, Agency for Healthcare Research and Quality. (2013a). *Noninvasive Technologies for the Diagnosis of Coronary Artery Disease in Women: Future Research Needs (Effective Health Care Program).* AHRQ / CreateSpace Independent Publishing Platform.

U.S. Department of Health and Human Services, Agency for Healthcare Research and Quality. (2013b). *Screening for Asymptomatic Coronary Artery Disease: A Systematic Review for the U.S. Preventive Services Task Force: Systematic Evidence Review Number 22.* AHRQ / CreateSpace Independent Publishing Platform.

Wang, M. (2020). *Coronary Artery Disease: Therapeutics and Drug Discovery (Advances in Experimental Medicine and Biology, Book 1177).* Springer.

Weber State University – Dumke College of Health Professions. (2021). *Acute Myocardial Infarction.* Weber State University. https://www.weber.edu/casestudies/myocardial-infarction-page-1.html

Willerson, J.T., and Holmes, Jr., D.R. (2015). *Coronary Artery Disease (Cardiovascular Medicine).* Springer.

World Health Organization. (2021). *Cardiovascular Diseases (CVDs).* World Health Organization. https://www.who.int/news-room/fact-sheets/detail/cardiovascular-diseases-(cvds)

CHAPTER 10 Congestive Heart Failure

Congestive heart failure (CHF) is a collection of symptoms that may be caused by mechanical or myocardial abnormalities as well as disturbances of heart rhythm. It eventually affects nearly every organ system in the body. Most cases of CHF involve systolic dysfunction of the left ventricle. People with type 2 diabetes mellitus are 2–4 times more likely to develop CHF than those without diabetes. CHF must be considered as the diagnosis for any adult patient presenting with dyspnea and/or respiratory failure. Complications of the disease often affect the lungs, including obstructive sleep apnea, pleural effusions, and pulmonary edema. The mortality rate for CHF is worse than for many types of cancer.

HEART FAILURE

Heart failure (HF) involves ventricular dysfunction that may be either left-sided or right-sided. Left ventricular failure results in fatigue and shortness of breath. Right ventricular failure results in an accumulation of fluid in the abdomen and peripheral areas of the body. Also, the ventricles may be affected individually or simultaneously. Diabetes mellitus increases the risks for coronary artery disease, resulting in CHF. With diabetes, there is often hypertension and atherosclerosis because of elevated blood lipids, and both of these conditions are related to HF. It is commonly understood that being overweight or obese, physically inactive, and having hypertension and high cholesterol is related to type 1 or type 2 diabetes, and these are also risk factors that lead to the development of HF.

Epidemiology

Globally, about 26 million people are affected by HF every year. Global rates of hospitalizations for CHF have not changed significantly in prevalence or incidence over the past 27 years. There are some statistics available for specific countries. For example, the Australian Bureau of Statistics documented in 2018 that their country had 110,000 people with HF, which appears to be lessening every year. Nearly twice the amount of Australians with HF were men. HF in Australia accounts for nearly 1 of every 50 deaths, and more women actually die from the disease than men. In China, current trends for increased rates of hypertension, high cholesterol, and type 2 diabetes mellitus are expended to increase deaths from cardiovascular events by 21.3 million. In the United States, there are more than 960,000 new cases of HF annually, and overall about 6.5 million people are living with some degree of HF.

Etiology and Risk Factors

Cardiac performance can be impaired by cardiac as well as systemic factors, which can also cause or worsen HF. Cardiac causes of HF include cardiomyopathy, MI, myocarditis, some chemotherapy drugs, aortic stenosis, mitral regurgitation, bradyarrhythmias, tachyarrhythmias, atrioventricular node block, left bundle branch block, ischemia, amyloidosis, chronic fibrosis such as systemic sclerosis, and hemochromatosis. Systemic causes of HF include diabetes mellitus, anemia, hyperthyroidism, Paget disease, aortic stenosis, and hypertension. Diabetes and HF are interlinked since having one of these conditions increases the likelihood of developing the other. Failure of the LV most often develops in hypertension, ischemic heart disease, aortic regurgitation, mitral regurgitation, aortic stenosis, most types of cardiomyopathies, and congenital disorders that include patent ductus arteriosus with large shunts, or ventricular septal defects. Failure of the RV is usually due to previous LV failure or by a severe lung disorder. Additional causes include multiple pulmonary emboli, pulmonary arterial hypertension, RV infarction, tricuspid regurgitation or stenosis, mitral stenosis, pulmonary artery or pulmonary valve stenosis, arrhythmogenic RV cardiomyopathy, pulmonary venous occlusive disease, or congenital disorders including **Ebstein anomaly** and **Eisenmenger syndrome**. Also, RV failure is mimicked by volume overload with increases systemic venous pressure in overtransfusion or polycythemia, obstruction of the vena cavae, acute renal injury with water and sodium retention, and hypoproteinemia that causes peripheral edema and low plasma oncotic pressure.

Biventricular failure is caused by amyloidosis, **Chagas disease**, or viral myocarditis since these affect the entire myocardium. It can also be caused by chronic LV failure that results in RV failure. A persistently high cardiac output (CO) can cause high-output HF. This may evolve into an inability to maintain adequate output. Conditions that can increase CO include end-stage liver disease, severe anemia, beriberi, advanced **Paget disease, thyrotoxicosis**, arteriovenous fistula, and chronic tachycardia.

Pathophysiology

The force and velocity of heart contractions is described as *cardiac contractility*. Along with myocardial oxygen requirements and ventricular performance, cardiac contractility is determined by a variety of factors. These include preload, afterload, the rate of the heart and its rhythm. The product of **stroke volume** and

DOI: 10.1201/9781003226727-13

heart rate is the CO. Factors affecting CO include neurohumoral factors, peripheral vascular tone, and venous return. The loading condition, at the end of the heart's diastole and systole is called the **preload**. This is the amount of end-diastolic fiber stretching and volume. It is affected by the myocardial wall composition and the ventricular diastolic pressure. A good measure of preload is usually the LV end-diastolic pressure – especially when it is higher than normal. The force resisting myocardial fiber contraction at the beginning of systole is called the **afterload**. The relationship between preload and the heart's performance ability is described by the **Frank-Starling principle**. In normal conditions, systolic contractile performance is represented by the CO or the stroke volume, and is equivalent to the preload in the normal physiological range.

When the heart is no longer able to provide body tissues with enough blood for metabolic activities, and there are cardiac-related increases in pulmonary or systemic venous pressures, organ congestion can result. This may be because of systolic or diastolic function abnormalities, but usually, there are abnormalities of both of these. A primary abnormality can be a change in the function of cardiomyocytes. Cardiac structural defects, rhythm abnormalities, and high metabolic demands also cause HF. With RV dysfunction, there is increased systemic venous pressure. Fluid moves to mostly the feet and ankles of patients able to walk, as well as the abdominal viscera. The liver is the organ that is most affected. Fluid accumulation (ascites) of the peritoneal cavity may occur.

With stress, neurohumoral responses aid in increasing heart function while maintaining organ perfusion and BP. However, continual activation of neurohumoral responses disrupts the balance between hormones that stimulate the myocardium or cause vasoconstriction, as well as the balance between vasodilating and myocardial-relaxing hormones. As we age, heart and cardiovascular changes reduce the threshold for HF to be expressed. There is more myocardial interstitial collagen, and the myocardium becomes stiffer. Myocardial relaxation is longer. There is a large reduction in diastolic LV function, even in healthy older adults. There is a slight decline in systolic function. Decreases in myocardial and vascular responsiveness to beta-adrenergic stimulation impair cardiovascular responses to greater workloads. Peak exercise capacity is greatly decreased. The carbon dioxide at peak exercise decreases, but not as much. This decline can be reduced if an individual regularly exercises. Therefore, older people are more likely to develop HF symptoms because of stress from systemic disorders or even slight cardiovascular events.

Clinical Manifestations

The amount of damage to the LV and RV influences the signs and symptoms of HF. Severe LV failure may result in pulmonary edema or cardiogenic shock. The most common symptoms of LV failure are dyspnea and fatigue because of increased pulmonary venous pressures. There may be low CO during rest, and an inability to change the CO during exercise. Usually, dyspnea occurs during exertion but is relieved by rest. As HF progresses, dyspnea may occur at rest and during the night, sometimes with coughing. If dyspnea occurs as the patient lies flat or soon after, and is quickly relieved by sitting up, this is described as **orthopnea** – indicating advanced disease. With **paroxysmal nocturnal dyspnea** (PND), the dyspnea awakens the patient a few hours after going to bed. It is only relieved by sitting up for 15–20 minutes. When HF becomes severe, **Cheyne-Stokes respirations** may occur – during the day or night. The sudden **hyperpneic** phase of these respirations can awaken the patient from sleep. Cheyne-Stokes respirations are linked to low CO, while PND is linked to pulmonary congestion. In HF, sleep apnea and other breathing disorders are common, and can worsen HF. Because of greatly reduced cerebral blood flow and hypoxemia, the patient may have chronic irritability and impaired mental performance.

The most common symptoms with RV failure include fatigue and ankle swelling. There may be a "fullness" of the neck or abdomen. Liver congestion can cause right upper quadrant abdominal discomfort. Stomach or intestinal congestion causes anorexia, early satiety, and bloating of the abdomen. If there is severe biventricular failure, skeletal muscle wasting may occur. This can reflect increased catabolism because of higher cytokine production. If a patient has extreme cardiac **cachexia**, the likelihood of death is increased. For older patients, atypical manifestations include confusion, delirium, falling, nighttime urinary incontinence, sudden declines in function, and sleep disturbances. HF can worsen any concurrent cognitive impairment or depression. Tachycardia and tachypnea may occur with LV failure. Severe LV failure may cause the patient to be visibly cyanotic or dyspneic, hypotensive, and agitated or confused due to hypoxia and insufficient cerebral perfusion. Some of these symptoms occur more often in older patients. Severe hypoxemia is reflected by central cyanosis that affects all of the body. Low blood flow with increased oxygen extraction is signified by peripheral cyanosis of the lips, fingers, and toes.

RV failure is signified by foot and ankle non-tender peripheral pitting edema, in which pressure by the examiner's fingers leaves imprints that are visible and palpable, and may be very deep. The liver is enlarged and may be pulsatile, and is palpable below the right costal margin. Abdominal swelling and ascites develop. The jugular venous pressure is elevated. An increased jugular venous pressure during inspiration is known as the **Kussmaul sign**, which indicating right-sided HF. If the liver is congested, it may be enlarged or tender. Hepatojugular or abdominal-jugular reflux may be present. Auscultation can detect murmur of tricuspid regurgitation or the RV third heart sound of the left sternal border. These findings are both changes during inspiration.

Diagnosis

Diagnostic methods include X-rays, ECG, and echocardiography. Blood tests help to identify the cause of HF and any systemic effects. HF may be suggested by orthopnea, exertional fatigue or dyspnea, edema, pulmonary crackles, tachycardia, a third heart sound, and jugular venous distention. However, these developments are usually not seen early in the disease course. Such symptoms are also caused by recurrent pneumonia, chronic obstructive pulmonary disease (COPD), and even old age or obesity. However, HF should be of accurate suspicion if there is a history of hypertension, MI, valvular disorders, or murmurs. There is moderate suspicion of HF in diabetic and older patients.

Chest X-rays include a cardiac **silhouette** that is enlarged, fluid in the major fissure, pleural effusion, and horizontal lines within the edges of the lower posterior lung fields. These are known as *Kerley B lines*. All of these factors indicate a chronic elevation of the left atrial pressure as well as long-term thickening of the intralobular septa from edema. There may also be upper lobe pulmonary venous congestion, along with alveolar or interstitial edema. An abnormal ECG increases the suspicion for HF and can identify the cause. This is especially true if ECG reveals left ventricular hypertrophy, previous MI, left bundle branch block, and rapid atrial fibrillation or another tachyarrhythmia. With chronic HF, a totally normal ECG is rare.

Echocardiography evaluates dimensions of the heart chambers, LV ejection fraction, valve function, LV hypertrophy, diastolic function, pulmonary artery pressure, pericardial effusion, and RV function. It can also detect intracardiac thrombi, calcifications, and tumors in the heart valves or mitral annulus. Radionuclide imaging can diagnose systolic and diastolic function, previous MI, or ischemia.

Treatment

It is crucial to diagnose and treat the underlying causative disorder. The short-term treatment goals include relief of symptoms and improvement of hemodynamics. There must be prevention of hypokalemia, kidney dysfunction, and symptomatic hypotension. Neurohumoral activation must be corrected. The long-term treatment goals include correction of hypertension, diabetes, improving cardiac function, prevention of atherosclerosis and MI, reducing hospitalizations, and improving quality of life as well as survival.

Dietary and lifestyle changes are indicated, as well as medications, devices, and for many patients, percutaneous coronary interventions, or surgery. Treatments are individualized in response to the causative factor, symptoms, medication response, and adverse effects of medications. Patients and caregivers must be educated about drug adherence, exacerbations, and linking causes to effects, such as dietary salt with weight gain or HF symptoms. Multidisciplinary teams are proven to improve outcomes and reduce hospitalizations, especially for the most severe cases of HF. Sodium restriction helps reduce fluid retention. Salt should not be used while cooking or added to cooked foods. Foods that are high in salt before preparation should be avoided. For severe HF, sodium is limited to less than 2 g/day by eating only low-sodium foods. Morning weight, measured daily, helps detect early accumulation of sodium and water. When weight increases more than 2 kg over several days, the patient can adjust the dose of diuretics. If weight gain continues or symptoms develop, the patient must consult a physician.

Intensive case management monitors drug adherence, unscheduled medical visits, and hospitalizations to identify the need for further intervention. A very specific diet is needed for diabetic patients or those with atherosclerosis. Patients must attain a body mass index (BMI) of 30 kg/m^2 or less, with an ideal range being 21–25 kg/m^2. Regular and light physical exercise is usually indicated to prevent skeletal muscles from losing adequate conditioning. Patients can dramatically improve when a variety of underlying conditions are successfully treated. Significant myocardial ischemia must be treated aggressively. Today's management of significant ventricular infiltration such as in amyloidosis has greatly improved, and newer treatments have greatly improved prognosis.

Long-term management for HF is achieved with diuretics, nitrates, digoxin, ACE inhibitors, beta-blockers, aldosterone antagonists, ARBs, and angiotensin receptor/neprilysin inhibitors.

If the sodium-glucose co-transporter 2 inhibitor called *dapagliflozin* is added, it can reduce complications and deaths if the patient has elevated natriuretic peptide levels. It has good effects in patients with diabetes mellitus or without. For arrhythmias, electrolytes are normalized, atrial and ventricular rates are controlled, and antiarrhythmic medications may be administered. For persistent sinus tachycardia, a beta-blocker given in increasing doses may be helpful. Atrial fibrillation with an uncontrolled ventricular rate is treated with a target resting rate being less than 80 beats per minute. Beta-blockers are used first, but rate-limiting calcium channel blockers are used with caution as long as systolic function is preserved. For some patients, digoxin is used to control heart rhythm or rate. A permanent pacemaker must be inserted for some patient.

Adequate treatment and correction of potassium and magnesium abnormalities reduce risks of ventricular arrhythmias. Antiarrhythmic medications may be needed for sustained ventricular tachycardia if it persists even with correction of causative conditions or optimal HF treatment. Amiodarone, beta-blockers, and dofetilide are the drugs of choice. Since amiodarone increases levels of digoxin and warfarin, their doses are decreased by half or stopped.

Drug toxicity with digoxin can occur even at therapeutic drug levels. Low doses of amiodarone are often used, with liver function and thyroid-stimulating hormone tests done every 6 months. Chest X-rays and pulmonary function tests are done once per year to assess pulmonary fibrosis, when there are abnormal previous chest X-rays or significantly worsened dyspnea.

Prevention

To prevent HF and heart disease, avoiding tobacco products, regular physical exercise, a heart-healthy diet, maintaining a healthy weight, good quality sleep, stress management, and regular health screenings for BP, cholesterol, and type 2 diabetes are essential.

Prognosis

The prognosis of HF is usually poor unless the cause can be corrected. After the first hospitalization, 5-year survival is only about 35%, no matter what the ejection fraction is. For overt chronic HF, deaths are based on ventricular dysfunction and symptom severity. Generally, patients experience slow deterioration of health, with occasional severe exacerbations, and eventual death. Modern therapies sometimes prolong life. For some patients, death is sudden, without warning or any worsening of symptoms.

CLINICAL CASE

1. What are the systemic causes of HF?
2. With aging and more myocardial interstitial collagen, what is the outcome?
3. What does the presence of orthopnea indicate in HF?

A 74-year-old woman with type 2 diabetes was hospitalized because of shortness of breath, orthopnea, and ankle edema. Over the past few weeks, she had suffered from dyspepsia and her physician found a new heart murmur that had not been present previously. The patient was experiencing tachycardia, though her resting blood pressure was 110/70 mm Hg. Late inspiratory crackles were heard in both lung fields. Chest X-ray confirmed cardiomegaly and interstitial edema. Echocardiography showed left ventricular end-diastolic distension and apical dilatation. There was vigorous contraction of the posterior wall. Though the left atrium was of normal size, there was high-velocity mitral regurgitation.

ANSWERS

1. The systemic causes of HF include diabetes mellitus, anemia, hyperthyroidism, Paget disease, aortic stenosis, and hypertension. Diabetes and HF are interlinked since having one of these conditions increases the likelihood of developing the other.
2. With aging and more myocardial interstitial collagen, the myocardium becomes stiff and myocardial relaxation takes longer. There is a large reduction in diastolic LV function, even in healthy older adults, and a slight decline in systolic function. Decreases in myocardial and vascular responsiveness to beta-adrenergic stimulation impair cardiovascular responses to greater workloads and peak exercise capacity is greatly decreased.
3. If dyspnea occurs as the patient lies flat or soon after, and is quickly relieved by sitting up, this is orthopnea, and indicates advanced disease.

CARDIOMYOPATHY

A **cardiomyopathy** is a primary myocardial disorder. It is different than structural cardiac disorders, including congenital heart disorders, coronary artery disease, or valvular disorders. There are three main types of cardiomyopathies which include *dilated, hypertrophic*, and *restrictive* cardiomyopathies. *Dilated cardiomyopathy* is myocardial dysfunction that results in HF, with ventricular dilation and systolic dysfunction. *Hypertrophic cardiomyopathy* is a congenital or acquired disorder, with extreme ventricular hypertrophy and diastolic dysfunction, lacking increased afterload – it may be caused by **coarctation** of the aorta, systemic hypertension, or valvular aortic stenosis. *Restrictive cardiomyopathy* involves noncompliant ventricular walls, which resist diastolic filling. When one ventricle is affected it is usually the LV. However, both ventricles can be affected. An ischemic cardiomyopathy can occur with severe CAD, with or without infarction. It is not a primary myocardial disorder. Cardiomyopathies are signified by signs and symptoms of HF, based on systolic, diastolic, or combined dysfunction. Diabetic cardiomyopathy is cardiac dysfunction with structural, functional, and metabolic alterations even though coronary artery disease may be absent.

Epidemiology

Dilated cardiomyopathy develops in patients of all ages, but is most common in adults younger than age 50. Approximately 10% of cases are in people over age 65. Estimated global prevalence is between 1 in every 250–2,500 people. Unlike most of the world in which dilated cardiomyopathy is relatively rare, it is a major cause of HF throughout Africa. In the United States, dilated cardiomyopathy affects men 3 times more than women. It also affects African Americans 3 times more than Caucasians. Approximately 5–8 of every 100,000 people develop dilated cardiomyopathy annually.

Hypertrophic cardiomyopathy affects 1 of every 500 people. It has been documented in more than 50 countries. In India and China, up to 2 million people are affected, and in the United States, about 700,000 people have hypertrophic cardiomyopathy. The average age for the diagnosis of hypertrophic cardiomyopathy is 39 years, but it has been diagnosed in infants and in people older than 80. It often appears during a person's late teens or early 20s. The condition is slightly male predominant (about 60% of cases). For unknown reasons, hypertrophic cardiomyopathy affects people of mixed racial or ethnic groups (51% of cases), followed by Caucasians (42%).

Restrictive cardiomyopathy is the least common type of cardiomyopathy. It makes up less than 5% of all cases of cardiomyopathy and usually affects older adults. Men and women are equally affected. It is even less common in children. There is no significant racial or ethnic predilection.

Etiology and Risk Factors

Pathogenic causes of *dilated cardiomyopathy* include coxsackievirus B, Chagas disease from *Trypanosoma cruzi*, and HIV infection. Both type 1 and type 2 diabetes increase the risk for developing cardiomyopathy. With diabetes, cardiomyopathy is related to features that include lower diastolic compliance, interstitial fibrosis, and myocyte hypertrophy. Additional causes are prolonged tachycardia, thyrotoxicosis, **toxoplasmosis**, and **beriberi**. Toxic substances include alcohol, organic solvents, ions of heavy metals, and chemotherapeutic agents such as doxorubicin and trastuzumab. Acute dilated cardiomyopathy is triggered by sudden emotional stress. This is usually reversible, as is dilated cardiomyopathy caused by prolonged tachycardia. One example is acute apical ballooning cardiomyopathy in which the apex is usually affected along with some segments of the left ventricle, resulting in regional wall dysfunction and occasionally focal dilation. Genetic factors are implicated in 20%–35% of cases. More than 60 genes have been documented.

Most cases of *hypertrophic cardiomyopathy* are inherited. There are more than 1,500 gene mutations inherited in an autosomally dominant pattern, but spontaneous gene mutations also occur. The phenotypic expression is widely varied. In rare cases, hypertrophic cardiomyopathy is acquired as part of conditions such as **acromegaly, neurofibromatosis**, and **pheochromocytoma**. In a small number of cases, symmetric hypertrophy has occurred. Approximately 66% of patients have obstructive physiology, either during exercise or at rest.

Restrictive cardiomyopathy is not always a primary disorder and is usually of unknown cause. However, it can develop because of genetic or systemic disorders. Some disorders such as **amyloidosis** and **hemochromatosis** also affect other tissues. In rare cases, amyloidosis affects the coronary arteries. Nodal conduction tissue can also be affected by **Fabry disease** and sarcoidosis. **Löffler syndrome** occurs in the tropics, starting as an acute arteritis accompanied by eosinophilia. Then, a thrombus forms on the endocardium, and AV valves, which progresses to fibrosis.

Pathophysiology

Dilated cardiomyopathy occurs without other disorders that are able to cause the myocardium to be dilated. These include severe occlusive CAD, hypertension, and valvular heart disease. Sometimes, dilated cardiomyopathy starts with acute myocarditis (usually of viral origin). There is a latent phase of various lengths, then diffuse necrosis of the myocardial myocytes because of an autoimmune reaction to myocytes altered by the virus, and then, chronic fibrosis. The myocardium is dilated, thinner, and hypertrophied as a compensatory mechanism. This often results in functional tricuspid or mitral regurgitation as well as atrial dilation. Dilated cardiomyopathy affects both ventricles in most cases, less often affecting just the LV, and only rarely affecting just the RV. When chamber dilation and dysfunction progress, mural thrombi can form because of stasis of blood. The acute myocarditis and late chronic dilated phases are often complicated by cardiac tachyarrhythmias. Atrioventricular block may also develop. As the left atrium becomes dilated, atrial fibrillation often occurs.

In *hypertrophic cardiomyopathy*, the myocardium is abnormal in its cells and myofibrils. *Restrictive cardiomyopathy* involves endocardial thickening or myocardial infiltration in one or both ventricle – usually the left ventricle is affected with one-sided disease. There may be myocyte death, infiltration of the papillary muscle, compensatory myocardial hypertrophy, and fibrosis. The mitral or tricuspid valves may become dysfunctional, causing regurgitation. In the AV valve, functional regurgitation may be caused by myocardial infiltration or thickening of the endocardium. When the nodal and conduction tissues are damaged, the SA and AV nodes malfunction. This can cause various amounts of block of both nodes. The primary hemodynamic outcome is diastolic dysfunction. The affected ventricle becomes rigid and noncompliant. There is impaired diastolic filling and a high filling pressure. Pulmonary venous hypertension develops. Systolic function may be greatly impaired if the compensatory hypertrophy of fibrosed or infiltrated ventricles is insufficient. If mural thrombi form, systemic emboli can develop.

Clinical Manifestations

Dilated cardiomyopathy usually develops gradually, except with acute apical ballooning cardiomyopathy, acute myocarditis, and tachyarrhythmia-induced myopathy. There is atypical chest pain in about 25% of cases and other symptoms are based on the affected ventricle. Exertional dyspnea and fatigue are caused by left ventricular dysfunction because of low CO and increased LV diastolic pressure. Peripheral edema and neck vin distention are caused by RV failure. Less often, the RV is mostly affected in a patient of younger age. Atrial arrhythmias and sudden death from malignant ventricular tachyarrhythmias are often seen.

Hypertrophic cardiomyopathy often causes death in younger athletes. It can cause unexplained syncope and never be diagnosed during life. Symptoms between ages 20 and 40 are usually due to exertion but can be varied. They include chest pain that usually resembles typical angina, dyspnea, palpitations, and syncope. Systolic function is adequate, so fatigue is uncommon. Most symptoms come from abnormal diastolic function. Syncope may occur after exertion due to either worsening outflow obstruction with increased contractility, or due to atrial or ventricular arrhythmias. Syncope indicates a higher risk of sudden death. The BP and heart rate are often normal. Increased venous pressure seldom causes any manifestations. With the obstructive type of hypertrophic cardiomyopathy, there is an audible systolic ejection-type murmur that does not radiate out to the neck. It is most easily heard at the left sternal edge, in the third or fourth intercostal space. At the apex, a mitral regurgitation murmur may be heard, because of distortion of the mitral apparatus. The LV outflow ejection murmur may be increased by a **Valsalva maneuver**. This reduces venous return as well as LV diastolic volume.

Restrictive cardiomyopathy causes exertional dyspnea, PND, orthopnea, and peripheral edema. A fixed CO rate causes fatigue because of resistance to ventricular filling. Atrial and ventricular arrhythmias as well as AV block are seen, but angina and fainting are rare. The signs and symptoms closely resemble constrictive pericarditis. During physical examination, the precordium is quiet. There a low-volume yet rapid carotid pulse, with pulmonary crackles. Sometimes there is a murmur due to functional mitral or tricuspid regurgitation.

Diagnosis

Dilated cardiomyopathy is diagnosed based on patient history and physical examination, plus excluding other causes of ventricular failure. These include primary valvular disorders, systemic hypertension, and MI. When there is no obvious cause, family history should be taken carefully, identifying anyone related to the patient that have early-onset heart disease or HF. There should be discussion of anyone in the family that suddenly died from a heart-related condition. Many facilities screen first-degree family members for cardiac dysfunction by using echocardiography, chest X-rays, ECG, and cardiac MRI. For some individuals, an endo-myocardial biopsy is performed.

If a patient has chest pain or acute symptoms of dilated cardiomyopathy, serum cardiac biomarkers are measured. Elevation of troponin is common along with HF, primarily with decreased kidney function. When HF exists, serum **natriuretic peptides** are usually elevated. If there is no obvious cause, iron-binding capacity, serum ferritin, fasting blood glucose, and thyroid-stimulating hormone levels are assessed. For some cases, serologic tests are performed to check for coxsackievirus, echovirus, HIV, *Toxoplasma*, and *T. cruzi*. A chest X-ray will show cardiomegaly that commonly affects all heart chambers. Right-sided pleural effusion is more common than on the left side, and is often present with interstitial edema and increased pulmonary venous pressure.

Electrocardiogram may reveal nonspecific ST-segment depression, with inverted T waves or low voltage, and sinus tachycardia. Pathologic Q waves may or may not be present in the precordial leads. This simulates a previous MI. Also common are atrial fibrillation and left bundle branch block. On echocardiography, there are hypokinetic and dilated heart chambers. This technique can rule out any primary valvular disorders. With dilated cardiomyopathy, segmental wall motion abnormalities may be present, since the condition can be irregular. A mural thrombus may also be seen. Today, cardiac MRI has become more popular and available, and provides detailed images of the structure and function of the myocardium. An MRI with gadolinium contrast can reveal abnormal myocardial tissue textures, or a "scarred" pattern, such as with late gadolinium enhancement (LGE). This can be diagnostic for active myocarditis, Chagas disease, muscular dystrophy, or sarcoidosis.

Positron-emission tomography (PET) is sensitive for diagnosing cardiac sarcoidosis. Coronary angiography can exclude CAD as being causative of LV dysfunction if the diagnosis is doubted following noninvasive tests. Chest pain and cardiovascular risk factors are often related to CAD, and older patients are more likely to have this disease. During catheterization, both ventricles can be biopsied. This is done selectively, if results are anticipated to influence treatment. Endomyocardial biopsy is used if there is suspected eosinophilic myocarditis, giant cell myocarditis, or sarcoidosis.

Hypertrophic cardiomyopathy is diagnosed based on the common murmur and the patient's symptoms. A history of unexplained fainting or a family history of sudden death that is unexplained prompts diagnosis. In any young athlete, unexplained fainting should always increase suspicion. Though they cause similar symptoms, hypertrophic cardiomyopathy must be distinguished from aortic stenosis and CAD. Infiltrative cardiac disorders such as amyloid heart disease and Anderson-Fabry disease can mimic hypertrophic cardiomyopathy. The best noninvasive tests include ECG and two-dimensional echocardiography, with or without MRI. Chest X-rays are usually normal since the ventricles are not dilated, but the left atrium can be enlarged. For sustained arrhythmias or syncope, the patient should be hospitalized. For high risk patients, exercise testing and 24-hour ambulatory monitoring may be effective. However, it is hard to identify these patients.

On ECG, there is usually the voltage criteria for LV hypertrophy. Extremely deep septal Q waves are often present along with asymmetric septal hypertrophy. Hypertrophic cardiomyopathy may produce a QRS complex in V1 and V2 that simulates an earlier septal infarction. There are usually abnormal T waves. Usually, there is a deep symmetric T-wave inversion. An ST-segment depression is common – especially with the apical obliterative subtype. The P wave is usually broad and notched. A biphasic P wave may indicate left atrial hypertrophy. There is increased incidence of a preexcitation phenomenon that is of the **Wolff-Parkinson-White syndrome** type that can cause palpitations. Bundle branch block is often seen. The 2-D Doppler echocardiography technique can determine the severity of hypertrophy and the amount of outflow tract obstruction, which are used to monitor effects of medical or surgical treatments. Cardiac catheterization is performed if invasive therapy is being considered. There is usually no significant stenosis of the coronary arteries. However, older patients may also have CAD. Genetic biomarkers do not identify people at high risk or affect treatment, though genetic testing may help in the screening of family members.

Restrictive cardiomyopathy is considered when there is HF and preserved ejection fraction. This is especially true if a systemic disorder that can cause restrictive cardiomyopathy has already been diagnosed. Required studies include ECG, chest X-ray, and echocardiography. An ECG is usually nonspecific. In chest X-rays, the heart is normal or small, but may be enlarged if there is late-stage amyloidosis or hemochromatosis. Normal LV ejection fraction is seen in echocardiography. Elevated LV filling pressures are often suggested in Doppler imaging of cardiac tissues.

If diagnosis is still not clear, an MRI can reveal abnormal myocardial texture when there is myocardial infiltration, such as by amyloid or iron. An MRI and cardiac CT can find pericardial thickening. This helps to diagnose the similar pericardial constriction that mimics restrictive cardiomyopathy. When required, cardiac catheterization and endomyocardial biopsy can be diagnostic. A biopsy can find endocardial fibrosis and thickening as well as iron or amyloid infiltration of the myocardium, and chronic myocardial fibrosis. If Fabry disease is present, biopsy can find inclusions in the vascular endothelial cytoplasm. Various tests and biopsies of different organ systems that causes restrictive cardiomyopathy must be done. These include fat pad biopsy (for amyloidosis) and liver biopsy or iron tests (for hemochromatosis).

Treatment

Initial treatments of *dilated cardiomyopathy* involve correcting treatable causes such as acute Chagas disease, toxoplasmosis, hemochromatosis, diabetes mellites, beriberi, or thyrotoxicosis. If HIV infection is present, antiretroviral therapy (ART) is very important. Immunosuppression is only used for patients that have had a biopsy indicating the presence of eosinophilic myocarditis, giant cell myocarditis, or sarcoidosis. Other treatments are also used for HF such as ACE inhibitors, aldosterone receptor blockers, beta-blockers, ARBs, ARNIs, hydralazine/nitrates, digoxin, and diuretics. Patients with idiopathic dilated cardiomyopathy respond very well to the standard treatments for HF. They usually respond better to these than patients that have ischemic heart disease. For peripartum dilated cardiomyopathy, ACE inhibitors and ARBs must be avoided because they can harm the fetus. These drugs are also not indicated while breastfeeding. Previously oral anticoagulation was used in other types of cardiomyopathies to prevent mural thrombus. Medical treatment reduces risks of arrhythmia, but implantable cardioverter-defibrillators can prevent death from sudden arrhythmia when there is continually reduced ejection fraction even with medical therapy. These devices may be required if AV block continues or develops in the chronic dilated phase. A popular choice is called dual-chamber implantable cardioverter-defibrillator (ICD) with a pacemaker backup. Left ventricular assist devices (LVAD) may be an alternative option. Patients under age 70 are given priority for heart transplantation because of the scarcity of donor hearts.

The treatment of *hypertrophic cardiomyopathy* is based on the disease's phenotype. Without obstruction, there is usually a stable course with no significant symptoms. Some patients have symptoms of HF because of diastolic dysfunction. Treatment usually involves beta-blockers and calcium channel blockers with heart rate-limiting effects that have a lower ability to dilate the arteries – such as verapamil. These drugs

can be used alone or together. As the heart rate is slowed, the diastolic filling period is lengthened. This can increase LV filling when there is diastolic dysfunction. For the obstructive phenotype, treatment is also focused on reducing the outflow tract gradient. This can be accomplished via the negative inotropic effects of the nondihydropyridine calcium channel blockers, beta-blockers, and disopyramide, which seems to be the most effective drug for patients that have a resting gradient. The beta-blockers are the best at reducing the gradient that occurs with exercise.

Invasive treatment is needed for patents with symptoms from significant outflow tract gradients 50 mm Hg or higher, even with medical therapy. Surgical myectomy can provide low death rates during surgery and excellent results. An alternative, used for older patients and those at high surgical risk, is percutaneous catheter alcohol septal ablation. Any drug that reduces preload decreases the size of the heart chambers and makes the signs and symptoms worse. These drugs include diuretics, nitrates, ACE inhibitors, and ARBs. Vasodilators also worsen ventricular diastolic function by increasing the outflow tract gradient, resulting in reflex tachycardia. The inotropic drugs worsen outflow tract obstruction. They do not relieve high end-diastolic pressure and can cause arrhythmias. These drugs include catecholamines and digitalis glycosides. A newer drug that may be beneficial is mavacamtem, an oral cardiac myosin inhibitor. The drug also reduces LV outflow tract obstruction and increases exercise tolerance.

An ICD should, in most cases, be placed if the patient has had syncope or sudden cardiac arrest, as well as when continual ventricular arrhythmia is confirmed. Defibrillators may not be required without these manifestations. Previously, it was advised that patients with hypertrophic cardiomyopathy avoid competitive sports. Today, it is recommended that diagnosed athletes have a comprehensive evaluation and discuss possible risks with a person that is an expert on the condition. For the dilated congestive phase, treatment is the same as for dilated cardiomyopathy with predominant systolic dysfunction. With asymmetric septal hypertrophy, genetic counseling is suggested.

For *restrictive cardiomyopathy*, diuretics can be used for edema or pulmonary vascular congestion. They must be give carefully since they can lower preload. Noncompliant ventricles require preload in order to maintain CO. Digoxin cannot greatly change hemodynamic abnormalities. It can cause serious arrhythmias if amyloidosis is present, since extreme digitalis sensitivity often occurs. For elevated heart rate, beta-blockers or rate-limiting calcium channel blockers may be used carefully, only in low doses. Nitrates and other agents that reduce afterload are not useful since they can cause extreme hypotension. For an early diagnosis, treatment of certain types of amyloidosis, hemochromatosis, *Löffler syndrome*, and sarcoidosis may be helpful.

Prevention

Dilated cardiomyopathy is not preventable. To prevent or reduce its complications, the general recommendations for cardiomyopathies are suggested. These include avoiding smoking, only drinking alcohol in moderation, avoiding cocaine and illegal drugs, a low-sodium diet, maintaining a healthy weight, exercising as part of a physician-recommended program, getting adequate rest and sleep, and managing stress. There is also no known prevention for hypertrophic cardiomyopathy. However, genetic testing is recommended to screen for the condition in families. Likewise, restrictive cardiomyopathy is not preventable.

Prognosis

Dilated cardiomyopathy has had a poor prognosis, but this has improved with use of beta-blockers, ACE inhibitors, mineralocorticoid receptor antagonists, implantable cardioverter-defibrillators, and cardiac resynchronization therapy. Within the first year, about 20% of patients die. After that, about 10% of patients die each year. Between 40% and 50% of deaths are sudden because of an embolic event or a **malignant arrhythmia**. Prognosis is improved if compensatory hypertrophy can preserve ventricular wall thickness. However, prognosis is worsened if there is extensive thinning of the ventricular walls, as well as dilation of the ventricle. When well-compensated with treatment, patients with dilated cardiomyopathy can remain stable for many years.

Hypertrophic cardiomyopathy is fatal in about 1% of adult cases every year, but is higher for pediatric patients. Sudden death is the most common outcome. Less often, patients experience chronic HF. There is a higher risk for sudden death with family history of this condition, cardiac arrest, or chronic ventricular arrhythmias. Additional higher risks are with patient history of unexplained fainting, cardiac arrest, or chronic ventricular arrhythmias. The prognosis of *restrictive cardiomyopathy* is poor, since diagnosis is usually made late in the disease course. Care is symptomatic and supportive for most cases. Patients with restrictive cardiomyopathy cannot tolerate the treatments used for dilated cardiomyopathy.

CLINICAL CASE

1. What is the definition of dilated cardiomyopathy?
2. What features are implicated when dilated cardiomyopathy occurs in someone with diabetes mellitus?
3. How are implantable cardioverter-defibrillators able to help patients with dilated cardiomyopathy?

A 61-year-old man was hospitalized because of fainting without any obvious cause. His heart rate was normal. Previously, his health had been classified as class III dyspnea after exertion without angina. His previous history included type 2 diabetes mellitus. Over the past 3 years, he had recurring episodes of feeling faint but not actually fainting. Dilated cardiomyopathy had been diagnosed with a LV ejection fraction of 20%. The patient was taking captopril, carvedilol, furosemide, and an oral anticoagulant. In the hospital, the patient's BP was 100/60 mm Hg with a heart rate of 76 BPM. There was a complete left bundle branch block. An electrophysiology study revealed inducible ventricular tachycardia. The chosen therapy was a dual-chamber ICD with a pacemaker backup, known as a DDD-ICD. After several months, the patient's condition was downgraded to class II and there were no more episodes of fainting.

ANSWERS

1. Dilated cardiomyopathy is myocardial dysfunction that results in HF, with ventricular dilation and systolic dysfunction.
2. With diabetes mellitus, cardiomyopathy is related to features that include lower diastolic compliance, interstitial fibrosis, and myocyte hypertrophy.
3. Implantable cardioverter-defibrillators can prevent death from sudden arrhythmia in patients with dilated cardiomyopathy when there is continually reduced ejection fraction, even with medical therapy. These devices may be required if AV block continues or develops in the chronic dilated phase.

PULMONARY EDEMA

Pulmonary edema involves a rapid movement of plasma fluid from the pulmonary capillaries into the interstitial spaces and alveoli. There is acute, severe LV failure, with alveolar flooding and pulmonary venous hypertension. The condition develops because of a sudden increase in LV filling pressure. Diabetic pulmonary edema may be related to cardiovascular disease or complications as well as the use of medications to control diabetes.

Epidemiology

Cases of pulmonary edema related to CHF are increasing in prevalence, most likely as a secondary effect because of global aging of the population. Incidence is highest in older adults. Globally, pulmonary is very common along with HF and low ejection fraction. An estimated 75,000–83,000 people experience pulmonary edema out of every 100,000 that have HF and low ejection fraction. Only about half of all patients discharged after hospitalization for HF with pulmonary edema will survive for 1 year. Mortality rates at 6 years of follow-up are at 85% of patients. Males are affected more often than female, and most are over age 65. There is no specific racial or ethnic predilection.

Etiology and Risk Factors

Approximately 50% of all cases of pulmonary edema are a result of acute coronary ischemia. Sometimes the condition is due to decompensation of extreme HF, which includes HF with preserved ejection fraction due to hypertension. The remainder of cases are due to arrhythmia, acute volume overload that is often linked to IV fluids, or an acute valvular disorder. Often, patients that do not follow their medication or dietary regimens develop pulmonary edema. Primary risk factors include MI, hypertensive heart disease, dilated cardiomyopathy, and valvular dysfunction. Additional risk factors include arrhythmias, congenital heart disease, diabetes mellitus, excessive alcohol use, and sleep apnea. Pulmonary edema that complicates diabetic ketoacidosis may be caused by increased permeability of the pulmonary capillary membranes and abnormal intravascular colloid/hydrostatic forces. Other risk factors include high altitudes, narcotic overdose, and pulmonary embolism.

Pathophysiology

An abnormal increase in extravascular lung water can be caused by physiologic changes that include an imbalance of **Starling force**, changes in valvular capillary membrane permeability, and lymphatic insufficiency. Fluid flux across capillary walls is normally controlled by a balance between hydrostatic and osmotic pressure gradients, between the interstitial space and capillaries. With cardiogenic pulmonary edema, the most common pathophysiological mechanism is an increase in pulmonary capillary pressure.

Clinical Manifestations

Pulmonary edema causes anxiety because of a sensation of suffocation, severe dyspnea, and restlessness. Often, there is coughing that produces a reddened sputum, cyanosis, pallor, and extreme sweating. There may be frothing from the mouth, but extreme **hemoptysis** is rare. While the BP can be variable, the pulse is rapid but of low volume. Significant hypertension indicates that the cardiac reserve is increased. A dangerous sign is hypotension in which the systolic BP is lower than 100 mg Hg. Over both lung fields, inspiratory fine crackles are dispersed anteriorly and posteriorly. Severe cardiac asthma may develop, causing wheezing. Efforts to breathe are noisy and often complicate auscultation of heart sounds. A merger of the third and fourth heart sounds, known as a **summation gallop**, may develop. Signs of RV failure may occur, including neck vein distention and peripheral edema.

Diagnosis

Pulmonary edema causes signs and symptoms that can mimic an exacerbation of COPD. The edema may be the primary symptom when the patient has no history of cardiac disorders. An immediate chest X-ray is usually sufficient for diagnosis and reveals extreme interstitial edema. If the diagnosis is still not confirmed, the serum brain natriuretic peptide (BNP)/N-terminal (NT)-prohormone BNP levels can be measured. They are elevated if pulmonary edema is present, but are normal if COPD is exacerbated. Other evaluations include blood tests, ECG, and pulse oximetry. The blood tests include cardiac biomarkers, BUN, electrolytes, and creatinine. For extremely ill patients, arterial blood gas measurements are taken. To determine the cause of pulmonary edema and select the best treatment, echocardiography may be done. Other factors to evaluate include severe hypoxemia and carbon dioxide retention, which is a late and severely negative sign of secondary hypoventilation.

Treatment

Treatment of pulmonary edema begins with 100% oxygen administered via a nonrebreather mask. The patient is kept in an upright position.

Furosemide is given by IV or continuous infusion. Nitroglycerin is administered sublingually, followed by an IV drip that is titrated upwards every 5 minutes as needed. Intravenous morphine has been used for severe anxiety and to reduce the breathing difficulties, but today is used mostly palliatively since studies have shown it is linked to worsened outcomes. If there is significant hypoxia, noninvasive ventilatory assistance is given by using bilevel positive airway pressure. Tracheal intubation and mechanical ventilation are needed if there is carbon dioxide retention or the patient is non-alert or not fully conscious.

Additional treatments are based on the cause of pulmonary edema. If there is rapid atrial fibrillation, cardioversion is done. Intravenous beta-blockers, digoxin, or careful use of calcium channel blockers can slow the ventricular rate. Intravenous vasodilators are used for severe hypertension. For acute MI or another acute coronary syndrome, treatments include thrombolysis or direct percutaneous coronary angioplasty, with or without stenting. The fluid status is usually normal before pulmonary edema develops. Therefore, diuretics may be not useful when patients have acute decompensation of chronic HF, and can precipitate hypotension. When systolic BP is lower than 100 mg Hg or there is shock, IV dobutamine and counterpulsation with an intra-aortic balloon pump may be needed. Direct-current cardioversion is used for ventricular or supraventricular tachycardia. Newer drugs are available but do not improve outcomes greatly, and can even be implicated in the death of the patient. These include intravenous BNP (nesiritide), ibopamine, levosimendan, pimobendane, and vesnarinone. Once the patient is stabilized, long-term treatment for HF is started.

Prevention

The prevention of pulmonary edema involves managing any existing heart or lung conditions. Patients are advised to control cholesterol and blood pressure via a heart-healthy diet, regular exercise, weight management, avoiding smoking, limiting alcohol and salt intake, and managing stress.

Prognosis

The prognosis of pulmonary edema is based on the cause, and the condition can resolve slowly or quickly. Breathing assistance may be required for a long period of time. Without treatment, prognosis is worsened, since the condition can be life-threatening.

COR PULMONALE

Cor pulmonale is defined as enlargement of the right ventricle because of a lung disorder (of the lung itself or its blood vessels) that results in pulmonary artery hypertension. The condition then leads to failure of the right ventricle. Cor pulmonale is chronic condition in most cases. However, it can be acute and even reversible. When diabetes mellitus is present, it increases the likelihood of the patient developing COPD.

Epidemiology

Global incidence of cor pulmonale is widely varied between countries, based on the prevalence of air pollution, smoking, and the risk factors for different lung diseases. Even though statistics show that COPD affects about 15 million people have COPD, exact prevalence of cor pulmonale is difficult to assess. This is because examination and testing are not highly sensitive in the detection of pulmonary hypertension and dysfunction of the RV. It is estimated that cor pulmonale makes up 7% of all types of adult heart disease. Deaths of patients that also have COPD are higher than in patients with COPD that do not have cor pulmonale. The disease makes up 10%–30% of hospitalizations for decompensated HF. Most patients that first develop cor pulmonale are in their 50s. It is more prevalent in males, partly because more men smoke tobacco products throughout the world than women. There is no clear indication that any specific racial or ethnic group has more cases of cor pulmonale.

Etiology and Risk Factors

Chronic cor pulmonale is usually due to COPD, but less common causes include chronic and unresolved pulmonary embolism, idiopathic alveolar hypotension, kyphoscoliosis, neuromuscular disorders affecting the respiratory muscles, obesity accompanied by alveolar hypoventilation, pulmonary veno-occlusive disorders or interstitial fibrosis, systemic sclerosis, and surgery or trauma that causes extensive loss of lung tissue. Diabetes mellitus is also implicated if it is present because it makes individuals 22% more likely to have COPD. Diabetes also harms the lungs by causing increased cases of pulmonary fibrosis, pneumonia, and asthma. With weakened lungs, the heart must work much harder, increasing likelihood for outcomes such as cor pulmonale. The only causes of acute cor pulmonale are injuries due to mechanical ventilation (often in patients with acute respiratory distress syndrome) and massive pulmonary embolization.

Pathophysiology

Pathophysiological mechanisms that influence the development of cor pulmonale include increased alveolar pressure, loss of capillary beds, medial hypertrophy in the arterioles, and vasoconstriction. Increased alveolar pressure may be due to mechanical ventilation. Loss of capillary beds may be caused by thrombosis in pulmonary embolism or because of bullous changes as part of COPD. Medial hypertrophy of the arterioles is often related to pulmonary hypertension caused by a variety of factors, and vasoconstriction can be caused by hypercapnia, hypoxia, or both. Afterload on the RV is increased by pulmonary hypertension. There is then an event cascade that is like the steps of LV failure. They include elevated end-diastolic and central venous pressure, with ventricular hypertrophy and dilation. Increased blood viscosity may increase demands upon the RV. The increased viscosity may be caused by hypoxia-influenced **polycythemia**. In rare cases, RV failure affects the LV when a septum is dysfunctional and bulges into the LV. This interferes with filling and results in diastolic dysfunction.

Clinical Manifestations

Cor pulmonale begins without symptoms except for dyspnea or exertional fatigue caused by an underlying lung disorder. With increased RV pressures, physical signs often include a left parasternal systolic lift, murmurs from functional tricuspid and pulmonic insufficiency, and a loud pulmonic component of the second heart sound. Later manifestations include distended jugular veins, hepatomegaly, leg edema, and an RV gallop rhythm of the third and fourth heart sounds.

Diagnosis

When any of the identified causes are present, cor pulmonale should be suspected. On chest X-rays, there is enlargement of the proximal pulmonary artery with distal arterial attenuation, and enlargement of the RV. On ECG, hypertrophy of the RV is linked to the amount of pulmonary hypertension. This is indicated by a QR wave and a dominant R wave, plus right axis deviation. Since pulmonary hyperinflation and bullae caused by COPD realign the heart, this means that diagnosis may be difficult via physical examination, X-rays, and ECG. To evaluate LV and RV function, echocardiography or radionuclide imaging is performed. Echocardiography assesses the systolic pressure in the RV, but may be limited because of the underlying lung disorder. For some patients, cardiac MRI can assess the heart chambers and their function. Right heart catheterization may be needed to confirm the diagnosis.

Treatment

The treatment of cor pulmonale is based on the cause, and to reduce hypoxia. It is important to diagnose and treat the condition before structural changes occur and cannot be reversed. Diuretics are only used for peripheral edema if there is LV failure plus pulmonary fluid overload. They must be used carefully since small preload decreases can worsen the disease. Pulmonary vasodilators are not effective. Digoxin is only effective if there is LV dysfunction, but it must be used with caution if the patient has COPD. Phlebotomy to decrease blood viscosity is not done unless there is significant polycythemia. For chronic cor pulmonale, long-term use of anticoagulants reduce the likelihood of venous thromboembolism.

Prevention

The prevention of cor pulmonale is based on lifestyle changes that protect the lungs and heart. Overall measures include regular exercise, a heart-healthy diet, maintaining a healthy weight, and avoiding smoking.

Prognosis

The prognosis for cor pulmonale is based on managing pulmonary hypertension. Without treatment, the condition is life-threatening.

KEY TERMS

- Acromegaly
- Afterload
- Amyloidosis
- Beriberi
- Cachexia
- Cardiomyopathy
- Chagas disease
- Cheyne-Stokes respirations
- Coarctation
- Dilated cardiomyopathy
- Ebstein anomaly
- Eisenmenger syndrome
- Fabry disease
- Frank-Starling principle
- Hemochromatosis
- Hemoptysis
- Hyperpneic
- Hypertrophic cardiomyopathy
- Kussmaul sign
- Löffler syndrome
- Malignant arrhythmia
- Natriuretic peptides
- Neurofibromatosis
- Orthopnea
- Paget disease
- Paroxysmal nocturnal dyspnea
- Pheochromocytoma
- Polycythemia
- Preload
- Restrictive cardiomyopathy
- Silhouette
- Starling force
- Stroke volume
- Summation gallop
- Thyrotoxicosis
- Toxoplasmosis
- Valsalva maneuver
- Wolff-Parkinson-White syndrome

REFERENCES

AHA Journals / Circulation. (2005). *Epidemiology and Etiology of Cardiomyopathy in Africa*. American Heart Association, Inc. https://www.ahajournals.org/doi/10.1161/circulationaha.105.542894

Bakris, G.L. (2012). *The Kidney in Heart Failure*. Springer.

Baliga, R.R., and Eagle, K.A. (2020). *Practical Cardiology: Evaluation and Treatment of Common Cardiovascular Disorders*, 3rd Edition. Springer.

Cleveland Clinic. (2021). *Restrictive Cardiomyopathy*. Cleveland Clinic. https://my.clevelandclinic.org/health/diseases/17427-restrictive-cardiomyopathy

DeMello, W.C., and Frohlich, E.D. (2010). *Renin Angiotensin System and Cardiovascular Disease (Contemporary Cardiology)*. Humana Press.

Domanski, M.J., Mehra, M.R., and Pfeffer, M.A. (2016). *Oxford Textbook of Advanced Heart Failure and Cardiac Transplantation (Oxford Textbooks in Cardiology)*. Oxford University Press.

Dumitrescu, S.I., Tintoiu, I.C., and Underwood, M.J. (2018). *Right Heart Pathology – From Mechanism to Management*. Springer.

Eisen, H. (2017). *Heart Failure: A Comprehensive Guide to Pathophysiology and Clinical Care*. Springer.

Estenson, J.G. (2015). *Cor Pulmonale – A Resource and Reference Guide for Patients and Health Care Professionals, Book 131*. Capitol Hill Press.

Felker, G.M., and Mann, D.L. (2019). *Heart Failure: A Companion to Braunwald's Heart Disease*, 4th Edition. Elsevier.

Garry, D.J., Wilson, R.F., and Vlodaver, Z. (2017). *Congestive Heart Failure and Cardiac Transplantation: Clinical, Pathology, Imaging and Molecular Profiles*. Springer.

Green, M., Krahn, A., and Alqarawi, W. (2020). *Electrocardiography of Inherited Arrhythmias and Cardiomyopathies – From Basic Science to Clinical Practice*. Springer.

Healthline. (2017). *Lifestyle Changes*. Healthline Media. https://www.healthline.com/health/cor-pulmonale#prevention

Henein, M.Y. (2010). *Heart Failure in Clinical Practice*. Springer.

Hosenpud, J.D., and Greenberg, B.H. (2006). *Congestive Heart Failure*, 3rd Edition. Lippincott, Williams, and Wilkins.

Jacob, E. (2013). *Medifocus Guidebook on: Congestive Heart Failure – A Comprehensive Guide to Symptoms, Treatment, Research, and Support*. Medifocus.com, Inc.

Jaski, B.E. (2015). *The 4 Stages of Heart Failure*. Cardiotext Publishing.

Kenny, T. (2007). *The Nuts and Bolts of Cardiac Resynchronization Therapy*. Blackwell Futura.

Klein, A.L., and Garcia, M.J. (2020). *Diastology: Clinical Approach to Heart Failure with Preserved Ejection Fraction*. Elsevier.

Lewin, M.B., and Stout, K.K. (2012). *Echocardiography in Congenital Heart Disease (Practical Echocardiography Series)*. Elsevier.

Mann, D.L. (2010). *Heart Failure: A Companion to Braunwald's Heart Disease*, 2nd Edition. Elsevier.

Maron, B.J., and Salberg, L. (2014). *A Guide to Hypertrophic Cardiomyopathy: For Patients, Their Families, and Interested Physicians*, 3rd Edition. Wiley-Blackwell.

Mayo Clinic. (2021a). *Dilated Cardiomyopathy*. Mayo Foundation for Medical Education and Research (MFMER). https://www.mayoclinic.org/diseases-conditions/dilated-cardiomyopathy/symptoms-causes/syc-20353149

Mayo Clinic. (2021b). *Pulmonary Edema*. Mayo Foundation for Medical Education and Research (MFMER). https://www.mayoclinic.org/diseases-conditions/pulmonary-edema/symptoms-causes/syc-20377009

Mayo Clinic. (2021c). *Strategies to Prevent Heart Disease*. Mayo Foundation for Medical Education and Research (MFMER). https://www.mayoclinic.org/diseases-conditions/heart-disease/in-depth/heart-disease-prevention/art-20046502

McCarthy, P.M., and Young, J.B. (2008). *Heart Failure: A Combined Medical and Surgical Approach*. Blackwell Futura.

MedicineNet. (2020). *At What Age Does Hypertrophic Cardiomyopathy Develop?* MedicineNet. https://www.medicinet.com/when_does_hypertrophic_cardiomyopathy_develop/article.htm

Mieszczanska, H.Z., and Budzikowski, A.S. (2018). *Cardiology Consult Manual*. Springer.

Nicholson, C. (2007). *Heart Failure: A Clinical Nursing Handbook, Book 17*. Wiley-Interscience.

Oxford Academic / European Heart Journal. (2017). *Affairs of the Heart: Outcomes in Men and Women with Hypertrophic Cardiomyopathy*. Oxford University Press. https://academic.oup.com/eurheartj/article/38/46/3441/4642969

Penn Medicine. (2021). *Pulmonary Edema*. Penn Medicine / The Trustees of the University of Pennsylvania. https://www.pennmedicine.org/for-patients-and-visitors/patient-information/conditions-treated-a-to-z/pulmonary-edema

Sinagra, G., Merlo, M., and Pinamonti, B. (2019). *Dilated Cardiomyopathy: From Genetics to Clinical Management*. Springer Open.

Smiseth, O.A., and Tendera, M. (2007). *Diastolic Heart Failure*. Springer.

Starr, M. (2014). *Heart Attacks, Heart Failure, and Diabetes*. New Voice Publications.

StatPearls. (2021). *Cor Pulmonale*. StatPearls. https://www.statpearls.com/articlelibrary/viewarticle/19975/

Toth, P.P., and Cannon, C.P. (2011). *Comprehensive Cardiovascular Medicine in the Primary Care Setting (Contemporary Cardiology)*. Humana Press.

Tsao, L., and Afari, M.E. (2020). *Clinical Cases in Right Heart Failure (Clinical Cases in Cardiology)*. Springer.

U.S. National Library of Medicine / National Institutes of Health / Cardiovascular Journal of Africa. (2007). *Race and Gender Representation of Hypertrophic Cardiomyopathy or Long QT Syndrome Cases in a South African Research Setting*. National Center for Biotechnology Information / U.S. National Library of Medicine. https://www.ncbi.nlm.nih.gov/pmc/articles/PMC3975543/

U.S. National Library of Medicine / National Institutes of Health / British Journal of Clinical Pharmacology. (1999). *Clinical Case Studies in Heart Failure Management*. National Center for Biotechnology Information / U.S. National Library of Medicine. https://www.ncbi.nlm.nih.gov/pmc/articles/PMC2014219/

VeryWellHealth. (2020). *What Is Restrictive Cardiomyopathy?* About, Inc. (Dotdash). https://www.verywellhealth.com/what-is-restrictive-cardiomyopathy-4082933

Wassermann, S. (2012). *Acute Cardiac Pulmonary Edema.* Literary Licensing, LLC.

Wiley Online Library / Journal of Internal Medicine. (2019). *Dilated Cardiomyopathy: From Epidemiologic to Genetic Phenotypes.* John Wiley & Sons, Inc. https://onlinelibrary.wiley.com/doi/full/10.1111/joim.12944

Williams, A.D., Capitanio, N., and Hayes, A. (2010). *Skeletal Muscle in Heart Failure and Type 2 Diabetes (Muscular System-Anatomy, Functions and Injuries).* Nova Biomedical.

CHAPTER 11 Stroke

A stroke occurs when a brain artery becomes blocked, or it ruptures. An area of brain tissue becomes necrotic as its blood supply is lost. This is known as a cerebral infarction. Approximately 14 million new strokes occur globally every year. Symptoms develop quickly. Most strokes are ischemic, usually caused by arterial blockage, and fewer are hemorrhagic, caused by arterial rupture. Transient ischemic attacks are like ischemic strokes, except that symptom usually resolve in less than 1 hour, and there is no permanent brain damage. Since diabetes mellitus increases risk factors for hypertension and high cholesterol, there are increased chances for having a stroke or heart attack. Adults with diabetes are about two times as likely to have a stroke or heart disease compared to adults without diabetes.

CLASSIFICATIONS

A *stroke* is clinically termed a *cerebrovascular accident* (CVA). Strokes are heterogeneous disorders signified by a focal, sudden interruption of blood flow within the cerebrum. They result in neurologic deficits. Most strokes are *ischemic*, but less often, *hemorrhagic* strokes occur. Strokes of either type constitute the fifth most common cause of death in the United States. There are approximately 14 million new strokes that occur globally every year. About 1 in 4 people over the age of 25 have some form of stroke. Nearly 60% of all strokes annually occur in people under age 70, with 52% occurring in men and 48% occurring in women. Strokes are also are the most common cause of neurologic deficits in adults. The arteries of the brain that are affected by strokes include those of the anterior and posterior circulation (see Figure 11.1). They may be the branches of the internal carotid artery (anterior circulation) or the branches of the vertebral and basilar arteries (posterior circulation). The anterior cerebral artery supplies the medial areas of the frontal and parietal lobes, along with the **corpus callosum**. The middle cerebral artery supplies large areas of the surfaces of the frontal, parietal, and temporal lobes. From the anterior and middle cerebral arteries – also called the **lenticulostriate arteries** – branches supply the anterior limb of the **internal capsule** and the **basal ganglia**. The brainstem, cerebellum, medial temporal lobe, and posterior cerebral cortex are supplied by the basilar and vertebral arteries. Bifurcation of the posterior cerebral arteries, from the basilar artery, supplies the medial temporal lobe including the **hippocampus**, occipital lobe, *geniculate* and mammillary bodies, and thalamus. There is a communication between the anterior and posterior circulation within the **circle of Willis**.

Ischemic Stroke

An *ischemic stroke* is usually the result of thrombosis or embolism. Ischemic stroke makes up at least 80% of all cases of CVAs. Sudden neurologic deficits occur because of focal cerebral ischemia. This is related to permanent brain infarction, which can be positively determined via diffusion-weighted MRI. Diabetes is a well-known modifiable risk factor for ischemic stroke.

Epidemiology

According to the World Stroke Organization, there were over 9.5 million new cases of ischemic stroke in 2016. However, over 67.5 million people either had a new ischemic stroke or had one previously. Nearly 60% of these occurred in people younger than 70 years of age. Approximately 61% of people currently living with complications of an ischemic stroke are under the age of 70. About 52% of cases of ischemic stroke occurred in men and 48% in women. In the United States, an estimated 636,000–795,000 cases of ischemic stroke occur annually. Between 82% and 92% of strokes in the United States are ischemic. At earlier ages, ischemic stroke causes more mortality and morbidity in men, but this reverses for women that are elderly. Risks of having a first stroke are nearly two times higher for African Americans than for Caucasians, and African Americans also have the highest rates of death from ischemic stroke. While overall death rates have been declining over decades, Hispanic Americans have seen an increase in death rates since 2013.

Etiology and Risk Factors

The most common causes of ischemic stroke, in descending order, include *atherothrombotic occlusion of large arteries*, cerebral embolism that is also described as an *embolic infarction*, non-thrombotic occlusion of small and deep cerebral arteries that is also called a **lacunar infarction**, and proximal arterial stenosis accompanied by hypotension that decreases cerebral blood flow within arterial areas described as **watershed zones**. This last and least common cause of ischemic stroke is referred to as **hemodynamic stroke**. The common causes of ischemic stroke are classified as the following, from most common to least:

■ *Cardioembolism* – Emboli can occlude any portion of the cerebral arterial tree and may originate as cardiac thrombi. The most common causes of this are atrial fibrillation, mitral stenosis as part of rheumatic heart disease, myocardial infarction, bacterial endocarditis with heart valve vegetations, prosthetic heart

DOI: 10.1201/9781003226727-14

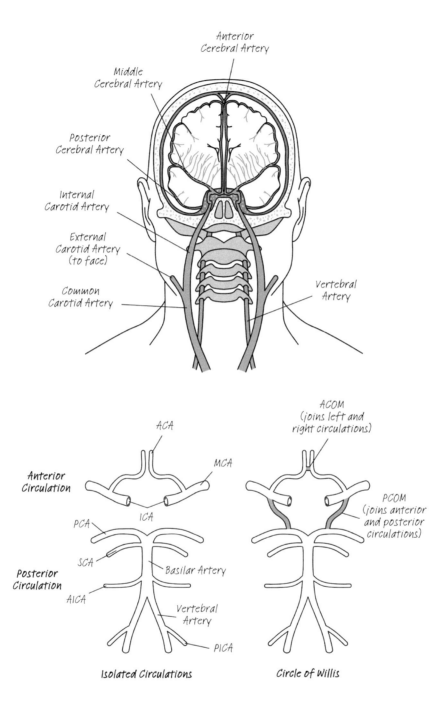

Figure 11.1 Arteries of the brain that are affected by strokes, including the anterior and posterior circulation. (With permission from Berger, W., and Berger, J. (2017). *Case Closed! Neuroanatomy*, 1st Edition. CRC Press/Taylor & Francis.)

valves, and mechanical circulatory assist devices such as a left ventricular assist device. Clots can also form after open-heart surgery or atheromas of the aortic arch or neck arteries. In rare cases, emboli from fractured long bones are made up of fat, or air from decompression sickness, or are venous clots moving from the right side of the heart through a patent foramen ovale with a shunt – known as *paradoxical emboli* – to the left side of the heart. Emboli can spontaneously dislodge or can occur after catheterization or other invasive cardiovascular procedures. In rare cases, an embolic stroke within the vertebral artery or its branches can result from thrombosis of the subclavian artery.

- *Cryptogenic* – There is no obvious cardioembolic, lacunar, or atherosclerotic basis.

- *Large-vessel atherosclerosis* – Affects the intracranial or extracranial arteries. An ulcerated atheroma is highly likely to result in thrombi. Atheromas occur in major cerebral arteries, often where there is turbulent blood flow, and especially at the bifurcation of the carotid artery. Most often, there is partial or complete occlusion by thrombi at the primary trunk of the middle cerebral artery and its branches. Less common occlusions occur in the large arteries of the brain base, deep perforating arteries, and small cortical branches. Occlusion also may occur in the basilar artery and the portion of the internal carotid artery between the **supraclinoid process** and the **cavernous sinus**.

- *Lacunar infarcts* – These are 1.5 cm or less in size and occur from nonatherothrombotic obstruction of smaller perforating arteries supplying deeper cortical structures. Usually, lipohyalinosis is the cause – this is when the small arteria media is degenerated and replaced by collagen and lipids. It is not proven whether emboli can cause lacunar infarcts. They are most often seen in older people with diabetes mellitus or uncontrolled hypertension.

However, there are some rarer causes of ischemic stroke. These include the following:

- *Vascular inflammation* – Resulting from acute or chronic meningitis, syphilis, or vasculitic disorders

- *Hypercoagulability disorders*–**Antiphospholipid syndrome** or **hyperhomocysteinemia**

- *Binswanger disease* – A progressive neurological disorder due to arteriosclerosis and thromboembolism

- *Fibromuscular dysplasia* – In which fibrous cells replace normal flexible cells of the arteries

- *Moyamoya disease* – Narrowing of the brain arteries that leads to blockages

- *Dissection* – Of the aorta or intracranial arteries

- *Hyperviscosity disorders* – Polycythemia, hemoglobinopathies, plasma cell disorders, or thrombocytosis

Sickle cell disease is a relatively common cause of ischemic stroke in children. All types of ischemic strokes are more likely when systemic perfusion is impaired. This may be from carbon monoxide toxicity, severe hypoxia or anemia, hypotension, or polycythemia. Strokes in watershed areas can occur since blood supply is usually low, especially with hypotension or stenotic major cerebral arteries. Rarely, vasospasm or venous sinus thrombosis has been linked to ischemic stroke. Vasospasm can occur after subarachnoid hemorrhage, during a migraine headache, or because of amphetamine or cocaine use. Venous sinus thrombosis can occur during an intracranial infection, after surgery, after childbirth, or because of a hypercoagulability disorder.

Modifiable risk factors that greatly contribute to an increased risk of ischemic stroke include cigarette smoking; hypertension; diabetes mellitus; dyslipidemia; abdominal obesity; insulin resistance; excessive alcohol use; insufficient physical activity; a diet high in calories, saturated fats, and trans fats; psychosocial stress such as depression; drugs such as amphetamines or cocaine; heart conditions – especially those that lead to emboli such as acute myocardial infarction, atrial fibrillation, and infective endocarditis; hypercoagulability; use of exogenous estrogen; and vasculitis. Risk factors for ischemic stroke that cannot be modified include previous stroke, the male gender, older age, the African American racial group, and family history of stroke.

Pathophysiology

When one brain artery has insufficient blood flow, there is often compensation by an efficient collateral system. This is especially seen between the vertebral and carotid arteries, by anastomoses at the circle of Willis. Less often, this occurs between the major arteries that supply the cerebral hemispheres. Collateral flow can be impaired by normal differences in the structure of the circle of Willis, atherosclerosis, different sizes of collateral blood vessels, and from acquired lesions. All of these increase the likelihood of brain ischemia occurring because of blockage of a single artery. Diabetes mellitus leads to ischemic stroke by causing vascular endothelial dysfunction, earlier arterial stiffness, thickening of the capillary basal membranes, and systemic inflammation. Patients with type II diabetes have arteries that are stiffer and decreased elasticity in comparison to those having normal glucose levels. Early structural impairment of the common carotid artery – primarily increased intima-medial thickness – is commonly associated with type 1 diabetes, and is an early sign of atherosclerosis.

Neurons can die when perfusion is less than 5% of normal for more than 5 minutes, however, the amount of damage is based on how severe the ischemia is. In mild cases, damage develops slowly. If perfusion is 40% of normal, brain tissue may not be totally lost until 3–6 hours have passed. Severe ischemia lasting for 15–30 minutes has the potential to destroy all brain tissue. Hyperthermia speeds up the damage, while hypothermia slows it down. For brain tissues that are ischemic but not irreversibly damaged, quickly restoring blood flow can reverse or reduce injury. Moderately ischemic areas called **penumbras** can be saved even if they surround areas of severe ischemia. Penumbras are present because of collateral blood flow. Ischemic injury is caused by the following:

- *Edema* – Resulting from inflammatory mediators such as interleukin-1B or tumor necrosis factor-alpha, and microvascular thrombosis; if severe or widespread, edema may increase intracranial pressure

- *Microvascular thrombosis* – A pathological occlusion of microvessels by thrombi rich in fibrin, platelets, or both

- *Apoptosis* – Programmed cell death

- *Infarction and cell necrosis* – From loss of adenosine triphosphate (ATP), loss of ionic homeostasis such as from altered amounts of intracellular calcium, excitatory neurotoxins such as glutamate, intracellular acidosis from lactate accumulation, and, as mediated by iron, free radicals that cause lipid peroxidative damage to cell membranes

Clinical Manifestations

The signs and symptoms of ischemic stroke are based on the area of the brain that is damaged. Neurologic deficits usually indicate which artery is affected, but not precisely. The abnormalities reach their maximal levels within only several minutes. This is typical of embolic strokes. In fewer cases, deficits evolve over 24–48 hours. This is called an *evolving stroke* and is usually an atherothrombotic stroke. In most evolving strokes, unilateral neurologic dysfunction develops without any fever, headache, or pain. They often begin in one arm and spread **ipsilaterally**. There is usually a step-by-step progression, with periods of stability. A stroke is referred to as *submaximal* when it is over, and later there is some residual function in the area of ischemia, indicating some tissue that is still viable, but at risk of being damaged.

Embolic strokes usually occur during the day and are often preceded by a headache, and then neurologic deficits. Thrombi occur more at night, with the outcome of the stroke seen upon awakening. Lacunar infarcts can cause classic syndromes that involve pure motor **hemiparesis**, ataxic hemiparesis, and pure sensory hemianesthesia. Aphasia and other signs of cortical dysfunction are not present. Multiple lacunar infarcts may cause multiinfarct dementia. As a stroke begins, a seizure can occur. This is more common with embolic strokes. Seizures can also occur even after months or years. Late seizures are caused by hemosiderin deposition or scarring at the area of ischemia. If the patient's condition deteriorates in 48–72 hours after clinical symptom onset – primarily progressive impairment of consciousness – this is usually due to cerebral edema, and not the infarct extending in size. Function usually improves in a few days unless an infarct is extensive. Additional improvement slowly occurs, for up to as long as 1 year.

Diagnosis

The diagnosis of ischemic stroke is based on sudden neurologic deficits related to a certain artery's location. Ischemic stroke is distinguished from **stroke mimics** which cause similar deficits. These include hemorrhagic stroke, hypoglycemia, postictal paralysis – usually involving weakness of the limb contralateral to the seizure focus – and in rare cases, migraine. With ischemic stroke, there are fewer developments such as headache, stupor, vomiting, or coma. There must be assessment of the parenchyma of the brain, blood, large arteries, and heart. It is difficult to differentiate between the types of stroke, but progression of symptoms, the start of onset, and the types of deficits are indicative. Neuroimaging and bedside glucose testing are always performed. History, examination, and neuroimaging are not enough to distinguish between embolic, thrombotic, and lacunar strokes. Therefore, tests are done to identify the causes and risk factors that are common and treatable.

To exclude intracerebral hemorrhage, epidural or subdural hematoma, or a tumor that is quickly growing or bleeding and causing symptoms, CT or MRI is done. Within a few hours, there may be only subtle CT evidence of an ischemic stroke, even when it involves the large anterior circulation. There may be effacement of the sulci or insular cortical ribbon. There can be a loss of the gray-white junction that is between the cerebral cortex and white matter. There may also be a density in the middle cerebral artery. Once there has been 6–12 hours of ischemia, hypodensities are visible, signifying medium to large infarcts. Smaller infarcts such as lacunar infarcts may only be seen via MRI. Highly sensitive for early ischemia, diffusion-weighted MRI can be performed immediately after the first CT.

When a cardiac cause of ischemic stroke is suspected, testing usually includes ECG, **Holter**

monitoring, serum troponin, and transthoracic echocardiography. When a vascular cause is suspected, the choice and sequence of tests are based on clinical findings and are highly individualized. Diagnostic options include the following:

- *Magnetic resonance angiography (MRA)* – Shows anterior circulation, plus excellent images of posterior circulation; this technique is preferred over CTA if the patient can keep still, to avoid motion artifacts; it is usually done urgently but should not delay intravenous tissue plasminogen activator (IV tPA) if it is needed

- *CT angiography (CTA)* – Shows anterior circulation, plus excellent images of posterior circulation; this also is usually done urgently but should not delay IV tPA if it is needed

- *Carotid and transcranial duplex ultrasonography* – Carotid duplex ultrasonography shows anterior circulation

- *Conventional angiography*

When there are thrombotic disorders causes of ischemic stroke, blood tests can be done. Routine tests usually include complete blood count (CBC), platelet count, fasting blood glucose, lipid profile, and prothrombin time/partial thromboplastin time (PT/PTT). Other tests include homocysteine measurement, antiphospholipid antibodies, antinuclear antibodies, erythrocyte sedimentation rate, rheumatoid factor, hemoglobin electrophoresis, syphilis serologic testing, and urinalysis for amphetamines or cocaine.

Treatment

The treatments of acute ischemic stroke usually require hospitalization. During the first evaluation and stabilization, a variety of supportive measures are often needed. These include the following:

- For decreased consciousness or bulbar dysfunction compromising the airway – ventilatory assistance and airway support.

- If there is a need to maintain oxygen saturation above 94% – supplemental oxygen.

- To correct hyperthermia – an antipyretic drug is used.

- To correct hypothermia – its cause must be ascertained as being stroke-related and then treated.

- Treating hypoglycemia or hyperglycemia to normalize blood glucose levels.

The perfusion of an area of the brain with ischemia may require high BP since autoregulation is lost. Therefore, the BP is not decreased except if there are signs of other end-organ damage, or the use of recombinant tissue plasminogen activator (tPA) with or without **mechanical thrombectomy** is likely needed. Signs of other end-organ damage include acute MI, aortic dissection, hypertensive encephalopathy, pulmonary edema, acute renal failure, and retinal hemorrhages. Lowering the BP by 15% within 24 hours after the onset of stroke is done if the BP is 220/120 mm Hg or higher on 2 readings taken 15 minutes apart. If the patient is a good candidate for acute reperfusion therapy, but the BP is higher than 185/110 mm Hg, the BP can be treated to lower it to less than this level with labetalol, nicardipine, or clevidipine. Nicardipine is given via IV infusion at first, increasing doses every 5–15 minutes. Labetalol is given in an IV bolus over 1–2 minutes and can be repeated one time. Clevidipine is given via the same method but the dose is titrated, doubling every 2–5 minutes to reach the desired BP.

Thrombolysis in situ is also known as angiographically directed intraarterial thrombolysis. It is used for thrombi and emboli, and may be used for major strokes if the symptoms started less than 6 hours previously. This is especially for strokes caused by large occlusions of the middle cerebral artery that cannot be treated with IV recombinant tPA. Up to 12 hours after the onset of symptoms, clots in the basilar artery can be intra-arterially lysed.

Mechanical thrombectomy is also called *angiographically directed intraarterial removal of a thrombus or embolus*, which uses a *stent retriever* device. This is done in larger stroke centers if the patient has had a recent large-vessel occlusion within the anterior circulation. It is not used in place of IV recombinant tPA within 4.5 hours of symptom onset for patients that are eligible and have had an acute ischemic stroke. The newer stent retrievers can reestablish perfusion in 90%–100% of cases. Today, clinical and imaging findings suggesting many tissues being at risk for infarction can justify mechanical thrombectomy later.

For the long-term treatment of ischemic stroke, supportive care is needed. This includes controlling hyperglycemia as well as far, to limit the amount of brain damage and improve future functionality. Before the patient eats, drinks, or attempts to swallow an oral drug, there must be screening for dysphasia. This helps identify any risks for aspiration. A speech-language pathologist or another healthcare practitioner that has been trained for this must perform the screening. After an acute stroke, enteral nutrition, if required, is started within 7 days after hospitalization. Early measures are done to prevent development of pressure ulcers. There must be attempts to prevent any secondary strokes. There is treatment of modifiable risk factors such as diabetes mellitus, hypertension, alcoholism, smoking, dyslipidemia, and obesity. Reduction of systolic BP may be of more effect if the target BP is below 120 mm Hg instead of the common level of below 140 mm Hg.

With use of warfarin, antiplatelet drugs have additive effects that increase bleeding risks. Aspirin is sometimes used with warfarin, but for only some high-risk patients. Clopidogrel can be used if the patient is allergic to aspirin. While taking clopidogrel, if the patient has a recurrent ischemic stroke or a coronary artery stent becomes blocked, there must be suspicion of impaired clopidogrel metabolism. During acute treatment, clopidogrel with aspirin is only given for less than 3 months. This combination is given before 30 days after stenting, usually up to a maximum of 6 months. When a patient cannot tolerate clopidogrel, ticlopidine can be used.

Prevention

The prevention of ischemic stroke includes lifestyle changes such as quitting smoking, consuming moderate amounts of alcohol, keeping weight at a healthy level, a cardiovascular-healthy diet, regular physical exercise, regular medical checkups, and preventing or treating underlying risk factors such as diabetes mellitus, hypertension, and hypercholesterolemia.

Prognosis

After an ischemic stroke, the progression of complications outcome are usually hard to predict during the first few days. A poor prognosis is suggested by older patient age, aphasia, impaired consciousness, and brainstem signs. A favorable prognosis is given for patients of younger age and when early improvements occur. About half of all patients with moderate to severe **hemiplegia**, and the majority of patients with less severe deficits have good sensory function. Over time, they are able to care for most basic needs and walk sufficiently well. About 10% of patients have a complete neurologic recovery. There is usually limits to the usability of the affected limb. The majority of deficits remaining after 1 year will be permanent. A stroke makes a person of high risk of additional strokes. Each stroke usually makes neurologic function worse. Approximately 25% of patients recovering from a stroke will have another in 5 years. Following an ischemic stroke, nearly 20% of patients die while hospitalized, and death rates increase with age.

CLINICAL CASE

1. What are the most common causes of ischemic stroke?
2. Which conditions may mimic strokes that resemble an ischemic stroke?
3. What is a mechanical thrombectomy, and its indication?

A 62-year-old woman was previously diagnosed with diabetes mellitus, hyperlipidemia, and hypertension. She was brought by her friend to a primary stroke center after experiencing sudden right-sided weakness. The patient had a left gaze preference, aphasia, right facial droop, right homonymous hemianopia, right hemiplegia, and dysarthria. A head CT scan was ordered. It revealed some hypodensity in the left middle cerebral artery. Then, a CT angiography was done, showing occlusion of the same artery. The diagnosis was mild ischemic stroke. The patient was given IV recombinant tPA (alteplase) at 2 hours after the symptoms had started. A mechanical thrombectomy was performed. One day later, the patient had only slight expressive aphasia and right facial droop, and after 3 months, had no neurological deficits.

ANSWERS

1. In descending order, the most common causes of ischemic stroke are atherothrombotic occlusion of large arteries, cerebral embolism (embolic infarction), nonthrombotic occlusion of small and deep cerebral arteries (lacunar infarction), and proximal arterial stenosis with hypotension that decreases cerebral blood flow in watershed arterial zones.
2. Stroke mimics of ischemic stroke include hemorrhagic stroke, hypoglycemia, postictal paralysis, and in rare cases, migraine.
3. Mechanical thrombectomy is also called angiographically directed intraarterial removal of a thrombus or embolus, which uses a stent retriever device. The newer stent retrievers are able to reestablish perfusion in 90%–100% of cases.

Hemorrhagic Stroke

A *hemorrhagic stroke* results from cerebral vessel ruptures, such as in *intracerebral hemorrhage* or *subarachnoid hemorrhage*. Hemorrhagic stroke makes up 20% of all cases of CVAs. Intracerebral hemorrhage is defined as focal bleeding from a vessel within the **parenchyma** of the brain, usually because of hypertension. This type of stroke usually occurs in the basal ganglia, cerebral lobes, cerebellum, or pons. However, it can occur in other areas of the brainstem or midbrain. Subarachnoid hemorrhage is sudden bleeding into the subarachnoid space, usually because of a ruptured aneurysm. Type 2 diabetes mellitus is associated with a higher incidence of hemorrhagic stroke.

Epidemiology

Intracerebral hemorrhage is the second most common stroke subtype, accounting for 10%–20% of all strokes. While it makes up 8%–15% of all strokes in the United Kingdom, United States, and Australia. It makes up 18%–24% of all strokes in countries such as Japan and Korea. Intracerebral hemorrhage is most common in low- and middle-income countries. Intracerebral hemorrhage occurs mostly in older adults (over age 75), with a slight male predominance, and in people of Asian heritage. Incidence is 52 cases of every 100,000 Asians, followed by 24 per 100,000 Caucasians, 23 per 100,000 Africans, and 19.6 per 100,000 people from a Hispanic background. However, in one study in the United States, African Americans had the highest incidence, with 49 cases per 100,000.

Subarachnoid hemorrhage caused by an aneurysm most often occurs between ages 40 and 65, but can occur at any age. Overall, it makes up about 5% of all types of stroke. Spontaneous subarachnoid hemorrhage occurs in about 1 of every 10,000 people annually, with females having 25% more cases than males. Approximately half of all patients are below 55 years of age. This is likely because most aneurysms occur relatively early, after the age of 40. The overall common age range is between 40 and 65. According to the Journal of Neurology, Neurosurgery, and Psychiatry, higher rates of subarachnoid hemorrhage occur in the countries of Japan (23 per 100,000) and Finland (20 per 100,000), low rates (4.2 per 100,000) occur in South and Central America. In the United States, subarachnoid hemorrhage disproportionately affects Mexican Americans more than any other racial or ethnic group.

Etiology and Risk Factors

An intracerebral hemorrhage is usually caused by a rupture of an arteriosclerotic artery that is small, after being weakened in most cases by chronic hypertension. This type of hemorrhage is usually single, very large, with severe outcomes. Less common causes include arteriovenous and other vascular malformations, congenital aneurysm, hemorrhagic brain infarction, mycotic aneurysm, excessive use of anticoagulants, primary or metastatic brain tumors, blood dyscrasia, intracranial artery dissection, a bleeding of vasculitic disorder, or moyamoya disease. A lobar intracerebral hemorrhage is a hematoma in the cerebral lobes, outside of the basal ganglia. They may be caused by angiopathy from amyloid deposits in the cerebral arteries. This is called *cerebral amyloid angiopathy* and is most common in older adults. There can be multiple and recurring lobar hemorrhages. Modifiable risk factors related to intracerebral hemorrhage include obesity, diabetes mellitus, cigarette smoking, and a diet high in saturated and trans fats as well as calories. Transient severe hypertension that leads to intracerebral hemorrhage may sometimes be caused by cocaine use, or the use of other sympathomimetic drugs.

In subarachnoid hemorrhage, the bleeding is located between the arachnoid and pia mater. Head trauma is the most common cause. However, traumatic subarachnoid hemorrhage is a distinctly separate disorder from nontraumatic subarachnoid hemorrhage. The cause of primary (spontaneous) subarachnoid hemorrhage is usually a ruptured aneurysm. In about 85% of patients, the aneurysm is classified as a congenital intracranial **saccular aneurysm**, or a **berry aneurysm**. The bleeding can resolve without treatment in some patients. Less common causes include arteriovenous malformations, bleeding disorders, and mycotic aneurysms.

Pathophysiology

The blood from an intracerebral hemorrhage gathers as a mass capable of dissecting through nearby brain tissues, and compressing them. This causes neuronal dysfunction. Intracranial pressure is increased by large hematomas. Transtentorial brain herniation may be caused by supratentorial hematomas and their resulting edema. The brainstem can be compressed, often resulting in secondary midbrain and pons hemorrhages. An intraventricular hemorrhage develops when the intracerebral hemorrhage ruptures into the ventricular system. Acute hydrocephalus may result. A cerebellar hematoma can expand, blocking the fourth ventricle, which also causes acute hydrocephalus. This hematoma can also dissect into the brainstem. A midline shift or herniation can be caused if a cerebellar hematoma is larger than 3 cm in diameter. When the brainstem is affected by herniation, intraventricular hemorrhage, hydrocephalus, dissection, or either midbrain or pontine hemorrhage, consciousness can be impaired, resulting in coma and death. The development of intracerebral hemorrhage because of diabetes mellitus is directly linked with the duration of the diabetes, due to the likelihood of chronic hypertension.

Subarachnoid hemorrhage causes aseptic meningitis. This usually increases intracranial pressure for days to weeks. Focal brain ischemia may be due to secondary vasospasm. Approximately 25% of affected patients develop signs of an ischemic stroke or transient ischemic attack. There is significant brain edema. Risks for vasospasm and infarction, known as *angry brain*, are highest between 72 hours and 10 days. Another common development is secondary acute hydrocephalus. Another rupture may occur. When it does, it is usually within 1 week. The incidence of nonaneurysmal subarachnoid hemorrhage is high in patients with type 1 diabetes. Of cerebrovascular deaths in this group of patients, 23% are due to hemorrhagic strokes. The association of type 2 diabetes with subarachnoid hemorrhage from a ruptured saccular intracranial aneurysm is unclear.

Clinical Manifestations

Intracerebral hemorrhage usually starts with a sudden headache that commonly happens during physical activity. The headache can be mild or absent in older patients. Often, the patient loses consciousness in only seconds or minutes. Other common symptoms include delirium, focal or generalized seizures, nausea, and vomiting. The neurologic deficits are usually sudden and very progressive. Large hemorrhages in the brain hemispheres cause hemiparesis. If they occur in the posterior fossa, cerebellar or brainstem deficits occur. These include conjugate eye deviation, ophthalmoplegia, pinpoint pupils, breathing that resembles snoring, and coma. In about 50% of patients, large hemorrhages are fatal in a few days. Those that survive experience a return to consciousness. Neurologic deficits slowly reduce as extravasated blood is resorbed. Since hemorrhage is not as destructive to brain tissue as an infarction, some patients have only a few neurologic deficits. If the hemorrhage is small, there may be focal deficits, but no impairment of consciousness. Headache or nausea may be only very slight. These hemorrhages can mimic an ischemic stroke.

With subarachnoid hemorrhage, the patient's headache is usually extreme and peaks within a few seconds. He or she may lose consciousness. This is usually immediate, but can occur after several hours. Extreme neurologic deficits may occur, becoming irreversible in minutes to several hours. Sensory function may be impaired. The patient may become very restless, and seizures can occur. Unless there is herniation of the cerebellar tonsils, the patient's neck is usually not stiff. Even so, aseptic meningitis causes moderate to severe meningismus within 1 day. There is usually vomiting and occasionally bilateral extensor plantar responses. There are often abnormalities of the heart or respiratory rates. During the first 5–10 days, continuing headaches, confusion, and fever are often seen. If there is secondary hydrocephalus, the patient may experience additional headache, motor deficits, and obtundation over weeks. If another bleed occurs, symptoms can recur, or new ones can emerge.

Diagnosis

The diagnosis of an intracerebral hemorrhage is based on sudden headache, focal neurologic deficits, and especially in high-risk patients, reduced consciousness. An intracerebral hemorrhage must be distinguished from hypoglycemia, ischemic stroke, subarachnoid hemorrhage, and seizures. Immediate blood glucose level measurement is required, as is immediate CT or MRI. Diagnosis is usually via neuroimaging. If no hemorrhage is seen but a subarachnoid hemorrhage is clinically suspected, a lumbar puncture is required. Within hours of the start of hemorrhage, CT angiography can reveal areas where the contrast agent extravasates into the clot – known as a *spot sign*. This indicates continuing bleeding. The hematoma is likely to expand, worsening the outcome.

The diagnosis of subarachnoid hemorrhage is based on the symptoms. Testing must be done quickly before irreversible damage occurs. Within 6 hours of the onset of symptoms, noncontrast CT is done. An MRI is just as sensitive but not as likely to be available quickly. If the volume of blood is small, or the patient is extremely anemic, with the blood being isodense with brain tissues, false-negative results can occur. When subarachnoid hemorrhage is suspected by not seen on imaging, or if neuroimaging is not available immediately, a lumbar puncture is done. This procedure is contraindicated if there is suspicion of increased intracranial pressure, since a sudden decrease in cerebrospinal fluid (CSF) pressure can reduce tamponade of a clot upon the ruptured aneurysm, resulting in additional bleeding. If subarachnoid hemorrhage is present, the CSF findings include excessive RBCs, increased pressure, and **xanthochromia**. However, RBCs in the CSF can be due to a traumatic lumbar puncture. This is suspected if the RBC count is lower in tubes of CSF drawn sequentially. Approximately 6 hours or longer after a subarachnoid hemorrhage, the RBCs experience **crenation**, and they lyse. This results in a xanthochromic CSF **supernatant**. The RBCs, when examined under a microscope, are crenated. These findings usually mean that a subarachnoid hemorrhage occurred before the lumbar puncture procedure. If doubt is still present, a hemorrhage should be suspected, or the lumbar puncture is repeated within 8–12 hours. Conventional cerebral angiography is done soon after the initial bleeding occurrence. Other options include magnetic resonance angiography and CT angiography. The two carotid and two vertebral arteries are all injected since as many as 20% of patients have multiple aneurysms. The multiple aneurysms occur more often in women.

Treatment

The treatment of an intracerebral hemorrhage involves supportive measures, plus control of all modifiable risk factors. Antiplatelet drugs and anticoagulants cannot be used. If the patient has taken anticoagulants previously, their effects are sometimes reversible by using fresh frozen plasma, prothrombin complex concentrate, platelet transfusions, or vitamin K. The drug called dabigatran can be 60% removed via hemodialysis. If the systolic BP is 150–220 mm Hg, it can be safely lowered to 140 mm Hg, if acute antihypertensive treatment is not contraindicated for the patient. When a patient has systolic BP is higher than 220 mm Hg, a continuous IV infusion of an antihypertensive is aggressively administered. This requires close monitoring of systolic BP. Nicardipine is given first, increasing in dosage every 5 minutes as needed so that systolic BP can be reduced by 10%–15%.

If there is a cerebellar hemisphere hematoma larger than 3 cm in diameter, a midline shift or herniation can occur. Surgical evacuation often saves the patient's life. If done early for a large lobar cerebral hematoma, the outcome may be equally as successful, though rebleeding is common and may increase the neurologic deficits. Early evacuation of a deep cerebral hematoma is usually not indicated, since the death rate is high during surgery and the neurologic deficits are often severe. Antiseizure drugs are usually only used if a seizure has occurred, and not as prophylactic agents.

For subarachnoid hemorrhage, the best available treatment is offered at comprehensive stroke centers. Hypertension is only treated if the mean arterial pressure is higher than 130 mm Hg. Intravenous nicardipine is titrated in the same way as for intracerebral hemorrhage. The patient is confined to bed rest, and there is symptomatic treatment of headache and restlessness. Anticoagulants and antiplatelet drugs are avoided. Oral nimodipine is given every 4 hours, for 21 days, to prevent vasospasm. However, the BP must be kept in the desired range, usually 120–185 mm Hg systolic. Also, with an accessible aneurysm, surgery can allow for it to be clipped or stented. This is especially preferred if the patient has an evacuable hematoma or acute hydrocephalus. When the patient can be aroused from unconsciousness, neurosurgeons usually operate within the first 24 hours.

Prevention

Intracerebral hemorrhage is linked to chronic hypertension, so controlling BP is an important way to reduce the risks of the condition's development. This involves managing stress, consuming a healthy diet, exercising regularly, avoiding smoking, limiting alcohol intake, and controlling diabetes mellitus. Treatment of other causative conditions can also prevent an intracerebral hemorrhage. Once an intracerebral hemorrhage has occurred, the initial goals of treatment are to prevent extension of the hemorrhage, and to prevent and manage secondary brain injury as well as other complications.

Prognosis

The prognosis of intracerebral hemorrhage is generally poor, since it is usually severe and has high rates of patient death. Often, family members must make a choice to limit or withdraw care. Prognosis is predicted by the available clinical grading systems. Care is often withdrawn within 2 days in the hospital, even though there has been evidence that early interventions could improve the prognosis. Recent guidelines suggest waiting more than 24 hours before making the decision to withdraw care.

Approximately 35% of subarachnoid hemorrhage patients die after an initial aneurysmal hemorrhage. About 15% more will die within several weeks due to another rupture. After 6 months have passed, second ruptures occur in about 3% of cases annually. The prognosis is generally the worst when an aneurysm is the cause. Prognosis is better if the cause was an arteriovenous malformation. The best prognosis is when angiography finds no lesion because the source of bleeding is small and has already sealed. Even with the best treatments, most survivors of subarachnoid hemorrhage have neurologic damage.

CLINICAL CASE

1. What is the definition of focal bleeding in the brain?
2. What are the modifiable risk factors related to intracerebral hemorrhage?
3. Are there methods that can help prevent intracerebral hemorrhage?

A 58-year-old male with type 2 diabetes mellitus presented to the emergency department because of sudden left arm weakness that had been present for 4 hours, and generalized headache. One year earlier, the patient had been diagnosed with hypertension, which was controlled fairly well with hydrochlorothiazide. However, in the hospital his BP was 160/110 mm Hg. A neurological examination revealed lower than normal muscle strength in his left arm as well as his left leg. Plain CT of the brain showed intracerebral hemorrhage. The patient was evaluated for nonoperative treatment, admitted to the ICU, and given IV labetalol. No additional neurological deficits developed, and he was put into the general medical ward within 36 hours.

ANSWERS

1. Intracerebral hemorrhage is defined as focal bleeding from a vessel within the parenchyma of the brain, usually because of hypertension. This type of stroke usually occurs in the basal ganglia, cerebral lobes, cerebellum, or pons, but can also occur in other areas of the brainstem or midbrain.
2. Modifiable risk factors related to intracerebral hemorrhage include obesity, diabetes mellitus, cigarette smoking, and a diet high in saturated and trans fats as well as calories. Transient severe hypertension that leads to intracerebral hemorrhage may sometimes be caused by cocaine use, or the use of other sympathomimetic drugs.
3. Controlling blood pressure is an important way to reduce the risks of developing intracerebral hemorrhage. This involves managing stress, consuming a healthy diet, exercising regularly, avoiding smoking, limiting alcohol intake, and controlling diabetes mellitus.

TRANSIENT ISCHEMIC ATTACK

A transient ischemic attack (TIA) involves symptoms of stroke that usually last for less than 1 hour. It is defined as focal brain ischemia, with sudden neurologic deficits. There is no visualization of any acute cerebral infarction when evaluation is done with diffusion-weighted MRI. The condition is similar to an ischemic stroke except that most TIAs last for less than 5 minutes. If deficits resolve in 1 hour, infarction is extremely unlikely. Deficits resolving between 1 and 24 hours usually have infarction. At this point, they are no longer considered to be TIAs. Within the first 24 hours, TIAs greatly increase risks of having an actual stroke. Hypertensive patients with diabetes mellitus have an increased frequency of transient ischemic attacks.

Epidemiology

Most cases of transient ischemic attacks occur in middle-aged or older adults. Global estimates are varied. For example, the estimated prevalence in the United Kingdom for a first TIA is 50 per 100,000 people. Age-adjusted incidence rates of TIA are estimated to be 72.2 per 100,000 people globally. The mean age of TIA patients is 66 years. The occurrence of TIAs is nearly even between men and women. There is no specific racial group, globally, with significantly higher cases of TIAs. Up to 500,000 people in the United States experience a TIA every year, and the other statistics resemble the global data – older age, and no significant male/female predilection. However, since African Americans have more frequent and severe hypertension, they also have the highest amounts of TIAs.

Etiology and Risk Factors

Most transient ischemic attacks are caused by emboli that usually come from the carotid or vertebral arteries. Rarely, TIAs occur from impaired perfusion caused by severe hypoxemia, a lowered oxygen-carrying capacity of the blood, or increased viscosity – especially in arteries of the brain that have become stenotic. Reduced oxygen-carrying capacity of the blood may be caused by extreme anemia or carbon monoxide poisoning. Increased viscosity may be due to severe polycythemia. Cerebral ischemia is usually not caused by systemic hypotension unless it is extreme or there is preexisting arterial stenosis. This is because autoregulation regulates blood flow in the brain, to be nearly normal over widely ranging systemic blood pressure. **Subclavian steal syndrome** involves a subclavian artery that is stenosed, proximal to the start of the vertebral artery. The stenosed artery "steals" blood from the vertebral artery. The blood flow becomes reversed in the vertebral artery. Since the vertebral artery supplies the arms during physical exertion, there are signs of vertebrobasilar ischemia. Sometimes, a TIA can occur in a child that has an extreme cardiovascular disorder producing emboli, or with very high hematocrit levels.

Modifiable risk factors for TIAs include cigarette smoking, diabetes mellitus, insulin resistance, dyslipidemia, hypertension, abdominal obesity, excessive alcohol use, insufficient physical activity, a diet high in saturated and trans fats as well as calories, depression and other psychosocial stress, acute MI, atrial fibrillation, infective endocarditis, hypercoagulability, and vasculitis use of amphetamines or cocaine. Unmodifiable risk factors for TIAs include family history of stroke, the male gender, older age, and a previous stroke.

Pathophysiology

Most transient ischemic attacks are pathophysiologically linked to microemboli originating in areas of atherosclerosis in the blood vessels of the neck. A blood vessel is obstructed, disrupting cerebral blood flow. The neurons cannot maintain aerobic respiration and the mitochondria switch to anaerobic respiration. There is low ATP and energy failure. Acidosis, ion imbalance, changes in glutamate levels, and depolarization occur. Intracellular calcium is increased. Cell membranes and proteins break down and free radicals are formed. This results in cell injury and death, and the TIA results.

Clinical Manifestations

With a transient ischemic attack, the neurologic deficits resemble those of strokes. **Amaurosis fugax** is transient blindness in one eye. This usually lasts for less than 5 minutes, and can occur if the ophthalmic artery is damaged by the TIA. Symptoms of TIAs begin quickly. They commonly last between 2 and 30 minutes and then completely resolve. It is possible for an individual to have several TIAs per day, or to have just 2–3 TIAs over several years.

Diagnosis

Transient ischemic attacks are diagnosed after they occur, based on the sudden neurologic deficits that indicate ischemia in an artery, yet resolve within 1 hour. If the patient has isolated peripheral palsy of a facial nerve, and impaired consciousness or unconsciousness, a TIA is not likely. They must be distinguished from conditions that cause similar symptoms, which include hypoglycemia, the **aura** of a migraine, and postictal (Todd) paralysis. Neuroimaging is needed since small hemorrhages, infarcts, and mass lesions cannot be clinically excluded. In most facilities, a CT is more immediately available. Unfortunately, CT is sometimes unable to visualize an infarct for more than 24 hours. Therefore, an MRI can be used to detect evolving infarcts within hours. Though not always available, a diffusion-weighted MRI is the best method to rule out infarcts if a TIA is suspected.

The cause of a TIA is evaluated the same way as for the causes of ischemic strokes. There are tests for cardiac sources of emboli, carotid stenosis, atrial fibrillation, and hematologic abnormalities. These tests include transesophageal echocardiography, transthoracic echocardiography, cardiac CT angiography, 24-hour Holter monitoring, ultrasonography, magnetic resonance angiography, electrocardiography, event recording (also called event monitoring), implantable loop recorders, and blood tests. Stroke risk factors are screened. Evaluation continues quickly, usually with the patient being hospitalized, since risks of an ischemic stroke are very high and they often happen quickly. Discharge of a patient must be carefully determined because it can be difficult to determine the safety of doing so. Within the first 24–48 hours, the risk of a stroke, whether major or minor, is highest. If any type of stroke is suspected to be likely, the patient is usually admitted for evaluation and telemetry.

Treatment

The treatment of a TIA focuses on stroke prevention, using antiplatelet drugs and statins. For some patients – especially with high risk of stroke but no neurologic deficits, carotid endarterectomy or arterial angioplasty, plus stenting, can be effective. If there are cardiac sources of emboli, anticoagulation is needed. Stroke may be prevented by modifying risk factors, if this is possible.

Prevention

The best way to prevent a transient ischemic attack is to eat a healthy diet, exercise on a regular basis, avoid smoking, and avoid excessive alcohol use. Good management of diabetes mellitus is also an essential method of preventing a TIA. Basically, anything that reduces the likelihood of developing atherosclerosis, hypertension, and high cholesterol helps to prevent a TIA. If a TIA has already occurred, these same changes help reduce risks of a recurring TIA or an actual stroke.

Prognosis

The prognosis for a transient ischemic attack is usually good since it generally leaves no permanent damage. However, prognosis can be worsened since a TIA is a warning sign for a future stroke. Patients, after a TIA, have a 13 times higher risk for a full blown stroke during the first year, plus a 7 times higher risk for the same over the next 7 years, compared to patients that never have a TIA. The risk of death, stroke, or MI over the next 5 years after a TIA is about 8.4%/year.

CLINICAL CASE

1. What is the age group of patients that most often experience TIAs?
2. How are TIAs diagnosed?
3. What are the complete treatment options for TIAs?

A 66-year-old diabetic woman experienced 20 minutes of left arm numbness and slurred speech, recovering completely without treatment. Her husband took her to the emergency department for evaluation. Previous medical history included a similar attack 2 weeks before, of nearly the same duration, but no medical treatment was sought at that time because the couple didn't think anything was seriously wrong. An MRI showed abnormal signals in the right precentral sulcus. A CT scan revealed a high-density lesion in the same area. However, the diagnosis was of a transient ischemic attack that was simply the first presentation of a subarachnoid hemorrhage. Over time, the patient's symptoms did not return, and another CT scan showed that the hemorrhage had completely resolved on its own. The patient was discharged but started on antiplatelet drugs and statins.

ANSWERS

1. The majority of cases of transient ischemic attacks occur in middle-aged or older adults. The mean age of TIA patients is 66 years.
2. TIAs are diagnosed after they occur, based on the sudden deficits that indicate ischemia in an artery, yet resolve within 1 hour. If the patient has isolated peripheral palsy of a facial nerve, and impaired consciousness or unconsciousness, a TIA is not likely. They must be distinguished from conditions that cause similar symptoms, which include hypoglycemia, the aura of a migraine, and postictal (Todd) paralysis. Neuroimaging is needed since small hemorrhages, infarcts, and mass lesions cannot be clinically excluded.
3. The complete treatment options for TIAs include antiplatelet drugs, statins, carotid endarterectomy or arterial angioplasty plus stenting, anticoagulation, and modifying risk factors.

KEY TERMS

- Amaurosis fugax
- Antiphospholipid syndrome
- Aura
- Basal ganglia
- Berry aneurysm
- Cavernous sinus
- Circle of Willis
- Corpus callosum
- Crenation
- Hemiparesis
- Hemiplegia
- Hemodynamic stroke
- Hippocampus
- Holter monitoring
- Hyperhomocysteinemia
- Internal capsule
- Ipsilaterally
- Lacunar infarction
- Lenticulostriate arteries
- Mechanical thrombectomy
- Parenchyma
- Penumbras
- Saccular aneurysm
- Stroke mimics
- Subclavian steal syndrome
- Supernatant
- Supraclinoid process
- Thrombolysis in situ
- Xanthochromia
- Watershed zones

REFERENCES

AAN.com – AAN Publications – Neurology. (2008). *Gender and Ethnic Differences in Subarachnoid Hemorrhage.* American Academy of Neurology / Wolters Kluwer. https://n.neurology.org/content/71/10/731

Aiyagari, V., and Gorelick, P.B. (2011). *Hypertension and Stroke: Pathophysiology and Management (Clinical Hypertension and Vascular Disorders).* Humana Press.

American Family Physician. (2004). *Transient Ischemic Attacks: Part II. Treatment.* The American Academy of Family Physicians. https://www.aafp.org/afp/2004/0401/p1681.html

Arce Puentes, D., and Cano, R.G.A. (2021). *Evaluation of the Patient with Transient Ischemic Attack: Application of the ABCD2 Score*. Our Knowledge Publishing.

Baker, D.M. (2008). *Stroke Prevention in Clinical Practice*. Springer.

Bendok, B.R., Naidech, A.M., Walker, M.T., and Batjer, H.H. (2011). *Hemorrhagic and Ischemic Stroke: Medical, Imaging, Surgical, and Interventional Approaches*. Thieme.

Bhopal, R.S. (2019). *Epidemic of Cardiovascular Disease and Diabetes*. Oxford University Press.

Biller, J. (2009). *Stroke in Children and Young Adults (Expert Consult)*, 2nd Edition. Saunders.

Boccardi, E., Cenzato, M., Curto, F., Longoni, M., Motto, C., Oppo, V., Perini, V., and Vidale, S. (2017). *Hemorrhagic Stroke – Emergency Management in Neurology*. Springer.

Bogousslavsky, J. (2005). *Stroke Management in Patients with Diabetes Mellitus or Metabolic Syndromes (Cerebrovascular Diseases)*. Karger Publishers.

Caplan, L.R. (2016). *Caplan's Stroke: A Clinical Approach*, 5th Edition. Cambridge University Press.

Carter Denny, M. (2020). *Acute Stroke Care (Manuals in Neurology)*, 3rd Edition. Cambridge University Press.

Centers for Disease Control and Prevention. *Stroke Statistics*. U.S. Department of Health & Human Services – USA.gov – CDC. https://www.cdc.gov/stroke/facts.htm

Chaturvedi, S., and Levine, S.R. (2008). *Transient Ischemic Attacks*. Blackwell Futura.

Corrigan, M.L., Escuro, A.A., and Kirby, D.F. (2013). *Handbook of Clinical Nutrition and Stroke – Nutrition and Health*. Humana Press.

Cureus. (2019). *Intracerebral Hemorrhage in a Patient with Untreated Rheumatoid Arthritis: Case Report and Literature Review*. Cureus. https://www.cureus.com/articles/21426-intracerebral-hemorrhage-in-a-patient-with-untreated-rheumatoid-arthritis-case-report-and-literature-review/metrics

Del Zoppo, G.R., Gorelick, P.B., and Eisert, W. (2010). *Innate Inflammation and Stroke (Annals of the New York Academy of Sciences)*. Wiley-Blackwell.

Gonzalez, R.G., Hiirsch, J.A., Lev, M.H., Schaefer, P.W., and Schwamm, L.H. (2010). *Acute Ischemic Stroke – Imaging and Intervention*, 2nd Edition. Springer.

Grotta, J.C., Albers, G.W., Broderick, J.P., Kasner, S.E., Lo, E.H., Sacco, R.L., Wong, L.K.S., and Day, A.L. (2021). *Stroke: Pathophysiology, Diagnosis, and Management*, 7th Edition. Elsevier.

Hacein-Bey, L. (2018). *Ischemic Stroke (Neuroimaging Clinics – Review Articles)*. Elsevier.

Health& Pty Ltd. (2021). *What Is the Outlook for a Transient Ischemic Attack?* Health& Pty Ltd. https://healthand.com/us/smart-search/answer/what-is-the-outlook-for-a-transient-ischemic-attack

Healthline. (2021a). *How to Prevent a Stroke*. Healthline Media. https://www.healthline.com/health-news/these-5-lifestyle-changes-can-help-prevent-a-second-stroke#5-important-lifestyle-changes

Healthline. (2021b). *Subarachnoid Hemorrhage*. Healthline Media. https://www.healthline.com/health/subarachnoid-hemorrhage

Hui, F.K., Spiotta, A.M., Alexander, M.J., Hanel, R.A., and Baxter, B.W. (2021). *12 Strokes: A Case-based Guide to Acute Ischemic Stroke Management*. Springer.

Johns Hopkins Medicine – Health. (2021). *Subarachnoid Hemorrhage*. The Johns Hopkins University, The Johns Hopkins Hospital, and Johns Hopkins Health System. https://www.hopkinsmedicine.org/health/conditions-and-diseases/subarachnoid-hemorrhage

Joseph, R. (2011). *Stroke & Brain Damage – Thrombi, Emboli, Hemorrhage, Aneurysms, Atherosclerosis, TIA, CVA, Disturbances of Cognition, Memory, Language, Visual Perception, Emotion, Physical Sensation*. University Press.

Larsen, H.R., Chambers, P., and Klughaupt, M. (2018). *Thrombosis and Stroke Prevention, 3rd Edition: The Afibber's Guide to Stroke Prevention*. International Health News.

Lee, S.H. (2018). *Stroke Revisited: Hemorrhagic Stroke*. Springer.

MacWalter, R.S., and Shirley, C.P. (2003). *Managing Strokes and TIAs in Practice*. CRC Press.

Mayo Clinic. (2021). *Transient Ischemic Attack (TIA)*. Mayo Foundation for Medical Education and Research (MFMER). https://www.mayoclinic.org/diseases-conditions/transient-ischemic-attack/symptoms-causes/syc-20355679

Medscape. (2020). *What Is the Incidence of Ischemic Stroke in the US and Globally?* WebMD LLC. https://www.medscape.com/answers/1916852-118708/what-is-the-incidence-of-ischemic-stroke-in-the-us-and-globally

Mohr, J.P., Wolf, P.A., Grotta, J.C., Moskowitz, M.A., Mayberg, M., and von Kimmer, R. (2011). *Stroke: Pathophysiology, Diagnosis, and Management (Expert Consult)*, 5th Edition. Elsevier.

NetCE, and Thompson, D. (2019). *Diabetes and Stroke: Making the Connection*. NetCE.

National Institutes of Health – National Library of Medicine – National Center for Biotechnology Information. (2013). *Transient Ischemic Attack and Minor Stroke Are the Most Common Manifestations of Acute Cerebrovascular Disease: A Prospective, Population-Based Study – the Aarhus TIA Study*. National Library of Medicine. https://pubmed.ncbi.nlm.nih.gov/23075482/

National Institutes of Health – National Library of Medicine – National Center for Biotechnology Information. (2011). *Prognosis in Intracerebral Hemorrhage*. National Library of Medicine. https://pubmed.ncbi.nlm.nih.gov/21769068/

National Institutes of Health – National Library of Medicine – National Center for Biotechnology Information. (1993). *Intracerebral Hemorrhage More Than Twice as Common as Subarachnoid Hemorrhage*. National Library of Medicine. https://pubmed.ncbi.nlm.nih.gov/8421201/

National Institutes of Health – National Library of Medicine – National Center for Biotechnology Information. (1990). *Prognosis of Transient Ischemic Attacks in the Oxfordshire Community Stroke Project*. National Library of Medicine. https://pubmed.ncbi.nlm.nih.gov/2349586/

National Institutes of Health – National Library of Medicine – National Center for Biotechnology Information. (1976). *Transient Ischemic Attacks: Pathophysiology and Medical Management*. National Library of Medicine. https://pubmed.ncbi.nlm.nih.gov/1264882/

NCBI. (2021). *Ischemic Stroke*. National Center for Biotechnology Information, U.S. National Library of Medicine. https://www.ncbi.nlm.nih.gov/books/NBK499997/

NCBI – PMC – US National Library of Medicine – National Institutes of Health – Journal of Stroke. (2017). *Epidemiology, Risk Factors, and Clinical Features of Intracerebral Hemorrhage: An Update*. https://www.ncbi.nlm.nih.gov/pmc/articles/PMC5307940/

NHS. (2021). *Prevention – Transient Ischaemic Attack (TIA).* Crown. https://www.nhs.uk/conditions/transient-ischaemic-attack-tia/prevention/

Oxford Academic – Endocrinology – Endocrine Society. (2018). *Age and Sex Are Critical Factors in Ischemic Stroke Pathology.* Oxford University Press. https://academic.oup.com/endo/article/159/8/3120/5051605

Park, J. (2017). *Acute Ischemic Stroke: Medical, Endovascular, and Surgical Techniques.* Springer.

Pendelbury, S.T., Giles, M.F., and Rothwell, P.M. (2009). *Transient Ischemic Attack and Stroke: Diagnosis, Investigation and Management.* Cambridge University Press.

Rajanikant, G.K., Gressens, P., Nampoothiri, S.S., Surendran, G., and Bokobza, C. (2020). *IschemiRs: MicroRNAs in Ischemic Stroke: From Basics to Clinics.* Springer.

Riggs, D. (2019). *Hemorrhagic Stroke: Pathophysiology and Interventions.* Hayle Medical.

Rolla, A.R., and Agarwal, S. (2019). *Clinical Atlas of Diabetes Mellitus.* Jaypee Brothers Medical Publishers Ltd.

Rothwell, P.M., Schulz, U.G., Malhotra, A., and Pendlebury, S.T. (2012). *Oxford Case Histories in TIA and Stroke.* Oxford University Press.

ScarySymptoms.com. (2021). *How Common Is a Transient Ischemic Attack?* ScarySymptoms.com. https://scarysymptoms.com/2015/09/how-many-americans-get-tia-every-year/

SCRIBD – Science & Mathematics. (2021). *Pathophysiology of TIA.* Scribd Inc. https://www.scribd.com/document/52530588/PATHOPHYSIOLOGY-OF-TIA

ShareCare.com (2021). *Can Intracerebral Hemorrhage Be Prevented?* Sharecare, Inc. https://www.sharecare.com/health/intracerebral-hemorrhage/can-intracerebral-hemorrhage-be-prevented

Spence, D., and Barnett, H.J.M. (2012). *Stroke Prevention, Treatment, and Rehabilitation.* McGraw-Hill Education / Medical.

Spiotta, A.M., and Crosa, R. (2019). *Ischemic Stroke Management: Medical, Interventional and Surgical Management.* Thieme.

Stroke – Volume 43, Issue 1. (2012). *Effects of Gender on the Phenotype of CADASIL.* American Heart Association, Inc. https://www.ahajournals.org/doi/10.1161/STROKEAHA.111.631028

Stroke.org / American Heart Association / American Stroke Association / Medtronic. (2021). *Case Study 1 & 2.* StrokeAssociation.org. www.stroke.org/-/media/stroke-files/ischemic-stroke-professional-materials/case-study-1-and-2-ucm_488417.pdf

UpToDate. (2021). *Spontaneous Intracerebral Hemorrhage: Treatment and Prognosis.* UpToDate, Inc. / Wolters Kluwer. https://www.uptodate.com/contents/spontaneous-intracerebral-hemorrhage-treatment-and-prognosis

Von Kummer, R., and Back, T. (2005). *Magnetic Resonance Imaging in Ischemic Stroke (Medical Radiology).* Springer.

Wiebers, D.O., Feigin, V.L., and Brown, Jr., R.D. (2019). *Handbook of Stroke,* 3rd Edition. Lippincott, Williams, and Wilkins.

World Stroke Organization. (2020). *World Stroke Organization (WSO): Global Stroke Fact Sheet 2019.* World Stroke Organization. https://www.google.com/url?sa=t&rct=j&q=&esrc=s&source=web&cd=&ved=2ahUKEwiIhcKvrvLxAhVPJt8KHS4uBp4QFjAAegQIBRAD&url=https%3A%2F%2Fwww.world-stroke.org%2Fassets%2Fdownloads%2FWSO_Fact-sheet_15.01.2020.pdf&usg=AOvVaw3OrW5kFX_6RG9D1fk_I2bP

CHAPTER 12 Psychosocial Aspects of Diabetes

Diabetes mellitus causes people to experience many changes in activities, lifestyle, relationships with others, and how to deal with medical and physical issues. Therefore, managing diabetes can have severe psychosocial consequences. The symptoms of diabetes can also mimic psychiatric disorders, making it difficult to formulate an accurate mental health diagnosis. Often, patients with diabetes are overwhelmed when they must follow the strict diet required for health, continually test blood glucose levels, and manage multiple medications. The chronic stress of diabetes mellitus can lead to depression, anxiety, panic, posttraumatic stress disorder, eating disorders, and even neurological outcomes. The direct relationship between diabetes and psychosocial distress is a real and significant factor that treating healthcare providers need to consider. Individuals with diabetes often need to make significant changes in their health behaviors and lifestyle in order to minimize the impact of this condition on their level of functioning. However, making these changes can be very difficult, especially without adequate support. Approaches to diabetes management can also be influenced by preexisting beliefs and cultural influences. A comprehensive understanding of all of these factors is therefore necessary in order to effectively address psychosocial aspects of diabetes care.

HEALTH BEHAVIOR

There are many challenges experienced by people diagnosed with diabetes mellitus. The American Diabetes Association considers Integrated Behavioral Healthcare the primary method of addressing these challenges. Behavioral health psychologists work closely with patients and focus on a variety of behavioral, emotional, and social factors commonly faced among individuals with diabetes. Unfortunately, the inclusion of behavioral health psychologists as part of diabetic treatment teams is not universal or widespread. This has occurred because of lack of awareness about the importance of incorporating behavioral counseling and costs involved. Although limited access remains a notable barrier to treatment, behavioral health therapists can focus on implementing and maintaining self-care methods which can be highly effective for diabetic patients. For example, behavioral counseling is quite successful in helping patients to achieve better weight and blood glucose control. The emotional support method described as BATHE (background, affect, trouble, handling, empathy) requires

less than 15 minutes per appointment and can be highly supportive of the patient's individual needs. If a patient is not able to be fully compliant with treatment goals, the therapist can directly deal with the problem toward finding a solution. Two primary areas of focus are maintaining self-care, including acceptance of and adherence to the prescribed treatment regimen, and managing emotional issues, which include distress and depression.

There are four categories of factors to consider when facilitating health behaviors and methods to change and improve them, as follows:

- *Motivators* – Factors that predispose the patient to action. These include perceived need and benefits of treatment, outcome expectancies, rewards and **incentives**, and cues to action.

- *Inhibitors and facilitators* – Factors that are barriers to action or resources for action. Barriers include lack of resources such as funding, skills, or support as well as various other internal or external obstacles to engaging in healthier behaviors.

- *Intentions* – A goal or objective that is often the driving force or ultimate cause of behavior change. The patient must intend to change and be willing to make the changes needed soon. A specific goal is required toward which they can work.

- *Triggers* – Events that bring the patient from predisposal into completing the needed action.

Changing behaviors can be very difficult for anyone. Therefore, the patient-centered approach provides opportunities for *empowerment*, which places the patient at the center of behavioral change to facilitate ownership and enthusiasm, and encourages utilization of personalized methods to make changes in behavior. These methods include collaborative goal setting, motivational interviewing, development of problem-solving skills, coping skills training, environmental change to reduce barriers to follow-through, behavioral contracting to improve accountability, methods of self-monitoring such as journaling, incorporation of incentives and rewards, and increasing or maintaining social support. Patients are more likely to initiate and follow through with behavior changes when they clearly see how making these changes will result in positive outcomes that are important to them. Being able to link a behavioral change to a patient's personalized goal if often more

DOI: 10.1201/9781003226727-15

powerful than simply explaining that a behavior change is healthier. For example, connecting an increase in regular exercise to being able to play with grandchildren for longer periods of time might be more salient to a patient than describing exercise as a means of better controlling blood sugar. Interventions can occur in a sequence that consists of five primary steps, known as the *5C intervention*. This includes the following:

- *Construction of a problem definition* – This starts with eliciting what the patient perceives as a major problem or focus of treatment to be addressed, which is discussed and defined specifically, breaking it down to small component parts, such as individualized meal portions.

- *Collaborative setting of goals* – This translates intentions into goals, which should be specific, measurable, action-oriented, realistic, and not overly challenging to the point of being unrealistic. An example of a specific goal might be not snacking after dinner. A measurable goal would be walking for 30 minutes three times per week. An action-oriented goal would be addressing the amount of exercise instead of the general goal of losing weight. A realistic but not overly challenging goal would be one that does not discourage the patient by being nearly impossible to achieve, but also is not so simple that there is no sense of accomplishment when it is successfully completed.

- *Collaborative solving of problems* – This involves identifying barriers and formulating strategies together between the patient and therapist. Barriers can be internal or external and include cognitions, emotions, social networks, resources, and physical environment. Interfering cognitions might be beliefs held by patients that treatments will or will not work. Emotional barriers might include lack of self-efficacy, which could result in lack of willingness to try to change. Limited social networks and support might be barriers as well. Insufficient resources might include lack of time or money. Issues pertaining to the physical environment might include insufficient facilities needed for behavioral change. Formulating strategies requires planning ways to overcome these barriers and to reproduce previous successes. Proactive strategies can eliminate barriers in advance. Reactive strategies can determine what to do if a new barrier is encountered. Previously encountered barriers are never described as "failures" but might be considered to be learning opportunities.

- *Contracting for behavioral change* – This begins by creating specific goals and strategies including the start time, in a written agreement known often as a *behavioral contract*. It describes what both the patient and the counselor will do. It makes responsibilities explicit toward maintaining accountability, but is not considered an enforceable document. The patient receives a copy to be used as a reminder. The patient should keep a written record of successes and relapses, plus their reasons, to identify successes and barriers. If the patient develops an increased interest or motivation in attaining goals, behavior change is easier. There is ongoing discussion about items that may need to be altered in the behavioral contract to ensure better outcomes. Rewards are determined and given out that do not oppose the success of behavioral change.

- *Continued support* – Since long-term behavioral support is most effective, it can include plans on how to handle relapses, since they happen to most patients. It is also essential to include positive self-reinforcements as part of emotional support.

Therapists working with diabetic patients must identify those suffering from distress related to their diagnosis of diabetes. They may be having difficulty accepting the disease, be overwhelmed by trying to manage it, not receiving adequate support from others, or worried about possible complications of the disease. Effective treatments are then applied to relieve this stress, such as cognitive-behavioral therapy. This is designed to help the patient identify negative and often unrealistic thoughts that lead to distress, poor motivation, and insufficient self-care. Instead, they learn positive methods of thinking and behaving that relieve distress, improve motivation, and promote self-care. Self-efficacy and a sense of "mastery" is promoted toward giving patients a better sense of control over their health and condition. Realistic expectations are encouraged, as is enhancement of motivation, initiative, and follow-through. Any patient suffering from a comorbid psychiatric disorder must also be identified. This may include depression (most commonly), and clinical eating and anxiety disorders. There may be a serious need to refer some patients for specialized mental health care beyond these behavioral health strategies specifically related to diabetes management.

LIFESTYLES

Patient lifestyles greatly influence the development and management of diabetes mellitus. Five primary lifestyle factors have been identified that lower the risk of developing diabetes. Type 2 diabetes is much more common than type 1. The five factors described here are focused on type 2 diabetes and include the following:

- *Healthy diet* – Especially plant-source foods and adequate dietary fiber

- *Maintaining an optimal body weight* – This provides the greatest protection against diabetes

- *Regular physical exercise as recommended by a physician* – Usually 30 minutes or more of moderate to vigorous aerobic exercise, and resistance exercise at least 2–3 times per week

- *Avoiding smoking*

- *Limiting alcohol use* – No more than 1 drink per day for women, and 2 drinks per day for men

Women with all five healthy lifestyle factors have an 84% lower risk of developing type 2 diabetes, and men have a 72% lower risk. Even among people with a family history of diabetes, which strongly increases risks for type 2 diabetes, lifestyle changes are largely able to prevent or delay development of the disease.

These recommended lifestyle factors help to reduce development of insulin resistance, which is central to type 2 diabetes. It occurs 10–20 years before onset of the disease. Low levels of insulin and high levels blood glucose actually worsen each other. There can be severe damage and additional health complications in the future, including cardiovascular disease, retinopathy, and neuropathy. Stress reduction and management are also extremely crucial. People with type 2 diabetes have much higher cortisol levels than those that are healthy, and cortisol is the "stress" hormone in the body. A chronic stress response results in hyperglycemia, which once becoming chronic, starts the damage to blood vessels while contributing to insulin resistance and dysfunction insulin secretion. Stress also impacts weight gain and results in poor eating behaviors. Type 2 diabetes also increases levels of inflammatory biomarkers. Therefore, reversing type 2 diabetes is linked to an extreme reduction in these biomarkers. One way to do this is through adequate sleep. The quantity and quality of sleep greatly predicts risks of developing or worsening type 2 diabetes.

CULTURE

Culture is a set of learned values, beliefs, customs, and behaviors that are shared by a group of interacting individuals. *Nationality* is an individual's country of origin. Each country has unique cultural groups. Each country has factors that influence culture, such as sociocultural history, language, economics, and government. The United States, England, Spain, Germany, and France have a multicultural foundation. Each cultural group uses its own language, and aspects include grammar and **pragmatics**. Different dialects may exist, which usually reveal cultural differences. Different languages may combine different cultures. *Race* is extremely different than culture.

Attitude is any of the major integrative forces in the development of personality that gives consistency to an individual's behavior. Attitudes are cognitive in nature, formed through interactions with the environment. They reflect the person's innermost convictions about situations good or bad, right, or wrong, desirable or undesirable. **Religions** are important to some cultures and individuals. They bond many attitudes, values, standards, and beliefs, while providing behavioral guidelines.

The term **cultural sensitivity** involves delivering health information that is based on cultural and ethnic norms, social beliefs, values, environmental, and historical factors that are unique to specific populations. There are important cultural factors to consider when working with individuals who have diabetes. To provide good diabetes education to people from all cultures, it is first essential to be aware of unique cultural sensitivities. To overcome cultural barriers, effective communication is essential. Limited proficiency with a country's language – especially with new immigrants from other countries – limits effective communication. Sometimes, illustrated graphic images must be used to communicate information. Professional interpreters may be needed in order to communicate. Cross-cultural communication is essential. Diabetes education programs implemented with culturally appropriate methods can improve patient knowledge, health behavior and status, as well as self-efficacy.

In various cultures, the use of insulin to treat diabetes is not a mainstay of treatment, and thus people may perceive insulin as not being totally safe. This may be influenced by cultural values, beliefs, religions, social factors, health literacy, and language barriers. Hispanics and Latinos who are diabetic may experience a lack of family support, which can delay the initiation of insulin treatment. Family members may convince them not to use insulin, since its use may actually be thought of as a burden upon the family, and interfere with daily life. Instead of insulin, prayer may be used as a way to manage diabetes and improve health, since diabetes is some-times viewed of us a type of "punishment" for behaviors that contradict religious beliefs. Some African Americans believe that insulin causes negative emotions and can interfere with daily schedules. Again, prayer may be used to cope with the disease and to help change unhealthy behaviors – instead of using insulin.

Despite these challenges to receiving treat-ment, type 2 diabetes is up to six times more common in people of South Asian descent, and up to three times more common in people of African and African-Caribbean descent. Today, India and China are considered to be the *dia-betes capitals* of the world. In the United States, African Americans and Hispanic Americans are more likely to have diabetes than non-Hispanic Caucasians. American Indians and Alaska Natives are more likely than other minorities to develop diabetes. Asian Americans and Pacific Islanders have a higher risk for diabetes than non-Hispanic Caucasians.

DIABETES AND MENTAL DISORDERS

Diabetes mellitus is related to a variety of men-tal disorders, and its effects upon psychiatric conditions are significant. The following sec-tions explain the relationships between diabetes and disorders that include depression, anxi-ety, panic disorder, posttraumatic stress disor-der, eating disorders in adolescents, delirium, dementia, and Alzheimer's disease (AD).

Depression

With either type 1 or type 2 diabetes, there is an increased risk of developing depression. Conversely, a person who has depression also has a higher chance of developing type 2 diabe-tes, of up to 60%. Diabetes is linked to emotional and mental health problems that can cause seri-ous problems with employment, productivity, and finances. Because lack of interest or motiva-tion is a common symptom of depression, indi-viduals with diabetes and depression might be less inclined to actively engage in healthy life-style behaviors to more effectively manage their diabetes as a direct result of their depressed mood. Fortunately, depression and diabetes can be simultaneously treated. Effective manage-ment of one of these conditions can positively affect the other.

Epidemiology

Depression may be about two times more com-mon in people with diabetes than in those without. Beyond depression specifically, a term called **diabetes distress** is used to describe a person's emotional response to living with and managing diabetes mellitus, since it is a life-threatening illness that must be continu-ally managed, which is often difficult to do. Diabetes distress is much more common than actual clinical depression in diabetic patients. People that inject insulin have more reported diabetes distress or depression than those tak-ing oral medications. Between 30% and 40% of adults with diabetes report significant levels of diabetes distress. More cases of diabetes dis-tress occur in younger middle-aged adults than in older adults. Women report more problems with depression and diabetes distress than men. Studies of diabetic-related depression in various racial or ethnic groups are lacking. Global data on documented cases of diabetic-related depres-sion have not been performed to any significant degree.

Etiology and Risk Factors

Depression can simply develop from the com-plexities and stressors of managing diabetes mellitus. Also, diabetes can cause other health complications that may worsen depressive symptoms. Depression often causes people to make poor lifestyle choices that are risk factors for diabetes. With its broad effects upon an indi-vidual's ability to perform and follow through with tasks, think, interact, and communicate, depression can interfere with multiple aspects of diabetes management. Common medica-tions such as beta-blockers and diseases such as hypothyroidism can cause depression or make it worse. Other common causes of depressed mood among individuals with diabetes include chronic pain, such as from diabetic neuropathy, and sleep abnormalities. Chronically high blood glucose may worsen depression as well.

Pathophysiology

There are no common genetic factors that explain the association between depression and diabetes. However, there is a definite pathophys-iological cycle between diabetes and depression. This is based on activation and disturbance of the body's stress system. Chronic stress activates the hypothalamus-pituitary-adrenal axis and the sympathetic nervous system. This increases production of cortisol in the adrenal cortex, plus the production of adrenaline and noradrena-line in the adrenal medulla. Chronic hypercor-tisolemia promotes insulin resistance as well as visceral obesity, leading to metabolic syn-drome and type 2 diabetes. Chronic stress and related hormones activate the fear system and the reward system – producing depression and cravings for food. Chronic stress also induces immune dysfunction, resulting in increased production of inflammatory cytokines. In large amounts, the cytokines interact with function of the pancreatic beta cells, leading to insulin resistance and type 2 diabetes. Inflammatory responses are also involved in the pathophysiology of depression. Therefore, stress and inflammation promote both depression *and* diabetes.

Whether diabetes mellitus or depression developed first, the cycle continues viciously without proper diagnosis and treatment of each of these conditions simultaneously. As an example of a diabetic patient who develops depression, the steps in the cycle are as follows:

- Poor diabetes management

- Complications start to occur

- The patient develops depressive signs, including extreme **mood swings**, indecisiveness, lack of motivation, lethargy, and low energy

- The patient engages in less social interaction, does not exercise as much or only engages in activities with low physical exertion, may develop unhealthy behaviors such as binge drinking or smoking, and consumes more processed foods since they are easier to access, and there is less need to spend a significant amount of time preparing meals with them

- All of these result in even poorer diabetes management and the cycle continues

For a patient who is not diabetic but is depressed, the cycle simply starts with the third step, which over time, decreases health status and leads toward type 2 diabetes mellitus.

Clinical Manifestations

A person with diabetes mellitus who develops depression may find it very difficult to exercise, follow medication regimens, adhere to a healthy diet plan, and manage his or her weight. Diabetes-related depression or distress therefore directly contributes to poor blood glucose management, increased hospitalizations, higher risks of long-term complications such as heart disease and retinopathy, and a reduced lifespan. The signs and symptoms of someone that has clinical depression as well as diabetes include:

- Depressed mood

- Loss of pleasure or interest

- Weight loss or gain

- Increased or decreased appetite

- Excessive sleep or insomnia

- Fatigue or loss of energy

- Reduced ability to concentrate or think; or indecisiveness

- Self-blame or guilt

Additional symptoms of depression include psychomotor agitation or retardation, and suicidal thoughts. Other symptoms of diabetes include blurred vision, dehydration, increased thirst, and frequent urination.

Diagnosis

To meet the criteria for clinical depression caused by diabetes or not, the patient must have four or more symptoms from the following list for at least 2 weeks:

- Depressed mood, most of the day, and nearly every day.

- Loss of interest in things or activities that were previously pleasurable.

- Disrupted sleep patterns, including waking up multiple times early in the morning, difficulty falling asleep, or difficulty staying asleep.

- There are guilty feelings about many things, as well as feelings of hopelessness.

- Low energy is experienced, with easy fatigue; this is compromised further by having poor sleep and appetite.

- There is an inability to focus on tasks; therefore, important decisions should be avoided until treatment for depression is underway.

- There are either increases or decreases in appetite, resulting in weight changes that can complicate diabetes further.

- Body movements can become altered; with psychomotor agitation, there is agitation and restlessness; with psychomotor retardation, there is excessive submissiveness and listlessness.

- If suicidal ideation develops – thoughts about or contemplations of committing suicide – the patient must seek treatment immediately.

Treatment

The management of concurrent diabetes and depression combines self-management, psychotherapy, medications, lifestyle changes, and collaborative care. Behavioral programs are successful in helping patients improve metabolic control, manage weight loss and other cardiovascular disease risk factors, and increase fitness levels. These programs increase the sense of well-being and improve quality of life, helping to alleviate depression. Psychotherapy has resulted in better diabetes management and improved depressive symptoms. Cognitive-behavioral therapy, which is based on the understanding that depression causes the patient to only notice negative things in life, is extremely successful in this regard. It teaches patients to avoid engaging in cognitive distortions, such as all-or-nothing thinking, creating strict and unattainable rules, and making "catastrophies" out of small problems in diabetes management. Family therapy and dialectical-behavior therapy have also demonstrated effectiveness for patients with diabetes-related depression or distress. Medications for diabetes and depression include the selective serotonin reuptake inhibitors, which are antidepressants that help regulate blood glucose. Lifestyle changes include getting regular exercise, healthy dietary modifications, and incorporating individualized stress reduction plans. Prolonged stress can result in high blood glucose. Stress management tools include getting regular exercise, meditation, adequate sleep, limiting alcohol and caffeine, and taking regular breaks from stressful work or situations. When a patient with diabetes and depression is supervised by a team of supportive caregivers, results are often improved. Unfortunately, only about 25%–50% of people with diabetes are actually diagnosed and treated for the related depression. Without treatment, depression usually gets worse and diabetes itself can be exacerbated as well. This often makes diabetic patients feel like they are continually failing in managing their disease. While this is not always necessarily true, it can negatively impact their motivation to follow treatment regimens correctly.

For diabetes distress, it is important to see an endocrinologist to manage the diabetes. Patients should also ask their physicians to refer them to mental health counselors that are experienced in dealing with diabetes distress or depression. Diabetes educators are also available for one-on-one meetings. Patients are advised to focus on one or two small management goals at a time for their diabetes, and not to focus on all goals simultaneously as this can be overwhelming. Diabetes support groups are available to share feelings and thoughts with people that are going through the same concerns. The *Behavioral Diabetes Institute* was developed to address the emotional needs of people with diabetes mellitus. It offers online information about diabetes, depression, and other common emotional issues that are related to diabetes. Treating diabetic depression or distress helps patients to generally feel better, have increased energy and better concentration, and improve interest and motivation toward living a longer, happier life.

Prevention

The prevention of diabetes mellitus has been previously discussed, but for prevention of the development of depression as a result of diabetes, psychoeducation and counseling is important as early as possible, since patients are at high risk of decreased psychological well-being. Mental and emotional difficulties develop quickly because of diabetes altering life routines. Psychotherapeutic methods such as cognitive-behavioral therapy, acceptance and commitment therapy, and cognitive analytic therapy are also important. These therapies can help patients by teaching them methods to accept and understand diabetes and the likely complications, even before they occur, so that mental and emotional health can be preserved. With better patient education, depressive symptoms can be prevented or at least reduced.

Prognosis

The prognosis of diabetes is worsened if depression is also present and not fully addressed. However, depression is underdiagnosed and often untreated in patients with diabetes. This obviously makes the prognosis for such patients worse, since the two diseases exacerbate each other over time. With proper treatment, the prognosis is vastly improved for most patients. It is advised that a multidisciplinary team be utilized to provide the most far-reaching care, and the best overall outlook.

CLINICAL CASE

1. Is there a link between diabetes mellitus and depression?
2. What is the pathophysiological cycle between diabetes and depression?
3. What types of psychotherapy are effective for diabetes-related depression?

A 67-year-old man with diabetes had lost his wife in 2 years ago, and had to be taken to the local emergency department because of severe hypoglycemia and confusion. He had taken an overdose of insulin. Once stabilized, he was referred for psychiatric evaluation. The patient denied any suicidal thoughts or alcohol abuse, stating that he had accidentally taken insulin lispro instead of insulin glargine. The hospital staff was skeptical of his description of what occurred, since he had experienced similar visits to the emergency department multiple times over the past 2 years. His explanation was always the same. After the psychiatric evaluation, he was not judged to be a suicidal risk. Outpatient mental health treatment, however, was initiated. His wide-ranging blood glucose levels were documented over time, and the patient later explained that when his blood glucose was high, he didn't want to eat, and that this increased his depression about managing his diabetes.

ANSWERS

1. With either type 1 or type 2 diabetes, there is an increased risk of developing depression. Also, a person with depression has a higher chance of developing type 2 diabetes, of up to 60%. Fortunately, depression and diabetes can be simultaneously treated. Effective management of one of these conditions can positively affect the other.
2. The pathophysiological cycle between diabetes and depression is based on activation and disturbance of the body's stress system. Chronic stress activates the hypothalamus-pituitary-adrenal axis and the sympathetic nervous system. This increases production of cortisol in the adrenal cortex, plus the production of adrenaline and noradrenaline in the adrenal medulla. Chronic hypercortisolemia promotes insulin resistance as well as visceral obesity, leading to metabolic syndrome and type 2 diabetes.
3. For diabetes-related depression, behavioral programs are successful in helping patients improve metabolic control, manage weight loss and other cardiovascular risk factors, and increase fitness levels. These programs increase the sense of well-being and improve quality of life, helping to alleviate depression. Psychotherapy has resulted in better diabetes management and improved depressive symptoms. Cognitive-behavioral therapy is extremely successful in this regard. Family therapy and dialectical-behavior therapy are also successful.

Anxiety

Anxiety is the result of a biological process to preserve and maintain wellness. However, at severe levels, anxiety can be extremely dangerous. Anxiety occurs when feelings of fear, apprehension, and distress become overwhelming, and completion of normal life activities, or even enjoying life, becomes very difficult. Persistent and excessive fear and worry develop, which are out of proportion to the cause of the situation. *Generalized anxiety disorder* is characterized by excessive, uncontrolled, and irrational worry about circumstances, events, or situations. It interferes with health, finances, family relationships, friendships, interpersonal relationships, and work. With diabetes mellitus, many people experience increased stress because of the long-term management of the disease. If concerns about the disease become intense, anxiety can result. People with diabetes are about 20% more likely to be diagnosed with anxiety than those without.

Epidemiology

While anxiety affects nearly everyone sometime in their lives, more than 4.5% of the global population has an actual anxiety disorder. They are more common in females than in males. With diabetes mellitus, anxiety most often affects younger patients, and for unknown reasons, people of Hispanic heritage appear more vulnerable as well. Diabetic patients are at least two times more likely to develop an anxiety disorder than nondiabetic patients. In a Taiwanese study over 4 years, the 1-year prevalence rates of anxiety disorders in diabetic patients was 128.8 per 1,000 people. Cumulative prevalence over the entire 4-year study increased to 289.9 per 1,000. In this study, a higher prevalence was seen in ages 65 or older, with females having more anxiety than males. People of a lower socioeconomic level also had more cases of anxiety. There have been no significant studies of diabetic-related anxiety in distinct racial or ethnic groups.

Etiology and Risk Factors

With diabetes mellitus, causes of anxiety may involve glucose monitoring and required finger prick tests, weight management, diet, hypoglycemic episodes, and long-term complications. Understanding that diabetes leads to heart disease, stroke, and kidney disease increases anxiety in many patients as well. In some studies, anxiety has been shown to actually be a significant risk factor for developing type 2 diabetes. Other causes of risk factors for anxiety include monitoring symptoms of diabetic retinopathy or neuropathy, wounds that heal slowly, and kidney damage.

Pathophysiology

Regardless of a person being diabetic or not, the development of anxiety follows a specific pathway. The sympathetic nerves alert the adrenal medulla to release adrenaline and a small amount of dopamine. The adrenaline induces release of the neurotransmitter epinephrine, boosting blood pressure and blood glucose. The glucose, with stored fatty acids, can be turned into quick energy by muscles. However, once this "rush" is over, the body experiences a "crash." The muscles – especially in the chest – feel tired and sore because of tension and rapid breathing. Hyperactivity of the amygdala, regardless of cause, indicates that an individual is not just experiencing a transient episode of anxiety, but may have an actual anxiety disorder warranting treatment.

Clinical Manifestations

The common symptoms of anxiety related to diabetes mellitus are very similar to those of general anxiety regardless of cause. They include nervousness, restlessness, tenseness, and feelings of danger, dread, or panic. The heart rate and breathing may become rapid. Sweating is increased or heavy. The muscles may twitch or tremble and the individual feels weak and lethargic. There is difficulty thinking clearly or focusing on specific thoughts. Often, insomnia develops. Digestive and gastrointestinal problems may include constipation, diarrhea, or gas. The individual may become likely to attempt to avoid anything involved in diabetes management that triggers anxiety. Some people experience obsessive thoughts or start compulsively performing certain behaviors. If a severe manifestation from diabetes has previously occurred, such as an amputation from a chronic wound that has not fully healed, the individual may develop a form of posttraumatic stress disorder as a result.

Diagnosis

Symptoms of anxiety and hypoglycemia can mimic each other. Therefore, it is important that a diabetic patient contact a physician to rule out hypoglycemia or other physiological sources of anxiety symptoms before referral to a mental health provider for anxiety. If an individual believes that anxiety has become significant because of diabetes, primary care physicians can ask a series of questions to assess the anxiety levels. There are also questionnaires available that can be used to assess these levels and prompt treatment decisions.

Treatment

Anxiety and actual anxiety disorders usually respond very well to treatment. Even so, according to the Anxiety and Depression Association of America, only about 36% of people are treated. Since anxiety as well as depression are linked to higher risks for premature death, treatment should occur. Cognitive-behavioral therapy that incorporates relaxation techniques such as deep breathing and progressive muscle relaxation is often very effective and can be used along with medications. The individual patient learns to identify and understand his or her anxious thoughts and behaviors, and then change or modify them toward reducing their anxiety and worry. Relaxation strategies can also be very effective in managing physiological symptoms of anxiety, such as increased heart rate, breathing rate, and muscle tension. Guided imagery, where a patient imagines a calm and peaceful scene or performs a "body scan" technique while engaging in slow diaphragmatic breathing and focusing on releasing tension in various muscle groups, can be useful in this regard. Medications include antidepressants and antianxiety drugs, most of which are compatible with diabetes medications. It is important that the physician assess the extent of the patient's diabetes and complications when determining the correct medications that should be used for anxiety.

Prevention

People with diabetes have additional stressors in their lives that can result in anxiety, stress, and worry. Mental stressors can cause increased blood glucose levels in type 2 diabetes, but can increase or decrease these levels in type 1 diabetes. Physical stressors increase blood glucose in both forms of diabetes. Therefore, there must be preventive patient education that discusses the impact of stress and why it is important to manage it. Prevention also includes screening for diabetes-related distress and depression, plus support groups with patients that have had anxiety, allowing for more sharing of information. Preventive measures can include physical exercises, meditation and mindfulness techniques, and keeping journals to document stressors and emotional reactions to them.

Prognosis

With adequate treatment, the prognosis of anxiety that accompanies diabetes mellitus is generally good. However, the presence of anxiety in diabetic patients worsens the prognosis of the disease. It increases noncompliance to treatments, and decreases quality of life while increasing death rates.

CLINICAL CASE

1. Which individuals are most affected by anxiety because of diabetes?
2. What may cause anxiety in diabetic patients?
3. Can symptoms of anxiety and hypoglycemia be similar?

A 50-year-old man previously diagnosed with anxiety is brought to the family physician by his wife. The man had fallen at home because he didn't see a coffee table due to a recent blurring of his vision. His wife describes other manifestations of his health, including confusion, forgetfulness, needing to go to the bathroom at least 3 times at night, tingling in his feet, an inability to walk as far as normal after dinner, and a cut on one leg that has not healed. The patient admits that the changes in his health are increasing his anxiety. After standard tests are done, he is diagnosed with type 2 diabetes mellitus. The physician discusses treatment options and explains that anxiety with diabetes is a common occurrence, and that with proper adherence to treatment, both conditions can respond well.

ANSWERS

1. With diabetes mellitus, anxiety most often affects younger patients, and for unknown reasons, people of Hispanic heritage. Diabetic patients are at least 2 times more likely to develop an anxiety disorder than nondiabetic patients.
2. With diabetes mellitus, causes of anxiety may involve glucose monitoring and required finger prick tests, weight management, diet, hypoglycemic episodes, and long-term complications. Understanding that diabetes leads to heart disease, stroke, and kidney disease increases anxiety.
3. Symptoms of anxiety and hypoglycemia can mimic each other. It is important that the patient contact a physician to rule out hypoglycemia before referral to a mental health provider for anxiety.

Panic Disorder

Panic disorder involves recurrent panic attacks, often accompanied by fears of future attacks. Panic attacks often have both emotional and physical components, such as feeling intense fear and having sensations of difficulty breathing or tightness in the chest. Because of the extreme discomfort associated with these symptoms, the affected individual may make behavioral changes in order to avoid any situation that could possibly instigate an attack. Panic is associated with worsened diabetes and functional losses. Panic is often comorbid with depression. It is important to address psychosocial disorders in patients with diabetes. A primary trigger of panic attacks, and in some patients, full-blown panic disorder, is repeated hypoglycemia. The fear of hypoglycemia is for some patients so severe that they avoid their self-management regimen to varying degrees. It is important to educate patients about the differences between the symptoms of hypoglycemia and the actual symptoms of a panic attack as well.

Epidemiology

Panic disorder often starts in early adulthood. It is less common in children and elderly individuals. Panic disorder affects 2%–3% of the global population annually, with women being affected about two times as often as men. Panic attacks generally affect up to 11% of the global population annually. There are no accurate statistics on how many people with diabetes also have panic disorder or panic attacks.

Etiology and Risk Factors

The cause of panic disorder is unknown. Panic reactions may be due to mistaking body sensations for situations that are life-threatening. Psychological factors such as environment, stress, and life transitions may be contributing factors. Triggers include major stress, medications, and physical condition or disorder. Substance abuse is also causative, and smoking tobacco may increase risks of panic disorder. Respiratory abnormalities are common with high levels of anxiety, and smoking worsens them. Caffeine also is linked to panic disorder because it increases heart rate. Certain medications can induce higher blood pressure. Risk factors for panic disorder include the female gender, age (18–35 years), medical history, and genetics. Hypoglycemia and panic disorder are linked in a very complicated way, but symptoms can be very similar. These shared symptoms include tachycardia, shakiness, irritability, difficulty concentrating, nausea, anxiety, and panic. Diabetic risk factors for panic attacks or panic disorder include higher A1c hemoglobin levels, increased diabetic complications, and disability.

Pathophysiology

Underlying mechanisms of panic attacks or panic disorder involve the hippocampus, anterior cingulate cortex, insula, amygdala, lateral prefrontal cortex, and periaqueductal gray matter. In a panic attack, there is usually elevated blood flow or metabolism. **Insula** hyperactivity is likely related to irregular norepinephrine activity. The periaqueductal gray matter is implicated in generating fear responses. There is an abnormally functioning "brain circuit" made up of the **amygdala**, central gray matter, ventromedial nucleus of the hypothalamus, and **locus coeruleus**. Often, there are lower than normal levels of gamma-aminobutyric acid (GABA). Hyperventilation is a component of panic, and results in the exhalation of excessive carbon dioxide. There may be a feeling of being unable to "catch their breath." The partial pressure of carbon dioxide is another mediator of panic disorder. Panic attacks may begin and worsen in association with diabetes progressing, increased complications, and loss of normal functioning. They are also accompany with depression in many patients.

Clinical Manifestations

The signs and symptoms of panic attack may include sudden and intense fear or discomfort, accompanied by at least four of the following symptoms:

- Feelings of choking
- Fear of dying, losing control
- Numbness or tingling
- Abdominal distress or nausea
- Increased heart rate or palpitations
- Chest discomfort or pain
- Chills or flushing
- Sweating
- Faintness, dizziness
- Shortness of breath
- Shaking

Panic attacks are very uncomfortable. They may occur with any anxiety disorder. Most affected individuals anticipate future attacks and worry about their occurrence. This is called **anticipatory anxiety**. The patients may worry about a serious disorder of the brain, heart, or lungs, so visits to physicians or the emergency department are common. Repeated panic attacks in people that have diabetes mellitus may lead to worsened disease control, more severe complications, and a reduced quality of life. About half of diabetics with panic attacks also have some level of depression. The A1c hemoglobin levels are usually slightly higher if panic attacks occur than they are in people that do not have these attacks.

Diagnosis

The diagnosis of panic disorder is based on medical history, review of current medications, a complete physical examination, discussion of symptoms and concerns, and a psychiatric assessment. There is evaluation of whether panic attacks are unexpected and recurrent. The patient and physician discuss whether one or more panic attacks was followed by at least 1 month of worrying about another attack, or changing behaviors to avoid having another attack. There is evaluation of any medical disorders, such as diabetes, that may be causative, along with medications or other substances. The patient must be evaluated about the possibility of having another type of mental health disorder. Diagnostic tests include blood and urine tests, various imaging studies, and electrocardiogram.

Treatment

With frequent panic attacks and avoidance behaviors, drug therapy plus intensive psychotherapy is needed. Antidepressants, benzodiazepines, and combinations of these can be helpful. When antidepressants are used with benzodiazepines, it is usually as an initial treatment. The benzodiazepines are slowly decreased in dosage and often eventually discontinued or used more sporadically. Some patients respond well only to combination therapy. Psychotherapies include exposure therapy and cognitive-behavioral therapy are also used together. Exposure therapy helps patients to directly experience and confront feared situations in a controlled environment, and reduce avoidance until the fear is extinguished. Cognitive-behavioral therapy teaches how to recognize and change distorted thoughts and false beliefs, and modify behaviors to become more adaptive to situations. With diabetes, treatment may also involve relaxation training incorporating slow breathing techniques while monitoring CO_2 levels in order to prevent hyperventilation. Biofeedback is an additional therapeutic technique that can improve symptoms of anxiety or panic while reducing the respiratory rate. This method gives patients visible evidence of how they are improving, thus providing them with a sense of control over their symptoms. Breathing training is helpful in panic disorder whether there is or is not any concurrent respiratory problems.

Prevention

The prevention of panic attacks or panic disorder begins with understanding family history, stressful live events, substance abuse, neurological problems, and the presence of other psychological disorders. Preventive measures include eating a balanced diet, avoiding smoking and excessive caffeine, limiting alcohol use, avoiding illegal drugs, and adequately treating diabetes mellitus.

Prognosis

The prognosis of panic attacks or panic disorder that accompanies diabetes mellitus is generally good with proper treatment. Adequate medications and psychotherapy are effective in about 85% of cases. Nearly 65% of patients with panic disorder achieve remission within 6 months. It is important to manage symptoms and complications of diabetes in order to improve the overall prognosis.

Posttraumatic Stress Disorder

Posttraumatic stress disorder (*PTSD*) develops in some people after a dangerous, frightening, or shocking event. It is common after fire, sexual assault, physical violence, a car accident, earthquake, or military combat. It involves intrusive memories of the event, reactivity to possible threats, and nightmares. Often, there are reports of feeling anxious or frightened even in the absence of danger. A person with PTSD may experience an activation of chronic stress symptoms, triggering the physiological factors that lead to type 2 diabetes. Additional studies are needed concerning the link between these two conditions.

Epidemiology

Posttraumatic stress disorder affects approximately 9% of the worldwide population, with adults most often experiencing it. Women are more likely to develop PTSD than men, but only slightly. According to a 2015 study, women with PTSD have twice the risk for developing type 2 diabetes. This is, in part, due to the unhealthy behaviors associated with PTSD, which include poor diet, smoking, and substance use. There is no racial or ethnic predilection for the disorder. With PTSD, age-adjusted incidence of type 2 diabetes is 21 cases per 1,000 population in obese patients, but only 5.8 per 1,000 in those that are not obese. Without PTSD, age-adjusted

incidence of type 2 diabetes is 21.2 per 1,000 in obese patients, and only 6.4 per 1,000 in those that are not obese.

Etiology and Risk Factors

Posttraumatic stress disorder is caused by events that involve horror, helplessness or fear. The events may directly or indirectly involve the affected individual. Common causes of PTSD include natural or man-made disasters, sexual assault, and war. Risk factors include emergency situations, violent crimes, violence in general, kidnapping, fire, robberies, accidents, death of a loved one, legal problems, and severe medical conditions such as diabetes mellitus, cancers, and AIDS. Also, PTSD can either cause or worsen diabetes. It may be severe enough to require medication. This makes an affected individual even more likely to develop type 2 diabetes. Those with PTSD that are overweight or obese are also more likely to develop the disease.

Pathophysiology

The pathophysiology of PTSD is not completely understood. The size of the hippocampus is inversely related to PTSD and the success of its treatment. The smaller the hippocampus, the higher the risk of PTSD. During trauma, higher levels of stress hormones suppress the activities of the hypothalamus. This may be a major factor in the development of PTSD. There are also low levels of serotonin, contributing to anxiety, aggression, irritability, impulsivity, an inability to stop thinking about traumatic events, and even suicidal thoughts. Low levels of dopamine promote **anhedonia**, apathy, impaired attention, and motor deficits. High levels of dopamine promote motor deficits, restlessness, psychosis, and agitation. There is less-than-normal activity in the dorsal and rostral anterior **cingulate cortices** and ventromedial prefrontal cortex. These areas are linked to experiencing and regulating of emotions. The pathophysiological relationship between PTSD and diabetes mellitus is not fully understood. However, a sustained activation of the hormonal stress axis, because of chronic stress symptoms, is likely implicated.

Clinical Manifestations

People with PTSD usually have frequent and unwanted memories and nightmares of the traumatic event. Less frequently, transient waking dissociative states occur as flashbacks. These may cause reactions that resemble those that occurred in the original event. Symptoms may be delayed, occurring several months or years after the causative traumatic event. Patients with chronic PTSD are often depressed, have anxiety disorders, or abuse substances. They may be guilty about actions that occurred during the traumatic event, or because they survived when others died. With diabetes mellitus, PTSD is able to increase total cholesterol levels, LDL, cause weight gain, and therefore, increase the body mass index (BMI).

Diagnosis

The diagnosis of PTSD is based on a patient having had direct or indirect exposure to a traumatic event, and the symptoms that manifest afterwards. As with PTSD in diabetic patients, diagnosis is based on elevated blood glucose, elevated fasting capillary glucose, and elevated nonfasting plasma or capillary glucose. Diagnosis of PTSD with diabetes simply combines the signs and symptoms of PTSD with the standard diagnosis of diabetes mellitus.

Treatment

Psychotherapy and medications are used to treat PTSD. For the PTSD, medications used typically target the most prominent symptoms and may include selective serotonin reuptake inhibitors (SSRIs) and serotonin-norepinephrine reuptake inhibitors (SNRIs). Exposure therapy is used, in which the patient is exposed to normally avoided situations that trigger stress in a controlled environment until the emotional reaction is extinguished. *Eye movement desensitization and reprocessing* is a type of exposure therapy. The patient is asked to follow the moving finger of the psychotherapist as he or she imagines being exposed to the trauma. Many patients must learn how to relax and reduce their anxiety before they are ready for exposure therapy. Breathing exercises, mindfulness, and yoga are all helpful. Behavioral and cognitive-behavioral therapies have provided the best outcomes for PTSD.

Clinically significant improvement of PTSD symptoms are considered to be 20 or more points on the *PTSD checklist* within 1 year. For people whose PTSD symptoms do not greatly improve, about 18 of every 1,000 develop type 2 diabetes. For those whose PTSD improve, about 16 of every 1,000 develop type 2 diabetes. Therefore, therapy for PTSD is able to somewhat reduce the risk for developing type 2 diabetes when a person has PTSD. Patient education about the possible health benefits of PTSD treatment may encourage affected individuals to participate in psychotherapy sessions.

Prevention

Prevention for some causes of PTSD is possible. Patient education is able to help individuals choose healthier lifestyles and habits, which can prevent severe medical conditions such as diabetes or AIDS, which are linked to PTSD. Also, PTSD can also result in a worsening of diabetes. Obviously, nonpreventable causes of PTSD include many emergency situations, disasters, violent crimes, violence in general, kidnappings, fires, robberies, accidents, deaths of loved ones, legal problems, and severe medical conditions such as many cancers.

Prognosis

Since *posttraumatic stress disorder* is highly treatable, the prognosis is often very good. The best prognosis is given for patients that seek help earlier in the disease course. Though not curable, treatments for PTSD help patients to eventually heal and accept the traumatic events they have experienced. They learn how to live with their stress and continue with their lives. However, some people with PTSD do not seek treatment, in order to avoid confronting the trauma they witnessed. This has a poor prognosis regardless of whether the affected individual also has diabetes mellitus.

Delirium and Dementia

Delirium along with dementia is one of the most common causes of cognitive impairment. Affective disorders such as depression can also disrupt cognition. Delirium and dementia are separate disorders that can easily be confused. In both, **cognition** is disordered. The major difference is that delirium mostly affects *attention and orientation*, while dementia mostly affects *memory*. It is important to understand that delirium often develops in patients who have dementia. Delirium is acute, transient, and usually reversible. It is more common in the elderly. When occurring in younger patients, it is usually linked to drug use or life-threatening systemic disorders. Delirium is sometimes also called *toxic encephalopathy* or *metabolic encephalopathy*. Dementia is chronic, global, and usually irreversible deterioration of cognition. It can occur at any age, but mostly affects the elderly. More than 5 million Americans have the condition. Dementia is classified as Alzheimer's or non-Alzheimer's; cortical or subcortical; irreversible or potentially reversible; and common or rare. There are links between delirium, dementia, and diabetes. With diabetes, delirium is mostly related to hypoglycemia and only occurs rarely with hyperglycemia. Hyperglycemia as well as hypoglycemia over the long term can damage the brain, resulting in short-term cognitive impairment and long-term problems such as confusion and memory loss. Many scientists believe that some cases of AD are related to complicated effects of type 2 diabetes upon the brain. Since diabetes damages blood vessels, it is a risk factor for vascular dementia as well. The links between diabetes and other dementia subtypes such as Lewy body dementia or **frontotemporal dementia** are unknown.

Epidemiology

Poorly controlled diabetes mellitus is a possible trigger of delirium. Cases of delirium secondary to hypoglycemia in patients with diabetes are common. However, reports of secondary delirium with hyperglycemia are rare, and usually occur in type 1 diabetes. There is a higher prevalence of cognitive dysfunction in diabetic patients over age 60, especially with type 1 diabetes. Diabetes is associated with a 60% increased risk of all types of dementia. In women, there is a relative risk of 1.62 times higher than in men. Risks for dementia is also more common in women. The relative risk for vascular dementia is 2.34 in diabetic women and 1.73 in diabetic men. Deaths of patients with dementia and diabetes are also higher than for patients that have dementia but are not diabetic. Age of onset of dementia and death occur earlier with diabetes than without. Dementia occurs an average of 1.7 years early, and death occurs 2.32 years earlier in diabetic patients. There appears to be no racial or ethnic predilection for dementia with diabetes.

Etiology and Risk Factors

With diabetes mellitus, delirium is mostly caused by hypoglycemia or low insulin levels. These conditions are also risk factors for the development of delirium. Diabetic dementia is a common long-term outcome of excessive body weight. Type 2 diabetes almost doubles risks for developing dementia, and when it develops, it is often earlier in life. Diabetes is also a major risk factor for dementia.

Pathophysiology

Delirium may involve reversible impairment of cerebral oxidative metabolism, generation of cytokines, and multiple neurotransmitter abnormalities. Any type of stress causes upregulating of the sympathetic tone while downregulating the parasympathetic tone. This impairs cholinergic function, which contributes to the condition. The elderly have a higher vulnerability to reduced cholinergic transmission, increasing risks. No matter what the cause, there is impairment of the cerebral hemispheres, or the arousal mechanisms of the thalamus and brainstem reticular activating system. Neurologists often use the words "delirium" and "toxic metabolic encephalopathy" interchangeably.

Cognition deteriorates slowly, and can be resolved if treated adequately. Up to half of all patients who have mild cognitive impairment will develop dementia within 3 years. Drugs that worsen cognitive deficits include benzodiazepines, certain tricyclic antidepressants, antihistamines, antipsychotics, benztropine, and alcohol. For example, **Wernicke-Korsakoff syndrome** is a form of dementia caused by chronic, long-term alcoholism, which leads to vitamin B1 deficiency.

However, the leading cause of dementia is *AD*, which results from death of cerebral cortex cells. Abnormal proteins, believed to be *beta amyloids*, form lesions in the cerebral cortex that eventually disrupt and destroy surrounding cells. *Vascular dementia* is caused by atherosclerosis in the brain, in which inadequate blood flow supplies insufficient oxygen. Areas of dead tissue then form, and vascular dementia develops. This is usually linked to previous cardiovascular conditions such as diabetes, heart disease, hypertension, and high cholesterol. *Parkinson's disease* results in buildup of **Lewy bodies** in the brain, which eventually affect memory and cognition, causing dementia. *Lewy body dementia* usually affects people with no family history, and its causes are unclear. **Huntington's disease** also results in dementia, and is caused by a genetic mutation resulting in death of nerve cells in the basal ganglia.

Clinical Manifestations

The clinical manifestations of delirium are primarily difficulty in focusing, maintaining, or shifting attention. The patient may be disoriented to time, and sometimes to place or person. They may hallucinate. There is confusion about daily events and routines, along with changes in personality. The thought patterns become disorganized, and speech may by disordered, slurred, rapid, with neologisms, aphasic errors, or chaotic patterns. Symptoms change over minutes to hours, and may be reduced during the day but worse at night. Symptoms include fearfulness, **paranoia**, and inappropriate behaviors. The patient may be agitated, irritable, *hyperalert*, and hyperactive – then becoming lethargic, quiet, and withdrawn. The extremely elderly often become quiet and withdrawn, which is often mistaken for depression. Some patients alternate between the two states. There are common distortions of sleeping and eating patterns. Due to the cognitive disturbances, the patient has poor insight and impaired judgment. Other signs and symptoms are based on the cause.

The signs and symptoms of dementia develop slowly, usually beginning with loss of short-term memory and sometimes other cognitive abilities as well, such as language, attention, and executive functioning. Symptoms are divided into early, intermediate, and late classifications. Personality changes and altered behaviors can develop early or late in the progression of dementia. Based on the type of dementia, motor and other focal neurologic deficits occur at different stages. In vascular dementia, these occur early, while in AD, they develop late. Early symptoms of dementia include short-term memory impairment, with the learning and retaining of new information becoming difficult. The patient will have difficulty finding the right word when speaking, and experience mood swings and personality changes. It may become harder to handle daily living tasks such as remembering where objects were placed, handling banking activities, remembering to take medications, and even getting lost in a familiar location. There may be impairment of abstract though, judgment, or insight. The patient often becomes agitated, hostile, and irritable because of these changes. Other manifestations include agnosia, apraxia, and aphasia. *Agnosia* is impairment of identifying objects while sensory function is normal. *Apraxia* is impairment in performing learned motor activities while motor function is still intact. *Aphasia* is impairment of language use or comprehension. Family members of dementia patients often report odd behaviors along with emotional changes.

The intermediate stage of dementia involves reduction in memory of remote events but not a complete loss of this memory. The patient may need help with more basic daily tasks such as bathing, dressing, eating, and toileting. Personality changes may worsen, with the patient more easily becoming anxious, irritable, inflexible, self-centered, angry, passive, unaffected, depression, indecisive, and lacking in spontaneity. Patients often withdraw from social situations, and behavior disorders may develop. They may wander, become quickly hostile or uncooperative, and even physically aggressive. In this stage, there is loss of social and environmental cues, and the patient usually does not know where they are, the hour, the day, the month, or even the year. Patients get lost easily, even within their own homes. They are at higher risk of falling or experiencing accidents and often need 24-hour supervision for safety purposes. Psychosis may develop with hallucinations and delusions, and sleep patterns are often disrupted.

The late, severe stage of dementia makes the patient unable to walk, feed himself or herself, or perform other daily living activities. Incontinence develops, all memories are lost, and there may be an inability to swallow. The patient is at risk of pneumonia mostly because of aspiration, pressure ulcers, and undernutrition.

It is usually necessary to place the patient into a long-term care facility. Eventually, the patient will no longer speak. When the patient appears ill, it is up to physicians to determine treatments, because there will be no febrile or leukocytic reactions to infections. In most cases, the patient will develop an infection, go into a coma, and ultimately die.

Diagnosis

The two conditions must not be mistaken for each other – especially in the elderly. There is no definitive laboratory test to establish the cause of cognitive impairment. Therefore, it is essential to conduct a thorough patient history and physical examination, along with knowledge of baseline function of the patient. Clinicians often overlook delirium, especially in the elderly. The condition should be considered for any elderly patient with impaired attention or memory. The next diagnostic steps involve use of the *Diagnostic and Statistical Manual of Mental Disorders* (DSM) or *Confusion Assessment Method* (CAM). For a positive diagnosis of delirium, there must be the following two components in existence: Acute cognition change that fluctuates during the day, and inattention – the inability to focus or follow what is spoken. Also, one of the following two components must exist: Disturbance of consciousness or having disorganized thinking such as rambling statements, irrelevant conversation, or illogical idea flow.

A short-term memory test is first conducted, such as registering three different objects and then recalling them after 5 minutes. Dementia patients will forget such simple information within 3–5 minutes. The dementia patient will struggle to name just a few common objects. A dementia diagnosis requires at least one of the following: Aphasia, apraxia, **agnosia**, or an impaired ability to organize, plan, sequence, or think abstractly.

The presence of multiple cognitive deficits, especially in a patient with an average or higher level of education, suggests dementia. Laboratory tests include levels of B12 and thyroid-stimulating hormone. Sometimes, CBC and liver function tests are performed. Testing for HIV or syphilis may be indicated. Lumbar puncture can be done if a chronic infection or neurosyphilis is suspected. For initial evaluation of dementia, or after a sudden change in cognition or mental status, CT or MRI should be performed. Neuroimaging can identify metabolic disorders such as **Wilson's disease**. A formal mental status examination can be conducted, and in many cases, formal neuropsychological testing is beneficial to assist with differential diagnosis and treatment planning.

Treatment

Delirium can be resolved by treating causes such as infection or dehydration, and by addressing pain or drug use. Good nutrition and hydration should be provided, and deficiencies of thiamin or vitamin B12 corrected. Drug regimens should be simplified. Intravenous lines, bladder catheters, and physical restraints should be avoided, as much as possible. Family members should receive counseling about the effects of delirium, and told that it is usually reversible but this may take weeks to months after the acute illness is resolved.

Medications for delirium include haloperidol, which can reduce agitation and psychotic symptoms. Drugs must be administered with care because they have the potential to prolong or exacerbate delirium. Second-generation, atypical antipsychotics may be preferred due to fewer extrapyramidal adverse effects, but their long-term use in dementia patients can increase risks of stroke and death. Benzodiazepines have a faster onset of action than antipsychotics, but often worsen confusion and sedation in delirium patients. While these drugs are equally effective for agitation, the antipsychotics have fewer adverse effects. Benzodiazepines are preferred when delirium is caused by sedative withdrawal, and for those who cannot tolerate antipsychotics. Doses of these drugs must be reduced as quickly as possible.

For dementia, treatment begins with occupational and physical therapists evaluating the living place for safety, to prevent falls and accidents, manage behavior problems, and plan for the future progression of the disease. Medical social workers often get involved and can assist patients and families with developing a plan for monitoring and overseeing performance of activities of daily living to ensure safety and accuracy, while also managing any disruptive behaviors which may arise. For wandering patients, there are signal monitoring systems available, and a program called *Safe Return* into which they can be registered. The patient may ultimately need to be moved into a living facility that does not have stairs, or an assisted-living or skilled nursing facility.

The living area should be designed to help preserve the patient's feelings of self-control and dignity. Radio, television, and night-light are all good objects to keep the patient oriented and to focus attention. Exercise should occur once per day, which improves cardiovascular tone and overall balance, as well as reducing restlessness, manage behaviors, and improve sleep. Music and occupational therapy help maintain fine motor control, and provides nonverbal stimulation.

Prevention

There is a positive association between delirium and hypoglycemia in critically ill patients with diabetes mellitus, yet delirium is not associated with more extreme glucose variability. To prevent delirium in a diabetic patient, glucose levels must be monitored very closely. To prevent dementia, there must be optimized glycemic control, avoidance of hypoglycemia, and a maximization of time in a controlled range of blood glucose. Blood pressure, obesity, and depression must all be managed. Patients should have regular physical activity and stop smoking. Given that diabetes is a risk factor for development of dementia, patient education about diabetic-related dementia is essential. All diabetic patients over 65 years of age should be screened for dementia. Cognitive impairment must be monitored. Reversible endocrine, metabolic, and nutritional causes of dementia must be screened for. Caregivers and family members must be involved in helping diabetic patients regarding their mental, physical, and financial needs.

Prognosis

The prognosis for delirium in a diabetic patient can be good if the diabetes is well-managed. With poor control, delirium can manifest and remain, worsening the prognosis. Fortunately, since delirium mostly occurs in association with hypoglycemia, correcting that problem usually resolves delirium.

CLINICAL CASE

1. When does delirium usually occur in a diabetic patient?
2. What is the pathophysiology behind delirium?
3. For a positive diagnosis of delirium, which components must be present?

An 80-year-old woman with type 2 diabetes had been taking oral antihyperglycemic medications. When she decided to stop taking them, she developed confusion, agitation, delusional ideas of persecution, and impulsivity. She became unable to properly care for herself. A friend discovered her completely disoriented at home, and brought her to the emergency department. The patient was alert but didn't know the time of day, and kept asking the hospital staff where she was. She made several attempts to leave, saying that she had to go home to cook dinner. Physical examination showed nothing significant. She had no fever or neurological symptoms. Biochemistry revealed extremely high serum glucose and glycated hemoglobin (HbA1c). The patient was diagnosed with an acute confusional form dementia in the context of poorly controlled type 2 diabetes mellitus.

ANSWERS

1. Delirium is mostly related to hypoglycemia in a diabetic patient, and only occurs rarely with hyperglycemia. Over time, hypoglycemia and hyperglycemia can damage the brain, resulting in short-term cognitive impairment and long-term problems such as confusion and memory loss.
2. Delirium may involve reversible impairment of cerebral oxidative metabolism, generation of cytokines, and multiple neurotransmitter abnormalities. Stress causes upregulating of the sympathetic tone while downregulating the parasympathetic tone, impairing cholinergic function, and contributing to delirium.
3. For a positive diagnosis of delirium, there must be acute cognition change that fluctuates during the day, and inattention – the inability to focus or follow what is spoken. There must also be disturbance of consciousness or disorganized thinking such as rambling statements, irrelevant conversation, or illogical idea flow.

ALZHEIMER'S DISEASE

AD is a condition characterized by progressive mental deterioration, often with confusion, memory failure, disorientation, restlessness, agnosia, speech disturbances, and hallucinosis. It is the most common form of dementia among elderly people, with no cure. It is ultimately a fatal disease, because of its complications. The patient becomes totally dependent for all care, which heavily burdens spouses and family members. This disease is also called *senile dementia-Alzheimer type*. Diabetes mellitus can increase risks for AD, but this is not completely understood. Diabetes is known to increase the likelihood for developing vascular dementia, and many diabetic patients have brain changes that are signs of vascular dementia as well as AD. Mild cognitive impairment may precede or accompany AD. Therefore, effective prevention or treatment of diabetes may help prevent AD from developing. There is also a hypothesis that AD is triggered by a type of insulin resistance and insulin-like growth factor dysfunction in the brain, resulting in the creation of a condition sometimes referred to as *type 3 diabetes*.

Epidemiology

Diabetes mellitus increases risks for eventually developing AD and other dementias. Developing type 2 diabetes before the age of 60 doubles the risk for dementia. For every 5 years a person lives with diabetes, the dementia risk increases by 24%. For people aged 65 and older, one out of eight people have AD, and almost one of every two people over age 85 does. Nearly 500,000 people under age 65 have early-onset AD or other dementias. While there is generally no difference between the genders in prevalence or incidence, though executive function declines more quickly in older women that have type 2 diabetes. Though no clear epidemiology about specific racial or ethnic groups with diabetes + dementia has been well documented, since African American and Hispanic patients generally have higher occurrences of diabetes, the likelihood of them eventually developing AD is predicted to also be increased.

Etiology and Risk Factors

The exact causes of AD are not fully understood. The strongest risk factor for developing dementia and AD is advancing age. However, there are some reversible causes of dementia or cognitive impairment that are sometimes called pseudodementia. These include deficiencies of vitamin B12, folate, hypothyroidism, and depression. Risk factors include aging, low education level, **Down syndrome**, and positive family history. The other risk factor include smaller size of brain, head injuries, and lower levels of mental and physical activity in later life. Diabetes mellites, obesity, smoking, hyperlipidemia, and hypertension are also implicated.

Pathophysiology

Cerebral atrophy in the subcortical nuclei, hippocampus, and amygdala are characteristic features in Alzheimer's patients. Senile plaques, beta (ß)-amyloid deposits, and neurofibrillary tangles in the cerebral cortex as well as the subcortical gray matter are also found. Only upon autopsy are these revealed. There is a decreased cholinergic innervation, with variable decreases in other neurotransmitters. Degeneration of the locus ceruleus and amyloid angiopathy are observed. The overproduction of amyloid is linked to earlier onset AD, which occurs prior to the age of 65. The most common finding in Alzheimer's patients is loss of cholinergic neurons, which neurons use acetylcholine to communicate.

Clinical Manifestations

The signs and symptoms include disorientation, confusion, memory failure, restlessness, agnosia, speech disturbances, and difficulty with concentration and/or multitasking. Paranoia may be observed, such as in accusations of stealing or being threatened by others. Psychotic symptoms may be hallucinations or **delusions**. The patient may become verbally or physically aggressive. Patients are initially unable to handle complex daily tasks such as managing medications and finances, and driving. As the condition advances, they begin to have trouble completing more basic tasks such as feeding, dressing, toileting, or bathing. The majority of them must be moved to skilled nursing facilities with 24-hour care. The signs and symptoms may correlate with the location of brain atrophy. In AD, the parietal and temporal lobes are primarily affected. Therefore, memory and visuospatial task abnormalities are observed first. Language is preserved early in the disease until later stages.

Diagnosis

Diagnostic criteria consist of a failure in at least three cognitive functions, including memory, use of language, attention, executive functioning, and visuospatial skills. Changes in personality may also be observed. Measurement of biomarkers in blood and cerebrospinal fluid, as well as neuroimaging tests to characterize brain changes, are assessments recommended by the Alzheimer's Association. Diagnosis is assisted by full clinical evaluation and presentation history. Laboratory tests can help rule out possible causes of symptoms, and include thyroid function tests, plus checking for levels of serum folate and vitamin B12. Either a CT scan or an MRI scan of the brain is needed to rule out structural causes of dementia or other cognitive impairment. A mental status examination or formal neuropsychological evaluation can provide additional information regarding the extent and severity of cognitive impairments.

Treatment

Preserving and slowing further decline of cognition and physical functioning are the primary focuses of treatment. This is often accomplished in assisted-living or skilled nursing care settings, where efforts can also be made to minimize psychiatric and behavioral symptoms. The safety of patients is important. Family members and caregivers often benefit from attending support groups to learn information about the disease and how to navigate many of the associated challenges. The U.S. Food and Drug Administration has approved two different classes of medications for AD. These include *acetylcholinesterase inhibitors* and *N-methyl-D-aspartate receptor modulators*. They allow more acetylcholine to remain between nerve cells, increasing their communication with other neurons. They are generally used with caution in patients who are using digoxin, calcium channel blockers or beta-blockers.

Memantine is the only example of *N-methyl-D-aspartate receptor modulators* that is currently used. It works by blocking the effects of glutamate in the brain, which causes large amounts of calcium to move into the neurons, causing their death. Memantine, therefore, is useful because it reduces the effects of glutamate, but does not totally block its binding. The adverse effects of memantine are headache, confusion, dizziness, and constipation. Because the two classes of AD medications work in different ways, they can be used in combination.

Prevention

The prevention for AD may involve diets such as the Mediterranean diet, the similar *MIND diet*, and other healthy eating patterns such as the *DASH diet*. The MIND diet combines features of the Mediterranean and DASH diets, focusing specifically on brain health. The letters M-I-N-D stand for *Mediterranean-DASH Intervention for Neurodegenerative Delay*. It encourages consumption of berries, green leafy vegetables, nonstarchy vegetables, nuts, olive oil, whole grains, fish, beans, poultry, and 1 glass of wine per day. Foods to limit include butter, margarine, cheese, red meat, fried food, pastries, and sweets. The diet has also been shown to slow cognitive decline significantly during an average of 5 years. The effects of good diet improve cardiovascular health, which can reduce dementia risk. Good physical activity, control of blood pressure, and cognitive training also are known to help prevent development of dementia.

Prognosis

Prognosis of diabetes-related AD is severity of the dementia, and the treatment of diabetes. With adequate diet, exercise, and medication, the progression of dementias may be slowed. Outlook also varies based on how soon dementia was diagnosed, individual characteristics of overall health, and earlier treatment. The average life expectancy after a diagnosis of AD is 3–11 years, though some people have lived up to 20 years.

CLINICAL CASE

1. What is the link between diabetes and AD?
2. What are the diagnostic criteria for AD?
3. Which medications may be helpful for AD?

An 89-year-old diabetic man was brought to a Veterans Administration medical center. He was thin and frail, and exhibited agitation and confusion. His son said that his appetite had become poor and he had lost 32 pounds in the last year, going from 170 to 138 pounds. The medical team was alerted to the fact that the family had a history of AD affecting several relatives. The patient's blood urea nitrogen, creatinine serum, C-reactive protein, and LDL/HDL ratio were all high. His total protein, albumin, prealbumin, hemoglobin, hematocrit, and ferritin were all low. He had recently fallen and hit his right hip on a nightstand, and there was a thickness nonpressure wound. The patient was given antibiotics for infection involving his hip wound, plus the wound was debrided. Then there was a discussion of care for the patient, since he had lost most of his abilities for self-care. AD was suspected and evaluated via brief neuropsychological evaluation.

ANSWERS

1. Diabetes is known to increase the likelihood for developing vascular dementia. Many diabetic patients have brain changes that are signs of vascular dementia as well as AD. The disease may be triggered by a type of insulin resistance and insulin-like growth factor dysfunction in the brain, resulting in "type 3 diabetes."
2. Diagnostic criteria for AD consist of a failure in at least three cognitive functions. These include memory, use of language, visuospatial skills, personality, and calculating skills. Measurement of biomarkers in blood and cerebrospinal fluid, along with neuroimaging tests to characterize brain changes, are recommended.
3. The acetylcholinesterase inhibitors and N-methyl-D-aspartate receptor modulator may be helpful for AD.

KEY TERMS

- Agnosia
- Amygdala
- Anhedonia
- Anticipatory anxiety
- Cingulate cortices
- Cognition
- Cultural sensitivity
- Delusions
- Diabetes distress
- Down syndrome
- Frontotemporal dementia
- Huntington's disease
- Incentives
- Insula
- Lewy bodies
- Locus ceruleus
- Mood swings
- Paranoia
- Pragmatics
- Religions
- Wernicke-Korsakoff syndrome
- Wilson's disease

REFERENCES

American Association of Diabetes Educators. (2015). *Cultural Considerations in Diabetes Education.* AADE. www.diabetese-ducator.org/docs/default-source/default-document-library/cultural-considerations-in-diabetes-management.pdf?sfvrsn=0

American Diabetes Association / Diabetes Care. (2007). *Behavioral and Psychosocial Interventions in Diabetes – A Conceptual Review.* American Diabetes Association. https://care.diabetesjournals.org/content/30/10/2433

American Diabetes Association / Diabetes Care. (2003). *On the Association between Diabetes and Mental Disorders in a Community Sample.* American Diabetes Association. https://care.diabetesjournals.org/content/26/6/1841

American Diabetes Association/Diabetes Spectrum. (2016). *Cultural Differences and Considerations When Initiating Insulin.* American Diabetes Association. https://spectrum.diabetes-journals.org/content/29/3/185

American Diabetes Association / DiabetesSpectrum. (2006). *Case Study: Cognitive Impairment, Depression, and Severe Hypoglycemia.* American Diabetes Association. https://spectrum.diabetesjournals.org/content/19/4/212

Behavioral Diabetes Institute. (2015). *Breaking Free From Depression and Diabetes – 10 Things You Need to Know and Do.* Behavioral Diabetes Institute. https://behavioraldiabetes.org/xwp/wp-content/uploads/2015/12/BDIDepressionBookletFINAL.pdf

Calm Clinic. (2020). *What Is the Pathophysiology of Anxiety?* Calm Clinic. https://www.calmclinic.com/other/pathophysiology-of-anxiety

Centers for Disease Control and Prevention – Diabetes. (2021). *Hispanic/Latino Americans and Type 2 Diabetes.* U.S. Department of Health & Human Services / USA.gov / CDC. https://www.cdc.gov/diabetes/library/features/hispanic-diabetes.html

Centers for Disease Control and Prevention – Prevent Diabetes Complications. (2021). *Diabetes and Mental Health.* U.S. Department of Health & Human Services / USA.gov / CDC. https://www.cdc.gov/diabetes/managing/mental-health.html

Cleveland Clinic. (2021). *Bulimia Nervosa.* Cleveland Clinic. https://my.clevelandclinic.org/health/diseases/9795-bulimia-nervosa

Diabetes.co.uk – Diagnosis. (2019). *Diabetes and Ethnicity.* Diabetes Digital Media Ltd. https://www.diabetes.co.uk/diabetes-and-ethnicity.html

Diabetes.co.uk – Diabetes Complications. (2019). *Diabetes and Depression.* Diabetes Digital Media Ltd. https://www.diabetes.co.uk/diabetes-and-depression.html

Diabetes.co.uk – Emotions. (2019). *Psychological Support and Counselling for Diabetes.* Diabetes Digital Media Ltd. https://www.diabetes.co.uk/psychological-support-and-counselling-for-diabetes.html

Diabetes In Control. (2006). *Panic Attacks Exacerbate Diabetes Symptoms.* DiabetesInControl.com. http://www.diabetesincontrol.com/panic-attacks-exacerbate-diabetes-symptoms/

Endocrinology Consultant / PTSD. (2021). *The PTSD-Diabetes Relationship Is Not a One-Way Street.* HMP Global. https://www.consultant360.com/exclusive/endocrinology/diabetes/ptsd-diabetes-relationship-not-one-way-street

Everyday Health. (2020). *The Diabetes-Anxiety Connection: How to Spot the Signs and Find Relief.* Everyday Health, Inc. https://www.everydayhealth.com/diabetes/symptoms/diabetes-anxiety-connection-how-spot-signs-find-relief/

Healthline. (2021a). *Symptoms of Anxiety.* Healthline Media. https://www.healthline.com/health/diabetes/with-anxiety#symptoms

Healthline. (2021b). *Symptoms of Hypoglycemia vs. Panic Attack.* Healthline Media. https://www.healthline.com/health/diabetes/with-anxiety#hypoglycemia-vs-panic-attack

Healthline. (2021c). *Treatment for Anxiety.* Healthline Media. https://www.healthline.com/health/diabetes/with-anxiety#treatment

Healthline. (2018). *Tips for Dealing with Anxiety and Diabetes.* Healthline Media. https://www.healthline.com/health/diabetes/with-anxiety

Healthline. (2017). *The MIND Diet: A Detailed Guide for Beginners.* Healthline Media. https://www.healthline.com/nutrition/mind-diet

Mayo Clinic. (2021a). *Diabetes and Alzheimer's Linked – Diabetes May Increase Your Risk of Alzheimer's. But Blood Sugar Control, Exercise and a Healthy Diet May Help.* Mayo Foundation for Medical Education and Research (MFMER). https://www.mayoclinic.org/diseases-conditions/alzheimers-disease/in-depth/diabetes-and-alzheimers/art-20046987

Mayo Clinic. (2021b). *Diabetes and Depression: Coping with the Two Conditions.* Mayo Foundation for Medical Education and Research (MFMER). https://www.mayoclinic.org/diseases-conditions/diabetes/expert-answers/diabetes-and-depression/faq-20057904

Mayo Clinic. (2021c). *Diabetes and Depression: Coping with the Two Conditions – What's the Connection between Diabetes and Depression? How Can I Cope If I Have Both?* Mayo Foundation for Medical Education and Research (MFMER). https://www.mayoclinic.org/diseases-conditions/diabetes/expert-answers/diabetes-and-depression/faq-20057904

MedScape / Drugs & Diseases / Psychiatry / Panic Disorder Q&A. (2018). *What Is the Prognosis of Panic Disorder?* WebMD LLC. https://www.medscape.com/answers/287913-95582/what-is-the-prognosis-of-panic-disorder

National Institutes of Health / National Library of Medicine / National Center for Biotechnology Information. (2020). *Comorbidity of Hypoglycemia Anxiety and Panic Disorder in a Patient with Type-1 Diabetes – Combined Treatment with Cognitive-Behavioral Therapy and Continuous Glucose Monitoring (CGM) in a Psychosomatic Day-Treatment Center.* National Library of Medicine. https://pubmed.ncbi.nlm.nih.gov/32120406/

National Institutes of Health / National Library of Medicine / National Center for Biotechnology Information. (2017). *Depression Can Be Prevented by Astaxanthin Through Inhibition of Hippocampal Inflammation.* National Library of Medicine. https://pubmed.ncbi.nlm.nih.gov/28017669/

National Institutes of Health / National Library of Medicine / National Center for Biotechnology Information. (2013). *Relationship between Posttraumatic Stress Disorder and Type 2 Diabetes in a Population-Based Cross-Sectional Study with 2970 Participants.* National Library of Medicine. https://pubmed.ncbi.nlm.nih.gov/23497837/

National Institutes of Health / National Library of Medicine / National Center for Biotechnology Information. (2006). *Panic Episodes among Patients with Diabetes.* National Library of Medicine. https://pubmed.ncbi.nlm.nih.gov/17088162/

NCBI / PMC / U.S. National Library of Medicine / National Institutes of Health / American Diabetes Association / DiabetesSpectrum. (2016). *Cultural Differences and Considerations When Initiating Insulin.* National Center for Biotechnology Information / U.S. National Library of Medicine. https://www.ncbi.nlm.nih.gov/pmc/articles/PMC5001223/

NCBI / PMC / U.S. National Library of Medicine / National Institutes of Health / Innovations in Clinical Neuroscience. (2018). *Delirium and Psychotic Symptoms Associated with Hyperglycemia in a Patient with Poorly Controlled Type 2 Diabetes Mellitus.* National Center for Biotechnology Information / U.S. National Library of Medicine. https://www.ncbi.nlm.nih.gov/pmc/articles/PMC6040722/

NCBI / PMC / U.S. National Library of Medicine / National Institutes of Health / Journal of Medicine and Life. (2016). *The Association between Diabetes Mellitus and Depression.* National Center for Biotechnology Information / U.S. National Library of Medicine. https://www.ncbi.nlm.nih.gov/pmc/articles/PMC4863499/

NCBI / PMC / U.S. National Library of Medicine / National Institutes of Health / World Journal of Diabetes. (2014). *Psychological Aspects of Diabetes Care: Effecting Behavioral Change in Patients.* National Center for Biotechnology Information / U.S. National Library of Medicine. https://www.ncbi.nlm.nih.gov/pmc/articles/PMC4265866/

NIH – National Library of Medicine – National Center for Biotechnology Information. (2007). *Epidemiology and Course of Anorexia Nervosa in the Community*. National Library of Medicine. https://pubmed.ncbi.nlm.nih.gov/17671290/

NIH – National Institute of Mental Health. (2021). *Eating Disorders*. U.S. Department of Health and Human Services – National Institutes of Health – USA.gov. https://www.nimh.nih.gov/health/statistics/eating-disorders

Ohio State University College of Nursing. (2019). *Diabetes Mellitus Case Study*. The Ohio State University. https://u.osu.edu/dmcasestudy/patient-history/

OnTrack Diabetes – Depression & Anxiety. (2021). *Depression Diagnosis*. Remedy Health Media, LLC. https://www.ontrackdiabetes.com/related-conditions/depression-anxiety/depression-diagnosis

Oxford Academic – European Journal of Public Health. (2011). *Relationship between Post-Traumatic Stress Disorder and Diabetes among 150,180 Asylum Seekers in the Netherlands*. Oxford University Press.

ResearchGate / General Hospital Psychiatry. (2011). *Prevalence and Incidence of Anxiety Disorders in Diabetic Patients: A National Population-Based Cohort Study*. ResearchGate GmbH. https://www.researchgate.net/publication/50212912_Prevalence_and_incidence_of_anxiety_disorders_in_diabetic_patients_A_national_population-based_cohort_study

Sacramento Injury Attorneys Blog. (2019). *PTSD Can Either Cause or Aggravate Diabetes*. Edward A. Smith Law Offices. https://www.sacramentoinjuryattorneysblog.com/how-ptsd-can-either-cause-or-aggravate-diabetes/

Steve Grant Health. (2021). *Lifestyle Factors and Type 2 Diabetes*. Steve Grant Health. https://www.stevegranthealth.com/articles/movement/lifestyle-factors-and-type-2-diabetes/

The Breathing Diabetic. (2004). *Respiratory Feedback for Treating Panic Disorder*. The Breathing Diabetic. https://www.the-breathingdiabetic.com/meuret-et-al-2004

TheDiabetesCouncil.Com. (2021). *Diabetes & Depression: How To Deal with It*. TheDiabetesCouncil.Com. https://www.thediabetescouncil.com/diabetes-depression-how-to-deal-with-it/

The Diabetes Site – News. (2021). *Study Says People Who Get Treatment for Their PTSD Are Less Likely to Develop Diabetes*. The Diabetes Site and GreaterGood. https://blog.thediabetessite.greatergood.com/ptsd-diabetes/

Time / Health / Mental Health. (2021). *The Link between Mental Trauma and Diabetes*. Time USA, LLC. https://time.com/3656362/the-link-between-mental-trauma-and-diabetes/

Touch Endocrinology. (2020). *Prevention of Diabetes Dementia*. Touch Endocrinology / Crossref Event Data / The Association of Learned & Professional Society Publishers. https://www.touchendocrinology.com/insight/prevention-of-diabetes-dementia/

University of Massachusetts Medical School / UMass Memorial Health / Diabetes Center of Excellence. (2019). *The Impact of Integrated Behavioral Healthcare in Diabetes*. University of Massachusetts Medical School. https://umassmed.edu/dcoe/news–events/umass-diabetes-news/2019/07/behavior-health/

UpToDate. (2021). *Bulimia Nervosa in Adults: Clinical Features, Course of Illness, Assessment, and Diagnosis*. UpToDate, Inc. https://www.uptodate.com/contents/bulimia-nervosa-in-adults-clinical-features-course-of-illness-assessment-and-diagnosis

U.S. Department of Health and Human Services / NIH / National Institute of Diabetes and Digestive and Kidney Diseases / Diabetes Discoveries & Practice Blog. (2020a). *Diabetes Distress and Depression*. U.S. Department of Health and Human Services / National Institutes of Health / USA.gov. https://www.niddk.nih.gov/health-information/professionals/diabetes-discoveries-practice/diabetes-distress-and-depression

U.S. Department of Health and Human Services / NIH / National Institute of Diabetes and Digestive and Kidney Diseases / Diabetes Discoveries & Practice Blog. (2020b). *Helping Patients with Diabetes Manage Stress*. U.S. Department of Health and Human Services / National Institutes of Health / USA.gov. https://www.niddk.nih.gov/health-information/professionals/diabetes-discoveries-practice/helping-patients-with-diabetes-manage-stress

U.S. Department of Health and Human Services / National Institutes of Health. (2011). *Five Lifestyle Factors Lower Diabetes Risk*. National Institutes of Health. https://www.nih.gov/news-events/nih-research-matters/five-lifestyle-factors-lower-diabetes-risk

VeryWellMind. (2021). *The Connection between PTSD and Diabetes*. About, Inc. (Dotdash). https://www.verywellmind.com/ptsd-diabetes-risk-2797464

VeryWellHealth / Mental Health / Panic Disorder Guide. (2021). *How Panic Disorder Is Diagnosed*. About, Inc. (Dotdash). https://www.verywellhealth.com/panic-disorder-diagnosis-5114973

VeryWellMind / PTSD / Related Conditions. (2021). *The Connection between PTSD and Diabetes*. About, Inc. (Dotdash). https://www.verywellmind.com/ptsd-diabetes-risk-2797464

VeryWellHealth / Type 2 Diabetes / Hypoglycemia. (2021). *The Link between Blood Sugar and Anxiety*. About, Inc. (Dotdash). https://www.verywellhealth.com/blood-sugar-and-anxiety-5179339

WebMD. (2021). *What to Know about Depression and Diabetes*. WebMD LLC. https://www.webmd.com/diabetes/what-to-know-about-depression-and-diabetes

WebMD. (2020a). *Bulimia*. WebMD LLC. https://www.webmd.com/mental-health/eating-disorders/bulimia-nervosa/mental-health-bulimia-nervosa

WebMD. (2020b). *Can You Prevent Anorexia?* WebMD LLC. https://www.webmd.com/mental-health/eating-disorders/anorexia-nervosa/prevent-anorexia-nervosa

WebMD. (2019). *How Can I Prevent Panic Attacks?* WebMD LLC. https://www.webmd.com/anxiety-panic/how-prevent-panic-attacks

CHAPTER 13 Other Complications of Diabetes

It is well known that diabetes causes many complications that affect multiple organ systems. Aside from the most common complications affecting the eyes, kidneys, heart, blood vessels, and nervous system, there are many other complications that may occur. Of these, the most serious are infections such as pneumonia, and foot disorders that can ultimately result in gangrene and amputations. Today, one of the most serious considerations is that diabetic patients are much more susceptible to serious COVID-19 infections that nondiabetic.

PERIODONTAL DISEASE

Periodontal disease involves gum and bone infections, which are more common in diabetic patients. In advanced cases, it can cause painful chewing and teeth loss. Thickening of blood vessels around gums increase the risk of periodontitis. This is because the flow of nutrients and removal of harmful wastes from the mouth is reduced, weakening resistance of gum and bone tissue to infection. The early stage of periodontal disease is called *gingivitis*, in which the gums become swollen and red, and may bleed. The more serious form is called *periodontitis*, in which the gums pull away from the teeth, bone may be lost, and the teeth can loosen and fall out.

Epidemiology

According to the National Institute of Dental and Craniofacial Research in 2018, incidence of periodontal disease in adults has decreased overall. Today, 8.5% of adults between ages 20 and 64 have periodontal disease. When diabetes is under controlled, there is no higher incidence of periodontal disease than in nondiabetics. Periodontal disease is overall more common in men (56%) than in women (38%). The periodontal disease occurs most frequently in African Americans adults, Hispanic American adults, smokers, elderly individuals, or people with lower incomes and less education. According to the CDC in 2015, periodontal disease incidence increases with age. In elderly people over age 65, approximately 70% have this condition.

Etiology and Risk Factors

Many types of bacteria proliferate on glucose and other sugars. High glucose levels in the mouth fluids help them grow and encourage gum disease. Any diabetic who also smokes greatly increases the chances of periodontal disease by 20 times. Risk factors for periodontal disease include diabetes, smoking, poor oral hygiene, heredity, stress, crooked teeth, immunodeficiency, defective fillings, medications that cause dry mouth, improperly fitting bridges, and in women, hormonal changes.

Pathophysiology

Periodontal disease develops as inflammation of the gingiva, which extends into the underlying supportive structures of the **periodontium**. This is started by the presence of plaque on the surfaces of the teeth and related structures. Progression of periodontal disease is influenced by factors such as the host response, microorganisms, systemic health, and the genetic makeup of the individual. Diabetes mellitus and periodontitis cross-influence the clinical outcomes of both diseases. With diabetes, periodontal disease results in increased loss of tooth attachment, more alveolar bone loss, increased bleeding when the gums are probed, increased tooth mobility, and eventually, tooth loss. Basic structural changes that occur in the periodontium of someone with diabetes are tissue degeneration and the existence of calcified bodies, located in and around the small blood vessels of the gingiva.

Clinical Manifestations

With diabetes mellitus, reduced salivation is commonly seen, which may or may not include symptoms of a burning sensation inside the mouth or on the tongue. There may be enlargement of the parotid salivary glands. Gingivitis is signified by unhealthy or inflamed gums that may be red, swollen, and even bleed. Daily brushing and flossing, plus regular cleanings by a dentist, can prevent gingivitis. Periodontitis is gum disease that can change from mild to severe. The signs of gingivitis, by this time, have worsened, and the gums may pull away from the teeth. There is long-lasting infection between the teeth and gums, and chronic bad breath. Loosened teeth may move away from each other, and there are changes in the way the teeth fit together when biting. Periodontitis can be prevented via deep cleanings by a dentist and in severe cases gum surgery.

Thrush is a condition also known as *candidiasis*. White or red patches develop on the gums, tongue, cheeks, or roof of the mouth. Thrush is prevented via proper cleaning of dentures, removing dentures for part of the day or night, and soaking them in a prescribed medication. **Xerostomia** is another condition linked to diabetes mellitus, and is commonly known as *dry mouth*. There is insufficient saliva, increasing risks for tooth decay and gum disease. There

DOI: 10.1201/9781003226727-16

may be mouth pain, cracking of the lips, and sores or infections. Xerostomia results in problems chewing, eating, and even swallowing or talking. Humidifying devices increase moisture in the air surrounding the patient. There may be a need to avoid spicy or salty foods, since they can cause pain in a dry mouth. *Oral burning* may occur in the mouth because of hyperglycemia. There may be a bitter taste, and symptoms often worsen throughout the day. Oral burning may require changes in diabetes medications. Once the blood glucose is controlled, the condition resolves. Other symptoms in the mouth include sores or ulcers that do not heal, dark spots or holes in the teeth, loose teeth, pain while chewing, altered taste sensations, and chronic bad breath. Some patients have pain chronic pain in the mouth, face, or jaw.

Diagnosis

Periodontal disease is diagnosed during standard dental examinations and cleanings. The hygienist and dentist look for early signs and symptoms of the disease. They measure the depth of the tooth sockets, also called *pockets*. If this depth is 3 mm or more, periodontal disease may be present. Bone loss is also determined by taking dental X-rays.

Treatment

When a diabetic patient must have oral surgery, his or her meal schedule may need to be changed, as well as the dosing of insulin. Abscesses or acute infections should still be treated immediately. Healing after oral surgery may take longer for diabetics. Once periodontal disease is treated successfully, controlling blood sugar levels usually becomes easier. Diabetics must have dental checkups every 3–4 months. It is important to brush and floss every day to remove bacteria that cause gum disease. A dentist must be visited at least once per year, or more if there are any warning signs or risk factors present.

Prevention

The prevention of periodontal disease requires avoiding smoking, maintaining good oral hygiene, receiving regular dental checkups, using an electric toothbrush, using saline rinses, and eating a well-balanced, healthy diet. Smoking less than one-half a pack of cigarettes may increase risk of periodontal disease. Preventing periodontal disease requires brushing at least two times per day and flossing the teeth once per day, preferably before bed time. Regular dental cleanings remove accumulated tartar and treat advanced gum disease.

Prognosis

The prognosis for periodontal disease is based on the seriousness of the condition, earlier diagnosis and treatment, and whether the treatments are aggressive enough. Following the advice of dentists or periodontists provides the best chances for a good prognosis. Since periodontal disease is considered a complication of diabetes mellitus, prognosis is based on the severity of the diabetes, which influences the severity of the periodontal disease.

CLINICAL CASE

1. What are the stages of periodontal disease?
2. How are diabetes and periodontal disease related?
3. What is the prognosis of periodontal disease when diabetes is present?

A 65-year-old woman with type II diabetes mellitus went to her dentist because of loosening teeth. The patient had not seen a dentist for 3 years, and never flossed. She stated that she only brushed her teeth about once per day. She quit smoking 10 years ago. Examination revealed red gingival margins that were inflamed. There were four teeth missing, and more than half of the remaining teeth had generalized advance bone loss. The diagnosis was of advanced chronic periodontitis, with modifying factors including diabetes and a history of smoking.

ANSWERS

1. The early stage of periodontal disease is called gingivitis. The more serious form is called periodontitis, in which the gums pull away from the teeth, bone may be lost, and the teeth can loosen and fall out.
2. Diabetes mellitus and periodontitis cross-influence the clinical outcomes of both diseases. With diabetes, periodontal disease results in increased loss of tooth attachment,

more alveolar bone loss, increased bleeding when the gums are probed, increased tooth mobility, and eventually, tooth loss. Basic structural changes that occur in the periodontium of someone with diabetes are tissue degeneration and the existence of calcified bodies, located in and around the small blood vessels of the gingiva.

3. Since periodontal disease is considered a complication of diabetes mellitus, prognosis is based on the severity of the diabetes, which influences the severity of the periodontal disease.

INFECTIONS

Common infections that may affect a diabetic patient more severely than a nondiabetic patient include influenza and pneumonia caused by *Streptococcus pneumoniae*. Because of this fact, people with diabetes are recommended to receive immunizations for influenza and pneumococcal disease. Diabetic patients are also more likely to be infected with unusual organisms such as fungi or Gram-negative bacteria. Additional infections seen in diabetic patients include yeast infections, external otitis, and **zygomycosis**.

Epidemiology

Diabetic patients that contract influenza are six times more likely to require hospitalization than nondiabetic patients. In recent years, about 30% of adult influenza hospitalizations reported to the CDC occurred in people with diabetes mellitus. People with diabetes are approximately three times more likely to die from influenza and pneumonia. While pneumonia is always a serious condition, diabetics with pneumonia are more likely to be sick for a longer time, require hospitalization. Diabetes also makes people more likely to develop fungal infections, with **Candida albicans** being most common.

Pseudomonas aeruginosa is a Gram-negative bacterium that has been found to cause infections in 17.5% of people with diabetes. *Proteus*, a genus of Gram-negative **proteobacteria**, causes infections in about 14% of diabetic patients.

Etiology and Risk Factors

The influenza viruses travel via droplets in the air and can be directly inhaled or transferred to the recipient's eyes, nose, or mouth. People with type 1, type 2, or gestational diabetes that develop influenza are at a high risk of serious complications that may result in hospitalization or death. Risk factors for influenza, aside from diabetes, include very young or very old age, living or working in conditions with many other people, hospitalizations, any other immune system-weakening conditions, chronic illnesses,

long-term aspirin therapy in people under age 19, pregnancy, and obesity.

Risk factors for infections with diabetes mellitus are common and may be linked with fungal infections of the mouth, lower GIT, skin, feet, blood, and urogenital system. **Mycosis** is a serious problem and significant cause of death. Fungal infections are also seen in hemodialysis patients with diabetes, or in diabetic patients following pancreas or kidney transplantation.

Diagnosis

The early diagnosis of infection is essential, especially for diabetic patients, because spread of the disease can cause severe complications. Current diagnostic methods include medical history, physical examination, blood tests, specimen cultures, and chest X-rays.

Treatment

With diabetes, treatment of infection should begin early to relieve symptoms and speed up recovery as well as preventing serious complications. In severe cases, intravenous antibiotics are given. Treatments for fungal infections in diabetic patients are generally the same as in nondiabetics, usually involving antifungal medications.

Prevention

An influenza vaccination is very important for diabetic patients due to their higher risk of developing complications. Annual vaccinations are recommended, and should be of the injectable form, since diabetic patients generally should not receive the nasal spray form of the vaccine. The pneumococcal vaccine is an excellent method of prevention against pneumonia in diabetic patients. It can be administered at any time of the year. The vaccine is about 60% effective at reducing risks for acquiring pneumococcal pneumonia. It can be given to any patient aged 2 years or older with diabetes. There is no complete method of prevention for fungal or bacterial infections in diabetic patients, but good hygiene and management of diabetes may be somewhat preventive.

Prognosis

The prognosis of infectious disease in diabetic patients is poorer than in nondiabetic patients. The mortality rates are higher in diabetic patients.

For example, pneumonia in some cases can be life-threatening. Even with successful treatment, prognosis can be varied because long-term health issues can persist.

CLINICAL CASE

1. Which common infections may affect a diabetic patient more severely than a nondiabetic patient?
2. What are the dangers of pneumonia in a diabetic patient?
3. What is the treatment of pneumonia when a person has diabetes?

A 68-year-old man with diabetes was brought to the emergency department by his wife. His symptoms included fever, malaise, a productive cough, and right pleuritic chest pain. The patient also described dyspnea with any exertion. Upon examination, his blood pressure was 150/80 mm Hg, pulse was 94 beats per minute, and respirations were at 20 breaths per minute. There were signs of mild emphysema and crackles audible in the right chest. The patient was diagnosed with pneumonia via a chest X-ray.

ANSWERS

1. Common infections that may affect a diabetic patient more severely than a nondiabetic patient include influenza and pneumonia caused by *Streptococcus pneumoniae*. Because of this fact, people with diabetes are recommended to receive immunizations for influenza and pneumococcal disease.
2. People with diabetes are approximately 3 times more likely to die from influenza and pneumonia. Diabetics with pneumonia are more likely to be sick for a longer time, require hospitalization, or die.
3. The treatment of pneumonia focuses on curing the infection and preventing complications. Options include antibiotics, cough medications, fever reducers, and pain relievers. Hospitalization is often needed, especially for diabetic patients. Gram-negative bacterial infections can be treated with oral antibiotics such as cephalexin or clindamycin. In severe cases, IV antibiotics are given, which include ciprofloxacin, clindamycin, cilastatin, imipenem, piperacillin, or tazobactam.

SLEEP APNEA

Sleep apnea may be linked to diabetes, which can repeatedly stop airflow during breathing. Sleep apnea involves loud snoring and pauses in breathing. Overweight patients may have more fat deposits around their upper airways, which obstruct breathing. Untreated or undiagnosed sleep apnea has serious complications. These include diabetes, glaucoma, myocardial infarction, cancer, and cognitive or behavioral disorders.

Epidemiology

According to the American Academy of Sleep Medicine in 2019, more than 26 million adults in the United States have obstructive sleep apnea. Between 28.5% and 44.1% of adult Americans between the ages of 30 and 70 years have sleep apnea. According to the CDC, sleep apnea is most common, for unknown reasons, in the states of Michigan, Indiana, Ohio, New York, Maryland, West Virginia, Kentucky, South Caro

lina, Georgia, and Alabama (see Figure 13.1). In these states, it affects 42% of the population. The Wisconsin Sleep Cohort Study of 1993 revealed that during middle age, about 24% of men and 9% of women had sleep apnea. According to the American College of Chest Physicians in 2010, the prevalence of obstructive sleep apnea in obese patients was between 25% and 45%. Between ethnic groups, Hispanic and Chinese Americans have the highest rates of sleep apnea. Researchers believe that approximately 86% of obese people and type 2 diabetic patients have sleep apnea.

Etiology and Risk Factors

The actual connection between type 2 diabetes mellitus and sleep apnea remains unknown. However, it is known that diabetic patients have higher rates of sleep apnea than nondiabetic patients. It is also possible that the two conditions can actually cause each other. Risk factors include excessive weight, a thick neck

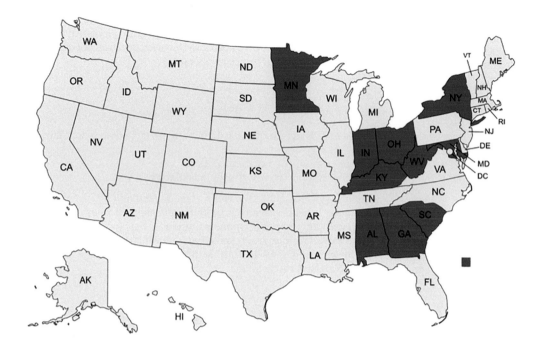

Created with mapchart.net

Figure 13.1 U.S. states with the highest rates of sleep apnea.

circumference, a narrowed airway, the male gender, older age, family history of sleep apnea, alcohol use, sedative or tranquilizer use, opioid use, smoking, congestive heart failure, hypertension, Parkinson's disease, polycystic ovary syndrome, hormonal disorders, previous stroke, and asthma.

Pathophysiology

The pathophysiology of sleep apnea involves recurrent upper airway collapse. This triggers hypopnea and apnea, resulting in impaired blood gas exchanges, sleep disruption, and systemic inflammation. Intermittent hypoxemia and sleep disruption are also two important factors in the pathogenesis of type 2 diabetes.

Clinical Manifestations

Signs and symptoms of obstructive sleep apnea and central sleep apnea somewhat overlap. The most common signs and symptoms include loud snoring, stopping breathing during sleep, gasping for air during sleep, waking up with a dry mouth, a morning headache, insomnia, hypersomnia, difficulty paying attention when awake, and irritability.

Diagnosis

Diagnostic tests for sleep apnea include nocturnal **polysomnography** and home sleep tests. In nocturnal polysomnography, the patient is monitored by equipment with regard to heart, lung, and brain activity, breathing, arm and leg movement, and blood oxygen levels. Home sleep tests measure similar activities but with less diagnostic relevance.

Treatment

Treatment for sleep apnea begins with losing weight, quitting smoking, and treating any existing allergies. Therapies include continuous positive airway pressure (CPAP), an automatically adjusting form of CPAP known as *auto-CPAP*, bilevel positive airway pressure (BPAP) devices, and oral appliances designed to open the throat by bringing the jaw forward. There may be a need to treat diabetes, heart, or neuromuscular disorders as well. Surgical treatments include *uvulopalatopharyngoplasty* to remove tissue from the rear of the mouth and top of the throat, often along with removal of the tonsils and adenoids. Some patients may require **bariatric surgery** to help with sleep apnea.

Prevention

Prevention of sleep apnea may be achieved by managing diabetes mellitus well, losing weight, exercising regularly, avoiding alcohol and medications that cause sleepiness since they also relax the muscles in the back of the throat, sleeping on the side or abdomen instead of on the back, and quitting smoking.

Prognosis

The prognosis of sleep apnea in diabetic patients is varied since sleep apnea makes it more difficult to manage diabetes. With pauses in breathing while asleep, increased blood carbon dioxide leads to insulin resistance, high blood glucose, chronic hypertension, higher incidence of heart problems or cardiovascular disease, and early morning headache.

CLINICAL CASE

1. Aside from diabetes, what are the risk factors for sleep apnea?
2. What are the diagnostic tests for sleep apnea?
3. Besides CPAP devices, what other treatments are available for sleep apnea?

A 61-year-old obese man with type 2 diabetes is evaluated by a physician for possible sleep apnea. He has no other complications of diabetes, but his wife reports chronic loud snoring, and the man states that he is sleepy all during the day, even though he regularly spends more than 8 hours per night in bed. In the past year, the patient has had trouble managing his plasma glucose levels. The patient was scheduled for a sleep study, which revealed that his sleep apnea was so severe that immediate CPAP therapy was needed. His energy levels improved immensely and he became able to exercise regularly – losing weight and improving his blood glucose levels.

ANSWERS

1. Other risk factors for sleep apnea include excessive weight, a thick neck circumference, a narrowed airway, the male gender, older age, family history of sleep apnea, alcohol use, sedative or tranquilizer use, opioid use, smoking, congestive heart failure, hypertension, Parkinson's disease, polycystic ovary syndrome, hormonal disorders, previous stroke, and asthma.
2. Diagnostic tests for sleep apnea include nocturnal polysomnography and home sleep tests. The patient is monitored by equipment with regard to heart, lung, and brain activity, breathing, arm and leg movement, and blood oxygen levels. Home sleep tests measure similar activities but with less diagnostic relevance.
3. Other therapies for sleep apnea include auto-CPAP, BPAP devices, oral appliances that open the throat by bringing the jaw forward.

DERMATOLOGIC DISORDERS

Diabetes affects every part of the body, including the skin. Often, skin abnormalities may be the first sign of diabetes mellitus. Fortunately, most skin conditions are preventable or easily treated if they are discovered early in their development. Diabetes makes it easier to develop bacterial or fungal skin infections as well as chronic itching. Other skin problems include diabetic dermopathy or blisters, **acanthosis nigricans**, and **eruptive xanthomatosis**. Bacterial infections include styes, boils, folliculitis, carbuncles, and infections around the nails. Fungal infections of the skin can cause blistering and scales, often in warm and moist skin folds. These are most common under the breasts, around the nails, between the fingers or toes, in the corners of the mouth, under the foreskin of uncircumcised men, in the armpits, and in the groin. Localized itching can be due to a yeast infection, poor circulation, or dry skin.

Epidemiology

Between 51% and 97% of people with diabetes mellitus experience a related dermatologic disorder. Bacterial skin infections affect about 16% of diabetes patients while fungal skin infections affect about 22%. The most common bacterial skin infection is a boil while the most common fungal skin infection are *tinea pedis* and **athlete's foot**. Chronic itching affects about 2.9% of the overall population, but is much more common with diabetes, at 11.3% of patients. Diabetic dermopathy affects 7%–35% of diabetic patients in varying amounts throughout the world. Approximately 36% of individuals with newly diagnosed type 2 diabetes have acanthosis nigricans. Necrobiosis lipoidica diabeticorum is rare, usually affecting adult diabetic women, but overall affecting only 0.3% of people with diabetes. Eruptive xanthomatosis is most common in younger men that have type 1 diabetes, but overall is extremely rare.

Etiology and Risk Factors

The most common cause of bacterial skin infections in relation to diabetes is *Staphylococcus aureus*. Fungal skin infections in diabetic patients are usually caused by *Candida albicans*. Diabetic blisters often occur with diabetic neuropathy. Acanthosis nigricans is the result of being very overweight or obese. Necrobiosis lipoidica diabeticorum, like diabetic dermopathy, is caused by blood vessel changes. Eruptive xanthomatosis is caused by poorly managed diabetes when there are high levels of cholesterol and fat in the blood.

Pathophysiology

Bacterial and fungal skin infections when diabetes is present have a variety of pathophysiological factors controlling their development. Diabetes causes reduced T lymphocyte responses and neutrophil function, lower secretion of inflammatory cytokines, glycosuria, humoral immunity disorders, angiopathy, neuropathy, hyperglycemia. Chronic itching may develop from damaged nerve fibers in the outer skin layers, linked to diabetic polyneuropathy or peripheral neuropathy. High levels of cytokines circulating through the body are inflammatory and can lead to itching.

Diabetic dermopathy may be related to local thermal trauma, reduced blood flow that causes impaired wound healing, or local subcutaneous nerve degeneration. Epidermal features include atrophy or flattening with **rete ridges** being obliterated, hyperkeratosis, and variable pigmentation of basal cells. Dermal changes include proliferation of fibroblasts, denser collagen, thickened collagen bundles, fragmentation or separation of collagen fibers, and dermal edema. Diabetic blisters may develop when diabetes is poorly controlled, though the actual pathophysiological processes are not fully understood. Eruptive xanthomatosis develops as a result of elevated triglycerides.

Clinical Manifestations

Bacterial skin infections linked to diabetes include styes, which are infections of the glands of the eyelid, boils, folliculitis – infections of the hair follicles, carbuncles – deep infections of the skin and underlying tissue, and infections around the nails. Inflamed tissues are usually hot, painful, red, and swollen. Fungal skin infections are signified by itchy rashes with moist, red areas that are surrounded by small blisters and scales. They develop in warm, moist folds of skin. Diabetic dermopathy often appears as light brown, scaly patches that are circular or oval and may be mistaken for age spots. Usually, the spots occur on the front of the legs, sometimes in varying amounts. The patches are not painful, do not itch, and remain closed. Diabetic blisters can develop on the backs of the fingers, hands, toes, feet, and less often, on the legs or forearms. They appear similar to burn blisters and can be quite large. However, they are painless and have no redness around their borders. Acanthosis nigricans involves tan or brown raised areas on the sides of the neck, armpits, and groin. It sometimes occurs on the hands, elbows, and knees. Necrobiosis lipoidica diabeticorum causes spots that are like diabetic dermopathy, but there are less of them. The spots are larger and deeper than those of diabetic dermopathy. The disorder can be itchy and painful, and the spots can open. Eruptive xanthomatosis involves pea-like skin enlargements that are firm and yellow. There is a red halo around each lesion, and they may be itchy. The condition is most common on the backs of the hands, feet, arms, legs, and buttocks.

Diagnosis

Bacterial and fungal skin infections are diagnosed clinically when diabetes is present. Diabetic dermopathy is diagnosed by observation to determine the shape, color, size, and location of lesions. Biopsies are not usually done because of the concern about slow wound healing. Blood tests, endoscopy, or X-rays may be needed to eliminate other causes besides diabetes. If biopsy is done, hyperkeratosis, leukocyte infiltration, and melanocyte proliferation may be seen.

Treatment

Bacterial and fungal skin infections are often treated with topical antibiotics. Chronic itching can be treated by limiting excessive bathing, especially when the humidity is low. Mild soap containing moisturizers and skin cream can be effective. Diabetic blisters heal on their own, usually without scarring, in approximately 3 weeks. The only treatment is to control blood glucose. Acanthosis nigricans is treated by losing weight and by creams that help improve the appearance of the dark skin spots. Treatment for necrobiosis lipoidica diabeticorum is not required unless the sores break open. Once diabetes is again under control, the lesions of eruptive xanthomatosis disappear.

Prevention

Skin infections in diabetic patients are preventable by practicing good skin care and controlling blood glucose.

Prognosis

The prognosis of dermatologic disorders is generally good. In diabetic patients, skin care is very important and early diagnosis is essential. In some skin infections that are severe, the outcome may be poor.

GASTROINTESTINAL PROBLEMS

Gastrointestinal complications of diabetes include gastroparesis, intestinal enteropathy, and nonalcoholic fatty liver disease. Some diabetic patients may develop esophageal manifestations. Diabetic neuropathy can be presented as abnormal peristalsis, impaired lower esophageal sphincter tone, and spontaneous contractions. Nonalcoholic fatty liver disease is also common with diabetes as well as obesity. The liver has features of alcohol-induced injury but without any history of significant alcohol consumption.

Epidemiology

Gastrointestinal complications of diabetes mellitus have become more common along with the increase in rates of diabetes. About 5%–12% of diabetic patients report having the symptoms of gastroparesis. It is more common in women than in men. With intestinal enteropathy, the prevalence of diarrhea is between 4% and 22% of diabetic patients. Constipation occurs in 20%–44% of patients, abdominal pain in 7.6%, and vomiting in 1.7%. With the worldwide increases in diabetes, nonalcoholic fatty liver disease is now the most common cause of liver damage in developed countries for people of all ages. It ranges in prevalence between 9% and 36.9% in various countries. About 20% of people in the United States have the disease, which predominates in Hispanic people more than other groups. In severely obese individuals, prevalence is more than 90%. It is prevalent in more than 60% of diabetics, but 20% or lower in normal-weight individuals.

Etiology and Risk Factors

Gastrointestinal complications of diabetes are often caused by abnormal GI motility, a result of diabetic autonomic neuropathy of the GI tract. Factors that contribute to diabetes-related reflux include hyperglycemia, obesity, and decrease bicarbonate secretion from the **parotid glands**. Gastroparesis is idiopathic in more than 50% of all cases, but autonomic neuropathy remains a significant cause of the condition in people with type 1 or type 2 diabetes. Between 30% and 50% of affected patients have had diabetes for years. The **vagus nerve** becomes damaged by years of high blood glucose, or insufficient transport of glucose into the cells. Constipation, as part of intestinal enteropathy, is caused by neuronal dysfunction in the large intestine as well as impairment of the gastrocolic reflex. If an individual has elevated hepatic transaminase levels, it is important to assess other possible causes of liver disease, which include hepatitis and **hemochromatosis**. The cause of nonalcoholic fatty liver disease is unknown but is often related to obesity and type 2 diabetes. All severely obese patients with diabetes have some amount of steatosis, and about 50% have steatohepatitis.

Pathophysiology

With gastroparesis, delayed gastric emptying may mostly be due to impaired vagal control. Other factors include impairment of inhibitory nerves that contain nitric oxide, damaged interstitial **Cajal cells**, and dysfunction of smooth muscles. There are three classifications of gastroparesis. *Mild gastroparesis* has symptoms that are relatively easy to control. *Compensated gastroparesis* can be partially controlled with antiemetic medications. *Gastric failure* involves refractory symptoms that persist regardless of treatment. Patients with diabetes may have accelerated or delayed intestinal enteropathy, alterations of gastric sensation, and impaired gastric accommodation. Antral hypomotility and **pylorospasm** due to vagal neuropathy can delay intestinal enteropathy. However, the relationship between impairment of gastric accommodation and rapid intestinal enteropathy has not been proven. Nonalcoholic fatty liver disease may progress to nonalcoholic steatohepatitis with various amounts of fibrosis and inflammation. Rarely, it leads to cirrhosis.

Clinical Manifestations

The esophageal manifestations of diabetic neuropathy result in dysphagia and heartburn, but only in a minority of patients. Gastroparesis causes nausea, vomiting, early satiety, bloating, postprandial fullness, and upper abdominal pain. Delayed gastric emptying is a contributing factor of poor blood glucose control. It may be the first sign of gastroparesis. Intestinal enteropathy can cause constipation, diarrhea, and fecal incontinence. Impaired motility of the small intestine can lead to stasis syndrome, resulting in diarrhea, which can be intensified by hypermotility due to decreased sympathetic inhibition, pancreatic insufficiency, malabsorption of bile salts, and **steatorrhea**. Fecal incontinence may result from abnormal internal and external anal sphincter function due to neuropathy. Most patients with nonalcoholic fatty liver disease are asymptomatic, but some have malaise or right upper-quadrant fullness. The disease can range from a slight elevation of liver enzymes to severe liver disease with fibrosis and nodular regeneration, but this development is rare.

Diagnosis

Gastroparesis is diagnosed after other causes are excluded, with postprandial gastric stasis confirmed by *gastric emptying scintigraphy*. This involves ingesting a technetium-labeled egg meal. Gastric emptying is measured by **scintiscanning** at 15-minute intervals over 4 hours. Retention of 10% or more of the meal at the end of 4 hours confirms gastroparesis. Other tests include **antroduodenal manometry**, a breath test using a nonradioactive isotope carbon-13 bound to a digestible substance, **electrogastrography**, MRI, and ultrasonography. Upper endoscopy or an upper GI series with small bowel assessment can rule out mechanical obstruction or other GI conditions. Ultrasonography is done if there are biliary tract symptoms or extreme abdominal pain.

Treatment

The treatments for gastroparesis require that patients stop taking any medications that worsen gastric dysmotility. They must control their blood glucose levels, consume more liquids, and eat smaller meals more often during the day. Any nutritional deficiencies must be corrected. Tobacco products must be avoided, and there must be a reduction in intake of insoluble dietary fiber, high-fat foods, and alcohol. Prokinetic agents such as erythromycin and metoclopramide may be effective in controlling symptoms. If reflux exists, it is managed by controlling blood glucose and using appropriate medications. Medications that delay gastric emptying include aluminum hydroxide antacids, anticholinergic agents, beta-adrenergic receptor agonists, calcium channel blockers, diphenhydramine, histamine H_2 antagonists, and proton pump inhibitors. If a patient has persistent nausea, antiemetics include ondansetron and promethazine.

In intestinal enteropathy, treatment of diarrhea is primarily empiric, to relieve symptoms, correct fluid and electrolyte imbalances, improve blood glucose control and nutrition, and manage underlying causes. Antidiarrheals must be used carefully since they can cause **toxic megacolon**. Constipation may alternate with diarrhea. Treatment includes adequate hydration, regular physical activity, and increased intake of fiber.

Sorbitol or lactulose may be helpful for constipation, and saline or osmotic laxatives may be required for more severe cases.

If a patient has elevated hepatic transaminase levels, gradual weight loss, control of blood glucose, and use of medications such as metformin or pioglitazone may be helpful. However, clinical benefits of aggressive treatment for nonalcoholic fatty liver disease are uncertain. Control of blood glucose is important in the management of most gastrointestinal complications, including this condition, as is gradual weight loss. Gemfibrozil and metformin can lower hepatic transaminase levels and improve results seen in ultrasonography.

Prevention

Idiopathic gastroparesis cannot be prevented. If the cause is known, treatment may be able to stop gastroparesis from progressing – such as strict blood glucose control. Better eating habits can also be preventative. Intestinal enteropathy can be prevented simply by avoiding any of the causative agents or factors. Nonalcoholic fatty liver disease, when due to diet or lifestyle, can be prevented by improving nutrition, eating smaller meals, reducing omega-6 fatty acid and fructose, and by choline supplementation. Also, treatment for obstructive sleep apnea may help prevent nonalcoholic fatty liver disease since hypoxic conditions are proven to damage the liver.

Prognosis

The prognosis for gastroparesis can be self-limiting with recovery in less than 1 year, though it sometimes takes longer than 2 years. If diabetic gastropathy is present, it usually progresses slowly, possibly becoming severe or even lethal. Intestinal enteropathy generally has a good prognosis with proper treatment. Nonalcoholic fatty liver disease that does not progress to fibrosis has a better prognosis than when it does progress. Obese patients have a worsened outlook than thinner patients. The prognosis is worsened if hypertension, chronic kidney disease, atrial fibrillation, myocardial infarction, ischemic stroke, cirrhosis, liver failure, or liver cancer also develop.

MUSCULOSKELETAL COMPLICATIONS

Musculoskeletal complications of diabetes include carpal tunnel syndrome, Dupuytren contracture, adhesive capsulitis, and sclerodactyly. *Carpal tunnel syndrome* is compression of the median nerve along its course through the carpal tunnel in the wrist. *Dupuytren contracture* is progressive contracture of the palmar fascial bands, resulting in finger flexion deformities. *Adhesive capsulitis* is commonly known as *frozen shoulder*, associated with shoulder pain and stiffness. *Sclerodactyly* is a localized thickening and tightness of the skin on the fingers or toes.

Epidemiology

Carpal tunnel syndrome is extremely common, mostly occurring in women between 30 and 50 years of age. Dupuytren contracture is also common, with higher incidence in men over age 45. Adhesive capsulitis affects 10%–46% of people with diabetes annually, and is much less common in nondiabetic individuals. Highest prevalence is between 40 and 70 years of age, with women affected in 70% of cases. There is no specific group of patients affected by sclerodactyly.

Etiology and Risk Factors

Carpal tunnel syndrome is related to other conditions besides diabetes, including rheumatoid arthritis, hypothyroidism, acromegaly, **amyloidosis**, and pregnancy-induced carpal tunnel edema. However, most cases are idiopathic, yet can be worsened by repetitive flexion and extension of the wrist. The autosomal dominant condition of Dupuytren contracture, with variable penetrance, is most common in patients with diabetes, alcoholism, or epilepsy. Specific causative factors are unknown. Causes and risk factors for primary adhesive capsulitis include diabetes, stroke, lung disease, connective tissue disease, thyroid disease, heart disease, and autoimmune disease. Secondary adhesive capsulitis develops after shoulder injury or surgery. Sclerodactyly is related to diabetes, scleroderma, and autoimmune disorders.

Pathophysiology

The pathophysiological mechanisms involved in carpal tunnel syndrome are complicated and not fully understood. In general, the syndrome is due to a fibrous hypertrophy of the synovial flexor sheath, and to repetitive wrist movements. The basic pathophysiology of Dupuytren contracture involves fibroblast proliferation and collagen deposition, leading to contractures of the palmar fascia. The pathophysiology of adhesive capsulitis has inflammatory and fibrotic components. Hardening of the shoulder joint capsule is implicated, due to scar tissue around the capsule. There may also be a reduction in synovial fluid, and later, inflammatory cytokines in the joint fluid. Eventually, there is dense collagenous tissue in the joint capsule. Sclerodactyly often progresses into ulceration of the skin of the distal digits, with atrophy of underlying soft tissues.

Clinical Manifestations

Signs and symptoms of carpal tunnel syndrome include hand and wrist pain, tingling, numbness, along the path of the median nerve. Sometimes, the entire hand is affected. The patient often wakes up at night with aching or burning pain, numbness, and tingling. Shaking the hand back and forth can relieve the pain and restore normal sensation. Later in the disease course, there may be **thenar atrophy**, and weakness of thumb opposition and abduction. Dupuytren contracture begins with tender palm nodules usually near the pinky or ring finger that gradually become painless. A superficial cord then forms, contracting the metacarpophalangeal joints and interphalangeal joints, resulting in arching of the hand. There may be fibrous thickening of the dorsum of the proximal interphalangeal joints. With diabetes, there can also be locked trigger fingers, systemic sclerosis, chronic reflex sympathetic dystrophy, and an **ulnar claw** hand.

Signs and symptoms of adhesive capsulitis include shoulder pain and limited range of motion. It may become impossible to make simple arm movements. The pain is usually dull or aching, and can worsen at night or with arm motions. There are three (and sometimes four) stages: Prodromal (sharp pain), freezing (chronic pain and loss of motion), frozen (adhesive), and thawing (recovery). There are three phases of skin changes with sclerodactyly: Edematous, **indurative**, and atrophic. It begins with puffy edema, morning stiffness, or arthralgias. Then there is skin thickening, pruritus, shiny and tight skin, loss of creases, and erythema. Late in the disease course, the skin becomes fragile and lax. The hand may assume a claw-like appearance.

Diagnosis

The diagnosis of carpal tunnel syndrome is via clinical evaluation and sometimes, nerve conduction testing. The *Tinel sign* is very suggestive, in which paresthesias are reproduced by tapping on the volar surface of the wrist above the site of the median nerve (see Figure 13.2). Wrist flexion (the *Phalen sign*) can reproduce tingling, as can direct pressure (the median nerve compression test). Nerve condition testing is done for severe symptoms, an uncertain diagnosis, or to exclude a more proximal neuropathy. Diagnosis of Dupuytren contracture is via clinical examination. Adhesive capsulitis is diagnosed by history and physical examination, excluding other shoulder conditions. The movement that is most severely prevented is external rotation of the shoulder. Imaging features can be seen on ultrasound or noncontrast MRI. There

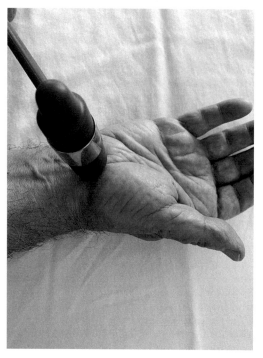

Figure 13.2 Tinel sign. (Provided by Jahangir Moini.)

may be fibrosis and thickening at the axillary pouch and rotator interval. **Hypoechoic material** around the long head of the bicep tendon is diagnostic. For sclerodactyly, diagnosis based on clinical examination.

Treatment

The treatment of carpal tunnel syndrome is with splinting, treating underlying disorders, and sometimes, injection of corticosteroids with anesthetics, and surgical decompression. Neutral wrist splints, often at night, as well as acetaminophen or NSAIDs may be helpful. Dexamethasone with lidocaine is often effective for mild disease, or when it occurs due to pregnancy. Surgical decompression may involve an open or endoscopic technique. Treatments for Dupuytren contracture include injection of corticosteroids before contractures develop, surgery if the contracture becomes disabling, and for some cases, injection of clostridial collagenase. Treatments for adhesive capsulitis include medications, occupational therapy, physical therapy, and surgery. Corticosteroids and NSAIDs may be helpful. Manipulation of the shoulder under general anesthesia can be used to break up the adhesions. Surgical capsular release is sometimes needed. Adjunctive treatments include acupuncture combined with shoulder exercises. While sclerodactyly is incurable, treatments can

be helpful, and include physical therapy, occupational therapy, ultraviolet light therapy, and surgery.

Prevention

Prevention of carpal tunnel syndrome includes monitoring hand and wrist pressure while working, bending, and stretching then hands while taking breaks from work (by making a fist and then opening the hands fully for 5–10 repetitions), avoiding bending the wrists all the way up or down, changing hand and wrist motions, improve posture, keeping adequately warm, making **ergonomic** changes, and occupational therapy. There are no ways to prevent Dupuytren contracture, but hand therapy and rehabilitee with thermoplastic night splints, plus regular physiotherapy exercises can be helpful.

Prognosis

Even after carpal tunnel surgery, less than 50% of patients report their hands returning completely to normal. There is often residual numbness or weakness. Total recovery is possible but may take up to 1 year. Dupuytren contracture progresses unpredictably, but surgery can usually restore normal finger movement. However, the disease recurs within 10 years in about 50% of cases. For adhesive capsulitis, range of motion and shoulder use usually improve slowly over time. A total or near-total recovery occurs in about 2 years. Though incurable, sclerodactyly usually has a good prognosis if treatment is given early and the hands do not form into a claw shape.

SEXUAL DYSFUNCTION

Erectile dysfunction (ED) is the inability to attain or sustain an erection for sexual intercourse. It is a complication of diabetes as well as vascular, neurologic, psychologic, and hormonal disorders. *Retrograde ejaculation* involves semen being ejaculated backward into the bladder instead of outward through the penis. *Decreased vaginal lubrication* is another condition related to diabetes, which results in vaginal dryness.

Epidemiology

ED affects up to 20 million American men, and was formerly known as *impotence*. Partial or complete ED affects over 50% of men aged 40–70, and increases in prevalence with aging. While the actual epidemiology for retrograde ejaculation's prevalence is not well documented, it is known that about 10%–15% of men undergoing prostate or bladder surgery later develop the condition. The epidemiology of decreased vaginal lubrication is also not well documented, but it is known to affect older women more often than younger women.

Etiology and Risk Factors

Primary ED is present when attaining or sustaining an erection has never been possible. Psychologic causes of primary ED include fear of intimacy, guilt, anxiety, or depression. Secondary ED is acquired later in life after previously having had normal function. It is the most common form, with more than 90% of cases having an organic etiology. Reactive psychologic difficulties may later develop, worsening the condition. Causes may be related to performance anxiety, stress, or depression. Psychogenic ED may involve a certain place, time, or partner. Organic causes of ED are usually vascular or neurologic disorders, often due to diabetes or atherosclerosis. Atherosclerosis of the cavernous arteries of the penis is highly common. Endothelial dysfunction is due to diabetes, smoking, and low testosterone levels. Neurologic causes include diabetic neuropathy. One of the most common causes of retrograde ejaculation is prostate surgery for noncancerous prostate enlargement. Other common causes include diabetes, certain drugs, spinal cord injuries, and major abdominal or pelvic surgery. Aside from diabetes, decreased vaginal lubrication may be due to hormonal changes related to menopause, pregnancy, or breastfeeding. It is also caused by irritation from contraceptive creams and foams, fear, and anxiety about sexual intimacy, OTC antihistamines, oral contraceptives, and reduced estrogen levels because of aging.

Pathophysiology

The pathophysiology of ED is either predominantly psychogenic or predominantly physical (organic). There may be direct inhibition of the spinal *erection center* by the brain, and excessive sympathetic outflow or increased catecholamine levels. Psychogenic ED can be generalized or situational. Organic ED can be vasculogenic, neurogenic, anatomic, or endocrinologic. Retrograde ejaculation is a disorder of ejaculatory function that results in anejaculation and fertility, due to heterogeneous conditions with different etiologies and treatments. The pathophysiology of decreased vaginal lubrication is based on altered serum estrogen levels.

Clinical Manifestations

The signs and symptoms of ED include difficulty in attaining or keeping and erection, and reduced sexual desire. Retrograde ejaculation is signified by semen going into the bladder instead of being ejaculated out of the body. An affected male may experience dry orgasms, cloudy urine after orgasm, and infertility. With decreased vaginal lubrication, the sexual

dyspareunia may develop since lack of sufficient lubrication may result in various degrees of pain during intercourse.

Diagnosis

Diagnosis of ED is based on clinical evaluation, screening for depression, and measuring testosterone levels. Evaluation for previous history of diabetes is important. Based on clinical suspicion, there may be a need to evaluate for occult diabetes, dyslipidemias, Cushing's syndrome, and thyroid disease. Retrograde ejaculation is diagnosed by finding a large amount of sperm in a urine sample taken shortly after orgasm. The diagnosis of decreased vaginal lubrication is based on dryness and pain during sexual intercourse, sitting, standing, exercising, and urinating.

Treatment

ED is treated initially by focusing on underlying causes such as diabetes. Medications include oral phosphodiesterase inhibitors. Vacuum erection devices or intracavernosal or intraurethral prostaglandin E1 may be needed. When other treatments fail, there can be a surgical implantation of a penile prosthesis. Behavior modifications such as diet changes and weight loss may be required. Unless infertility is a concern, retrograde ejaculation does not usually require treatment. Decreased vaginal lubrication is treated with artificial lubricants, and vaginal suppositories. Water- or silicone-based lubricants are recommended since oil-based lubricants can break down latex, reducing the effectiveness of condoms. The *American Society for Reproductive Medicine* recommends canola oil and mineral oil as fertility-preserving personal lubricants.

Prevention

Methods of preventing ED include quitting smoking, a healthy diet, avoiding excessive alcohol, maintaining a healthy weight, physical activity, and avoiding illegal drugs. Retrograde ejaculation is not totally preventable. Men requiring treatment for an enlarged prostate must consider less invasive surgeries such as transurethral microwave thermotherapy or transurethral needle ablation. Control of medical conditions that cause nerve damage may also aid in prevention. Diabetes medications must be taken as prescribed and appropriate lifestyle changes must be implemented. Prevention of vaginal dryness because of decreased lubrication requires the use of vaginal moisturizers such as K-Y Liquibeads or Replens, oral probiotic supplements that enhance vaginal health, and increased soy into the diet. There are also low-dose vaginal estrogen creams, tablets, and rings.

Prognosis

ED can be cured, and the long-term prognosis is usually good for 80%–95% of affected men. Some men benefit from the use of vacuum pumps and do not even require medication, improving prognosis. If caused by medications, retrograde ejaculation often resolves once they are stopped. If caused by surgery or diabetes, the condition is often not correctable. The prognosis for decreased vaginal lubrication is usually good as long as treatments or preventive measures are used.

CLINICAL CASE

1. Which subtype of ED is caused by diabetes mellitus?
2. How is ED diagnosed in a diabetic patient?
3. Aside from vacuum devices, how is ED treated?

A 64-year-old man with type 2 diabetes has had ED for 8 years. His complications include neuropathy, a previous myocardial infarction, and peripheral vascular disease. Since he takes about 14 different tablets every day, he states that he is not interested in a medication for his ED. The patient's urologist suggests a vacuum therapy device. The patient agrees to try it and the urologist gives him instruction on use and educates him about having an engaging conversation about the device with his wife. The patient followed this advice, and over time, found that the vacuum device improved his condition. The couple was happy that ED was no longer affecting their relationship.

ANSWERS

1. Organic causes of CD are usually vascular or neurologic disorders, often due to diabetes or atherosclerosis, with atherosclerosis of the cavernous arteries of the penis being highly common. Endothelial dysfunction is due to diabetes, smoking, and low testosterone levels. Neurologic causes include diabetic neuropathy.
2. Diagnosis of ED is based on clinical evaluation, screening for depression, and measuring testosterone levels. Evaluation for previous history of diabetes is important. Based on clinical suspicion, there may be a need to evaluate for occult diabetes, dyslipidemias, Cushing's syndrome, and thyroid disease.
3. ED is treated initially by focusing on underlying causes such as diabetes. Medications include oral phosphodiesterase inhibitors. Intracavernosal or intraurethral prostaglandin E1 may be needed. There can also be a surgical implantation of a penile prosthesis. Behavior modifications such as diet changes and weight loss may be required.

FOOT DISORDERS

Diabetes may damage the blood vessels that supply the peripheral nerves. Diabetic neuropathy is accumulated peripheral nerve damage. There are a variety of foot disorders that are seen in patients with diabetes mellitus. Foot ulcers and gangrene are examples of diabetes complications. Chronic diabetes can damage the blood vessels of feet. The nerves of the feet become greatly reduced in size and function.

Epidemiology

According to the National Institute of Neurological Disorders and Stroke, an estimated 20 million Americans have some type of peripheral neuropathy. Approximately 50% of diabetics have peripheral neuropathy. Diabetic foot ulcers with neuropathy, but without vascular disease, make up 60%–70% of cases. About 15%–20% of diabetic foot ulcers only involve vascular disease, and the same percentage involve both neuropathy and vascular disease. Diabetic foot ulcers occur in both type 1 and type 2 diabetes patients. About 5%–10% of patients have had foot ulcers or currently have them. About 1% of patients have had amputations. Foot ulcers precede more than 80% of amputations. Lifetime risks for developing foot ulcers in diabetic patients may be as high as 25%. The major risk factor for foot ulcers is distal symmetric neuropathy.

Etiology and Risk Factors

The cause of foot disorders due to diabetes is nerve damage (diabetic neuropathy). Lack of feeling leads to trauma and injury, often with poor healing. Risk factors for foot disorders include insufficient self-monitoring, insufficient hygiene, inadequate treatment of corns and calluses, incorrect trimming of toenails, walking barefoot, inadequate protection from extreme temperatures, inadequate exercise to maintain blood flow, and avoiding regular health checkups that include foot examinations.

Pathophysiology

Patients who have sensory neuropathies have impaired sensation of pain. Therefore, they not know of foot trauma caused by shoes that do not fit correctly, weight bearing that is improper, hard objects inside shoes, or athlete's foot and other infections. Since those with neuropathy cannot detect pain, they may walk in a way that causes trauma and necrosis to areas of the feet. According to the National Institute of Diabetes and Digestive and Kidney Diseases in 2018, 15% of diabetics develop foot ulcers, and of these, 12%–24% require amputation. The issue of diabetic foot ulcers is most concerning in Hispanic, African, and Native Americans since they have the highest prevalence of diabetes in the world.

Clinical Manifestations

Foot deformities can occur from motor neuropathy along with weakness of the intrinsic foot muscles. This can lead to high-pressure focal areas. Foot ulcers can occur when loss of sensation is combined with abnormally focused pressure. The most common areas of trauma include the great toe (where weight is borne while walking), the back of the heel, and the plantar metatarsal area. Symptoms of neuropathy include pain, numbness, and tingling in the hands and feet. There may be muscle weakness, gastroparesis, bowel problems, difficult bladder emptying, sexual dysfunction, and dizziness or lightheadedness when sitting up or standing up quickly. Once the feet began to experience peripheral neuropathy, blisters and sores can develop often without notice, progressing into severe complications leading to amputation. Diabetes-related nerve damage can also change the shape of the feet and toes. A rare condition called Charcot's foot damages the bones and tissues of the feet. The chronic pain of peripheral neuropathy may lead to anxiety, grief, and depression.

Gangrene is a condition involving tissue death and decay (see Figure 13.3). It is caused by lost blood supplies or by bacterial infections. Removing dead tissue – often by amputation – as well as with antibiotics, usually treats it. There are three different types of gangrene:

- *Dry gangrene* – From lost blood supply to affected tissues

- *Wet gangrene* – From bacterial infections, or in diabetics, a complication of foot ulcers

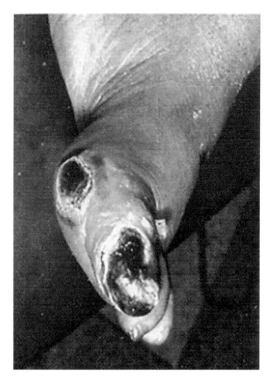

Figure 13.3 Gangrene.

- *Gas gangrene* – Usually caused by *Clostridium perfringens*, a bacterium that produces gas and toxins

People with diabetes are at higher risk of developing dry or wet gangrene, since they have damage to their blood vessels, and often, impaired abilities to fight infections. The toes, feet, lower limbs, hands, and sometimes fingers may be vulnerable to conditions that cause gangrene. Symptoms include numbness, coldness of the affected area, discoloration – from red to blue to black – and a foul-smelling discharge.

Diagnosis

All patients with diabetes must receive a complete foot examination annually. This must include assessments of foot structure, biomechanics, protective sensation, skin integrity, and vascular status. A somatosensory test, using the *Semmes-Weinstein monofilament* should be performed. This inexpensive device tests loss of protective sensation as the monofilament is held either with the hand or attached to a handle. When the other end of the monofilament presses against the skin, buckling or bending slightly, 10 g of pressure are delivered where it makes contact. The patient should report when he or she feels the monofilament, usually in four different sites on the foot. Just one incorrect response may indicate loss of protective sensation and higher risk of ulcers. Diabetics must wear correctly fitted shoes and inspect their feet every day for open sores, blisters, and fungal infections between the toes. Another person should assist if the patient's eyesight is poor.

Treatment

When a lesion is found, prompt medical attention is essential for preventing serious complications. In patients who have had previous ulcers, specially designed shoes are effective to prevent relapses. Since cold temperatures cause vasoconstriction, adequate foot coverings should be worn to keep the feet dry and warm. Toenails must be cut straight across in order to prevent ingrown nails from occurring. In diabetics, the toenails are often deformed and thickened – indicating the need to see a podiatrist. Smoking must be avoided since it results in vasoconstriction, contributing to vascular disease. For diabetics with foot ulcers and peripheral arterial disease, cardiovascular risk factors must be assessed. Growth factors can be used to treat ulcers that resist standard therapies, since they allow cells to communicate normally. This greatly affects cell proliferation and migration as well as synthesis of the extracellular matrix.

Basic principles of wound healing are used for diabetic foot ulcers. Healing can occur if the arterial inflow of blood is adequate, infections are treated correctly, and pressure is removed from wounds and the nearby surrounding areas. It is difficult for patients to avoid putting pressure onto ulcers when they have reduced peripheral sensation. Lack of pain allows pressure to be placed directly onto ulcers, stopping healing. A neuroischemic ulcer is the most difficult type to heal. Adequate noninvasive examination and arteriography must be performed for nonhealing diabetic foot ulcers if there is any doubt as to the patient's vascular status. Poor wound debridement must also be avoided. There is often extensive buildup of calloses from the patient putting pressure on an active ulcer. All dead and macerated tissue must be debrided and removed to allow for faster ulcer healing.

Prevention

The prevention of foot ulceration in diabetics, using relatively simple techniques, can reduce amputations by as much as 80%. Foot condition must be assessed early, and patient education is essential. At very least, foot assessments must occur annually, and for many patients, more often. Simple examinations can allow for problems to be assessed before they become serious. No exceptions are allowed – especially since type 2 diabetics may present with neuropathy, vascular disease, and/or foot ulcerations. Foot examinations must assess calluses, deformities, muscle wasting, and dry skin. Appropriate monofilaments must be used to assess pressure perception. A 128-Hz tuning fork is used to perceive vibration over the hallux of the foot. Lack of ankle reflexes is another predictor of foot ulceration.

Prognosis

Foot disorders are relatively common with long-term diabetes, and infections can develop even with careful monitoring. Prognosis depends on how early a foot wound was found, the presence of an infection, the extent of the infection, and how effective treatments may be. Prognosis is worsened with an uncontrolled infection, resulting in amputation.

CLINICAL CASE

1. How common are diabetic foot ulcers?
2. Where are the most common areas of trauma?
3. How important is the prevention of food ulceration in diabetic patients?

A 69-year-old man presented to his physician with a nonhealing diabetic foot ulcer. It had been present for nearly 2 months. The man was scheduled for 20 sessions of hyperbaric oxygen therapy. Even with the repeated treatments, the ulcer only healed slightly. Eventually, full closure of the foot ulcer was achieved with continuous diffusion of oxygen therapy. The procedure provided a continuous flow of humidified oxygen directly to the bed of the wound, resulting in full wound closure and pain relief.

ANSWERS

1. Diabetic foot ulcers with neuropathy but without vascular disease make up 60%–70% of cases. About 15%–20% of diabetic foot ulcers only involve vascular disease, and the

same percentage involve both neuropathy and vascular disease. Diabetic foot ulcers occur in both type 1 and type 2 diabetes. Foot ulcers precede more than 80% of amputations. Lifetime risks for developing foot ulcers in diabetic patients may be as high as 25%.

2. The most common areas of trauma include the great toe where weight is borne while walking, the back of the heel, and the plantar metatarsal area.

3. The prevention of foot ulceration in diabetics, using relatively simple techniques, can reduce amputations by as much as 80%. Patient education is essential. Foot assessments must occur at least annually, and for many patients, more often. No exceptions are allowed – especially since type 2 diabetics may present with neuropathy, vascular disease, and/or foot ulcerations.

KEY TERMS

- Acanthosis nigricans
- Amyloidosis
- Antroduodenal manometry
- Athlete's foot
- Bariatric surgery
- Cajal cells
- Candida albicans
- Dyspareunia
- Electrogastrography
- Ergonomic
- Eruptive xanthomatosis
- Hemochromatosis
- Hypoechoic material

- Indurative
- Mycosis
- Parotid glands
- Periodontium
- Polysomnography
- Proteobacteria
- Pylorospasm
- Rete ridges
- Scintiscanning
- Steatorrhea
- Thenar atrophy
- Thrush
- Toxic megacolon
- Ulnar claw
- Vagus nerve
- Xerostomia
- Zygomycosis

REFERENCES

American Academy of Periodontology / Perio.org. (2021). *Diabetes and Periodontal Disease*. American Academy of Periodontology / AAP Foundation. https://www.perio.org/consumer/gum-disease-and-diabetes.htm

American Diabetes Association / Clinical Diabetes. (2016). *Oral Manifestations of Diabetes*. American Diabetes Association. https://clinical.diabetesjournals.org/content/34/1/54

American Diabetes Association / Complications. (2021). *Skin Complications*. American Diabetes Association. https://www.diabetes.org/diabetes/complications/skin-complications

American Diabetes Association / Diabetes Care. (2010). *Barely Scratching the Surface*. American Diabetes Association. https://care.diabetesjournals.org/content/33/1/210

American Diabetes Association / Diabetes Spectrum. (2006). *Case Study: Sleep Apnea Diagnosis in a Man with Type 2 Diabetes – Improved Control*. American Diabetes Association. https://spectrum.diabetesjournals.org/content/19/3/190

American Family Physician. (2008). *Gastrointestinal Complications of Diabetes*. American Academy of Family Physicians. https://www.aafp.org/afp/2008/0615/p1697.html

BMC / Springer Nature / Diabetology & Metabolic Syndrome. (2016). *Skin Disorders in Diabetes Mellitus: An Epidemiology and Physiopathology Review*. BioMed Central Ltd. https://dmsjournal.biomedcentral.com/articles/10.1186/s13098-016-0176–y

British Journal of Diabetes and Vascular Disorders. (2014). *Diabetic Dermopathy*. British Journal of Diabetes and Vascular Disorders. http://www.bjd-abcd.com/index.php/bjd/article/viewFile/24/63

Centers for Disease Control and Prevention. (2021a). *Diabetes and Pneumonia: Get the Facts*. Centers for Disease Control and Prevention. https://www.cdc.gov/diabetes/projects/pdfs/eng_facts.pdf

Centers for Disease Control and Prevention. (2021b). *Influenza (Flu) / Diabetes*. U.S. Department of Health & Human Services / USA.gov / CDC. https://www.cdc.gov/flu/highrisk/diabetes.htm

Cleveland Clinic / Health Library / Disease & Conditions. (2021). *Gum (Periodontal) Disease*. Cleveland Clinic. https://my.clevelandclinic.org/health/diseases/21482-gum-periodontal-disease

Clinical Advisor / Clinical Challenge. (2018). *Case Study in Diabetes: Fungal Infections*. Haymarket Media, Inc. https://www.clinicaladvisor.com/home/features/clinical-challenge/case-study-in-diabetes-fungal-infections/

Healthline. (2019). *Type 2 Diabetes and Skin Health*. Healthline Media. https://www.healthline.com/health/type-2-diabetes/skin-problems#symptoms

Healthline. (2018). *Can Diabetes Cause Vaginal Yeast Infections?* Healthline Media. https://www.healthline.com/health/diabetes/diabetes-and-yeast-infections

Mayo Clinic. (2021). *Sleep Apnea*. Mayo Foundation for Medical Education and Research (MFMER). https://www.mayoclinic.org/diseases-conditions/sleep-apnea/symptoms-causes/syc-20377631

MyoAir. (2019). *Sleep Apnea Can Make Managing Diabetes More Difficult: What You Need to Know*. MyoAir. https://myoair.com/articles/sleep-apnea-can-make-managing-diabetes-more-difficult-what-you-need-to-know

NCBI / PMC / U.S. National Library of Medicine / National Institutes of Health / Indian Journal of Endocrinology and Metabolism. (2012). *Infections in Patients with Diabetes Mellitus: A Review of Pathogenesis*. National Center for Biotechnology Information / U.S. National Library of Medicine. https://www.ncbi.nlm.nih.gov/pmc/articles/PMC3354930/

NCBI / PMC / U.S. National Library of Medicine / National Institutes of Health / Journal of Medicine and Life. (2016). *The Association between Diabetes Mellitus and Depression*. National Center for Biotechnology Information / U.S. National Library of Medicine. https://www.ncbi.nlm.nih.gov/pmc/articles/PMC4863499/

NIH / National Library of Medicine / National Center for Biotechnology Information. (2020). *Malignant Otitis Externa Is Associated with Diabetes: A Population-Based Case-Control Study*. National Library of Medicine. https://pubmed.ncbi.nlm.nih.gov/31976744/

NIH / National Library of Medicine / National Center for Biotechnology Information. (2018). *Gastrointestinal Manifestations of Diabetes*. National Library of Medicine. https://pubmed.ncbi.nlm.nih.gov/33651548/

NIH / National Library of Medicine / National Center for Biotechnology Information. (2013). *Clinical Aspects of Fungal Infections in Diabetes*. National Library of Medicine. https://pubmed.ncbi.nlm.nih.gov/23923382/

NIH / National Library of Medicine / National Center for Biotechnology Information. (2006). *Common Pathogens Isolated in Diabetic Food Infections*. National Library of Medicine. https://pubmed.ncbi.nlm.nih.gov/18603922/

Quality Health. (2021). *Pneumonia and Diabetes*. QualityHealth.com. https://www.qualityhealth.com/diabetes-articles/pneumonia-diabetes

University of Michigan Health / Michigan Medicine. (2021). *Diabetes and Infections*. Regents of the University of Michigan. https://www.uofmhealth.org/health-library/uq1148abc

U.S. Department of Health and Human Services / NIH / National Institute of Diabetes and Digestive and Kidney Diseases. (2021a). *Diabetes, Gum Disease, & Other Dental Problems*. U.S. Department of Health and Human Services / National Institutes of Health / USA.gov. https://www.niddk.nih.gov/health-information/diabetes/overview/preventing-problems/gum-disease-dental-problems

U.S. Department of Health and Human Services / NIH / National Institute of Diabetes and Digestive and Kidney Diseases. (2021b). *Treatment for Gastroparesis*. U.S. Department of Health and Human Services / National Institutes of Health / USA.gov. https://www.niddk.nih.gov/health-information/digestive-diseases/gastroparesis/treatment

VeryWellHealth / Ear, Nose & Throat / ENT Disorders / Pneumonia. (2021). *Causes and Risk Factors of Pneumonia*. Dotdash. https://www.verywellhealth.com/pneumonia-causes-risk-factors-770691

VeryWellHealth / Type 2 Diabetes / Living With. (2019). *The Connection between Diabetes and Periodontal Disease*. Dotdash. https://www.verywellhealth.com/diabetes-and-gum-disease-connection-1059401

Diabetes mellitus – especially type 2 diabetes – has similar risk factors to those of cancer, linking the diseases together. With diabetes, cancer may be related to increased age, the male gender, the African American and non-Hispanic Caucasian racial or ethnic groups, being overweight or obese, a poor diet, lack of exercise, smoking, and excessive alcohol consumption. With diabetes, it is very important to have regular screenings for complications that include cancer. Treatments for cancer are often more difficult when diabetes is present. Outcomes of treatment are also affected since diabetic patients have generally poorer health than nondiabetic patients, and insufficient ability to combat the damage caused by cancer. Control of blood glucose levels is very important to help improve the effectiveness of treatments for any type of concurrent cancer.

THYROID CANCER

Thyroid cancer is one of the most common malignant endocrine tumors. It is subclassified as papillary, follicular, medullary and anaplastic carcinoma. Patients with diabetes are at a 1.34 times higher risk for thyroid cancer than those without diabetes. Thyroid cancer is most common between the ages of 20 and 50, and is three times more common in women than in men. Papillary carcinoma of the thyroid is a malignant epithelial tumor. Follicular carcinoma is the second most common type of thyroid carcinoma. It is encapsulated and has invasive growth. Medullary thyroid carcinoma (MTC) is the third most common of all thyroid tumors. Anaplastic thyroid carcinoma (ATC) is very aggressive and malignant. It is made up of undifferentiated follicular thyroid cells, which do not look like normal thyroid cells. Anaplastic carcinoma is considered to be a grade IV tumor.

Epidemiology

According to the American Cancer Society, estimates of cases of thyroid cancer in the United States for 2021 are 32,130 in women and 12,150 in men, totaling 44,280. Caucasians have the highest rates of thyroid cancer, while African Americans have the lowest rates. Globally, thyroid cancer affects about 0.4 of every 100,000 women, and 0.3 of every 100,000 men. Incidence of thyroid cancer has doubled globally since 1990. The prevalence of papillary carcinoma of the thyroid has increased since the year 1975, from 4.8 to 14.9 cases per 100,000 individuals. In the United States, it makes up about 45,000 new diagnoses every year. The annual prevalence of follicular thyroid carcinomas in the United States, in 2009, was 12 cases per 1 million women, and 5.5 cases per 1 million men. This form makes up 10%–15% of all thyroid cancers. Follicular carcinomas are very rare in children. Highest annual cases were in patients between the ages of 70 and 79 years. MTC makes up less than 2.5% of all malignant thyroid tumors. Because of its rarity, the global prevalence and incidence of MTC are not well documented. There is no racial or ethnic predilection, and no clear statistics as to which countries have more cases than others. Anaplastic carcinoma of the thyroid is also very rare, affecting less than 2% of thyroid cancer patients, but is responsible for 20%–50% of deaths. ATC affects 1–2 out of every 1 million people annually in the United States. The majority of patients are over age 65, and 90% of cases occur above the age of 50.

Etiology and Risk Factors

Exposure to ionizing radiation is the main cause of papillary thyroid carcinoma. Risk factors may include genetics, alcohol consumption, diabetes mellitus, dietary nitrites, excessive dietary iodine, obesity, and smoking. The actual causes of follicular thyroid carcinoma are unknown, but inadequate dietary iodine is a significant risk factor. Genetic factors are considerable for follicular thyroid carcinomas. The cause of MTC is not known, and there is no relationship to external ionizing irradiation of the head and neck. Often, the tumor develops along with Hashimoto's thyroiditis, but this is not fully understood. The etiology of ATCs is unclear. Risk factors include inherited cancer syndromes, including **Cowden's syndrome**, **Carney complex**, **Werner's syndrome**, and familial adenomatous polyposis.

Clinical Manifestations

Papillary carcinoma often is detected as a painless mass, with enlargement of the cervical lymph nodes. However, some patients may complain about neck pain, hoarseness, and dysphagia. Patients have also nodal metastases in the lateral neck. Follicular thyroid carcinoma is often a painless tumor, from less than 1 cm in diameter up to several centimeters. Large tumors cause dyspnea or dysphagia, and throat or neck soreness and pain. There may be unintended weight loss and night sweats. Cervical lymph node enlargement at diagnosis is not common. Sometimes, the first symptom is metastasis that can be signified by a lung nodule or a bone fracture. If a metastasis is diagnosed as being from the thyroid, a neck

DOI: 10.1201/9781003226727-17

examination will usually reveal a thyroid mass. In certain cases, findings of bone metastases prompt reexamination of an earlier resected thyroid mass that was believed to be an adenoma. There are also rare cases of functional follicular thyroid carcinoma related to hyperthyroidism. The majority of MTCs are painless. Extensive localized tumor growth causes upper airway obstruction plus dysphagia. With metastases, some patients experience flushing and severe diarrhea because of high circulating calcitonin levels and other products that result from the tumor. Patients may present with a firm neck mass that is fixed in one location. The tumor is widely infiltrative. Hoarseness, breathing problems, dysphagia, and pain are common symptoms, as well as dyspnea and vocal cord paralysis. Approximately 35% of patients initially present with distant metastasis to the lungs and bones.

Pathology

Papillary carcinoma may appear in one or both lobes. It is poorly defined, with a firm texture and a granular white cut surface. The size of the tumor is between 2 and 3 cm in diameter, with calcifications. The cytoplasm is eosinophilic. Psammoma bodies are classic features, which are round, calcified, and hard masses. There is a great amount of fibrous stroma, particularly at the advancing edge of the tumor. Often, there are multinucleated giant cells of a nonneoplastic histiocytic nature scattered throughout, which are easily found in cytology studies. Secondary cystic changes often occur, with most cysts being lined with papillary formations that aid in diagnosis.

Follicular thyroid carcinomas are solid and encapsulated. Some have cystic features. Hemorrhage may be seen in biopsied lesions. In extremely invasive tumors, there is prominent extension into the thyroid or extrathyroidal tissue. Structurally, these tumors are similar to follicular adenomas. Most pathologists diagnose them based on total thickness penetration of the tumor capsule. Invasion is not related to capsule rupture from surgical manipulation, and pseudoinvasion is caused by biopsy trauma. Most invasive follicular carcinomas are large in size. If there is a solid or trabecular growth pattern, the tumor must be distinguished from poorly differentiated thyroid carcinoma. Clear cell cytoplasm is most common, with oval or round nuclei and small nucleoli. Cytoplasmic clearing occurs because of lipid, thyroglobulin, glycogen, and mucin accumulation. It is important to exclude metastatic clear cell carcinoma that arises from the kidney, parathyroid tumors, and medullary thyroid carcinoma. The clear cell variant may be more aggressive than the classic form of follicular carcinoma, but this is not proven.

Medullary thyroid carcinomas are usually single, circumscribed and unencapsulated tumors with a gray-tan to yellow color. The size usually is 2–3 cm in diameter. Differently, the inherited tumors are usually multicentric and bilateral. For members of families with tumor syndromes, a full examination is required of the thyroid gland since gross tumors may not be visualized, and prophylactic thyroidectomies are often performed. Tumors less than 1 cm in diameter are identified incidentally from resected thyroid glands, or in patients with nodular thyroid disease after screening for calcitonin level changes. Cells are of various sizes, and may be round or spindle-shaped. The nuclei are round and have small nucleoli plus chromatin. The mitotic activity is low in most primary tumors. In fixed samples, cytoplasm is eosinophilic, with fine granules. Measurement of serum calcitonin is highly helpful. In MTC patients with palpable thyroid nodules, there may be cervical lymph node metastases. Nodal metastases often involve central compartment nodes. Hematogenous metastases are often to the lungs, bones, and liver.

ATC is the primary malignancy of the gland, and often spreads to regional lymph nodes as well as distant locations. The tumor is often large, multicolored, with necrosis and an infiltrative growth pattern. Vascular invasion is common, and involves penetration of the vessel walls by spindle cells, protruding into the lumina. The cells usually include epithelioid and spindle cells, plus giant cells that resemble osteoclasts, and tumor diathesis. Clusters of tumor cells are often infiltrated by neutrophils.

Diagnosis

Ultrasonography is a very helpful diagnostic method that reveals hypoechoic or isoechoic solid nodules. Thyroid scans using iodine-123 (^{123}I) result in most papillary carcinomas appearing hypofunctional. However, in rare cases they appear hyperfunctional. Ultrasound guides fine-needle aspiration biopsy of abnormal nodes. In some cases, CT and MRI can determine how much extrathyroidal extension is present. Cytological diagnosis of a follicular neoplasm demonstrates that thyroid cytology is limited, since follicular carcinoma diagnosis is based on demonstrating capsular invasion, vascular invasion, or both. Imaging studies include X-rays and CT scans. Early diagnosis of MTCs is essential to improve the chances for a cure.

Cervical ultrasonography helps confirm that a mass is within the thyroid, accurately defines its size, classifies it as cystic or solid, and determines whether additional nodules are present. Radionuclide scanning with radioiodine or technetium pertechnetate is helpful only in selected cases. There is cellularity via fine-needle aspiration, depending on which area of the tumor is biopsied.

Treatment

Total surgical resection via thyroidectomy, with or without isthmectomy, is the treatment of choice for papillary thyroid carcinomas. This includes dissection of any involved cervical lymph nodes. After total surgical resection, the patient must receive lifelong hormone replacement therapy. When a residual tumor cannot be removed, radiation therapy is needed. Chemotherapy options include cisplatin and doxorubicin. Antineoplastic agents are used to inhibit cell growth and proliferation in the case of metastases. Surgery is the treatment of choice for follicular thyroid carcinoma. After radioactive iodine treatment, the patient is placed on a 2-week low-iodine diet. Iodine-131 is used for ablation of thyroid tissue. Surgical resection and radiation therapy are the principal treatments for MTCs. Sometimes a total thyroidectomy is the best method to accomplish a cure if there are no distant metastases or extensive involvement of the lymph nodes. Most cases of ATCs are unresectable at presentation because of invasion of cervical structures. Surgery is not curative and should aim to secure the patient's airway. Often, radiation therapy and chemotherapy are administered.

Prevention and Early Detection

Since the actual cause of papillary thyroid carcinoma is unknown, it cannot be fully prevented. Reducing radiation exposure during childhood is suggested. Other preventive measures may include genetic testing, limiting alcohol consumption, treating diabetes mellitus, reducing dietary nitrites, having adequate dietary iodine, treating obesity, and avoiding smoking. For high-risk patients, surgical removal of the thyroid may prevent papillary thyroid carcinoma from developing. Better diagnostic methods are resulting in earlier detection of papillary thyroid carcinoma. There is no actual prevention for follicular thyroid carcinoma and the same risk reduction strategies exist as for papillary thyroid carcinoma. There are also no specific methods for its early detection. However genetic testing may be considered. There is no known method of prevention for medullary thyroid cancer. Newly identified *rearranged-during-transfection point mutations* have helped to detect MTC earlier than in previous decades, and new treatment guidelines have resulted. Screening methods are based on serum calcitonin levels, and for metastatic or recurrent MTCs, neck ultrasonography, chest CT, liver MRI, bone scintigraphy, and axial skeleton MRI are options. There is no known method of preventing anaplastic thyroid carcinoma. There is also no way to diagnose the disease early. By the time symptoms are present, there is often evidence that the carcinoma has spread to distant body sites

Prognosis

Prognosis is based on extent of the disease. Prognosis is further based on patient age at diagnosis, tumor size, staging, and distant metastases. There is increased mortality for patients between 40 and 45 years of age, as well as for tumors that are larger than 3 to 4 cm in diameter. Overall mortality rates are 1%–7%. The 5-year survival rate for papillary carcinoma is 97.9% in the United States. Globally, the survival rate is 96%. Extrathyroidal tumor extension worsens prognosis, with widespread extension being worse than only minimal extension. Prognosis is very poor for bone and visceral metastases. Other factors that worsen prognosis include tumor cell type, incomplete surgical excision, and the male gender. Total surgical resection is very important regarding prognosis. Recurrence within 10 years after initial surgery is usually related to increased mortality. Prognosis for follicular carcinomas is an excellent with capsular invasion, but not with vascular invasion. Tumors invading even only 1–2 vessels may show hematogenous metastasis. Prognosis is worsened with larger numbers of vessels being invaded. Distant metastases most often occur in the lungs, bones, brain, and liver. Prolonged survival is possible, when the tumor responds to radioactive iodine.

For medullary thyroid carcinoma, 5-year survival rates are 77% and 10-year survival rates are 65%, based on staging. Patient age is important along with staging to determine prognosis for MTCs. A poor prognosis is related to the presence of high calcitonin after surgical resection. When the tumor is more aggressive, the prognosis is poor. Vascular invasion also worsens outlook. The 1-year survival rate for anaplastic thyroid carcinomas is 10%–20%. Generally speaking, mortality rates are 90%. A primary presentation with a large, infiltrative tumor suggests a poor prognosis. There is a better outlook when the tumor is found incidentally during another surgery.

CLINICAL CASE

1. What are the subclassifications of thyroid cancer, and what is the link with diabetes?
2. How do medullary thyroid carcinomas usually appear?
3. What are the screening options for thyroid carcinoma?

A 69-year-old diabetic woman was taken to a cancer care facility because of suspected thyroid cancer. She was previously prescribed liraglutide for her diabetes, which she had taken over 18 months. Evaluation revealed that her calcitonin levels had been increasing over time. Fine-needle biopsy had revealed the cancer to be medullary carcinoma. A total thyroidectomy was performed successfully. It was found that two undetected papillary tumors had also been removed as part of the surgery. The patient fully recovered. She is cancer-free at 1 year of follow-up.

ANSWERS

1. Thyroid cancer is subclassified as papillary, follicular, medullary, and anaplastic carcinoma. Patients with diabetes are at a 1.34 times higher risk for thyroid cancer than those without diabetes.
2. Medullary thyroid carcinomas are usually single, circumscribed and unencapsulated tumors with a gray-tan to yellow color. The size usually is 2–3 cm in diameter.
3. The screening options for thyroid carcinoma are based on serum calcitonin levels and biopsy. For thyroid metastatic, neck ultrasonography, chest CT, liver MRI, bone scintigraphy, and axial skeleton MRI are options.

PANCREATIC CANCER

Pancreatic cancer is a highly invasive cancer of the digestive system. The most common type of pancreatic cancer is *ductal adenocarcinoma*. The majority of pancreatic cancers are exocrine tumors, forming from the ductal and acinar cells. Pancreatic endocrine tumors originate from the islet cells, and secrete several hormones. This type of tumor may also occur in the duodenum or lungs. To improve management and survival rates from pancreatic cancer, it is important to identify the clinical features and biomarkers that distinguish pancreatic cancer-related diabetes from type 2 diabetes. For patients that are middle-aged and have new-onset diabetes, MRI may be considered to assess pancreatic tumors.

Epidemiology

Pancreatic cancer is the ninth most common cancer in men, and the tenth most common cancer in women. Approximately 92% of pancreatic cancers are adenocarcinomas, which occur at a mean age of 55 years, and are more common in men. They affect more than 55,000 people annually in the United States alone, and are usually fatal. Pancreatic cancer accounts for 3% of all cancers in the United States. Incidence is about 13 per 100,000 people. The mortality is much higher in African Americans.

Globally, pancreatic cancer is the 12th most common cancer in men and the 11th most common cancer in women. There are about 460,000 new cases globally each year. The incidence of pancreatic cancer comprises 2.5% of all types of cancer, worldwide. Age-specific incidence rates increase vigorously at age 50–54. The countries with the highest rates of pancreatic cancer include Hungary, Uruguay, Moldova, Latvia, Japan, Slovakia, Estonia, Czech Republic, the United States, France, and Austria.

Etiology and Risk Factors

The clear cause of pancreatic cancer is not known. The most common risk factors for pancreatic cancer include obesity, diabetes, chronic pancreatitis, smoking, the male gender, and the African American ethnicity. Caffeine and alcohol use do not appear to be risk factors. However, some studies have shown that heavy alcohol use may cause chronic pancreatitis, which can impact the development of pancreatic cancer. Long-term diabetes is a risk factor for pancreatic cancer, increasing the likelihood of it developing by 1.5–2 times. The duration of the diabetes is also important. Those with diabetes for 5 years or longer are more likely to develop pancreatic cancer. Those with new-onset diabetes after the age of 50 have almost 1% higher likelihood of being diagnosed with pancreatic cancer within 3 years. Pancreatic cancer may cause cells to resist insulin, meaning that diabetes can be a symptom of the cancer.

Clinical Manifestations

The initial symptoms of pancreatic cancer are pain and weight loss. Upon diagnosis, about 90% of patients have locally advanced tumors that have affected the regional lymph nodes, liver, and lungs. Abdominal pain is severe and common, radiating to the back. An adenocarcinoma of the head of the pancreas may cause obstructive jaundice and itching. Splenomegaly and GI hemorrhage also occur. Up to 50% of patients with the cancer may develop diabetes mellitus. The cancer can shift production of digestive enzymes, causing malabsorption of foods, which resulting in bloating, gas, and foul-smelling diarrhea. Vitamin deficiencies and weight loss may occur.

Pathology

Adenocarcinomas of the pancreas often develop from duct cells. In general, ductal adenocarcinomas are poorly defined and firm. They have glandular structures within **desmoplastic stroma**. The tumors do not stain with endocrine markers. Microscopically, diagnosis is confirmed by staining. There is disorganization of the extracellular matrix, using hematoxylin and eosin (H & E) dyes. Similar conditions that can develop into pancreatic ductal adenocarcinoma include *intraductal papillary mucinous neoplasia* and *mucinous cystic neoplasia*.

Diagnosis

Diagnosis of pancreatic cancer begins with medical history and physical examination. Abdominal CT with contrast enhancement, endoscopic retrograde, ultrasound, magnetic resonance cholangiopancreatography, cholangiopancreatography, and a positron emission tomography are used to diagnose pancreatic cancer. Routine blood laboratory tests are performed, including liver function and tumor marker testing. Liver metastasis or bile duct obstruction may be diagnosed by elevated bilirubin, alkaline phosphatase, and surgical biopsy.

Treatment

Pancreatic cancers are considered to be unresectable when they are diagnosed, due to metastases. Based on tumor location, surgery is performed. External beam radiation therapy is often used. Chemotherapy and radiation combinations may be also used. If there are liver or distant metastases, chemotherapy may be used. For moderate to severe pain, oral opioids are administered. Pain control is more important than any concern about addiction. Long-acting preparations are good for chronic pain, and include transdermal oxymorphone, oxycodone, or fentanyl. Exocrine pancreatic insufficiency is treated with oral pancrelipase. Dosage is based on symptoms, the amount of steatorrhea, and dietary fat content. Proton pump inhibitors or H2-blockers may also be required. If diabetes mellitus is present, it must be monitored and controlled with care.

Prevention and Early Detection

Unfortunately, there is no method of preventing pancreatic cancer. However, steps that can be taken to reduce risks of its development include quitting smoking, a healthy diet, avoiding heavy use of alcohol, maintaining a normal body weight, and regular physical activity. There is no screening test that decreases the risk of dying from pancreatic cancer. However, for people with family history, genetic testing may be able to find gene changes that increase the risks for the disease. For those at high risk, endoscopic ultrasound or MRI may help to detect early pancreatic cancer.

Prognosis

The prognosis for pancreatic cancer is very poor. For most patients, the 5-year survival is less than 2 years, since so many have advanced disease by the time it is diagnosed.

CLINICAL CASE

1. How common are pancreatic adenocarcinomas?
2. What are the links between diabetes and pancreatic cancer?
3. What is the actual prognosis for pancreatic cancer?

A 72-year-old diabetic man was hospitalized because of symptoms that included loss of appetite, early satiety, abdominal pain, and jaundice. Imaging revealed a mass within the head of his pancreas. It was biopsied and found to be a low-grade adenocarcinoma. A biliary drain was inserted. After a few days the patient was discharged. A skilled surgical team evaluated the findings that had been collected. Seven days later, an open pylorus-preserving pancreaticoduodenectomy, with cholecystectomy, was performed. The tumor was a moderately differentiated ductal adenocarcinoma with negative margins. Surrounding lymph nodes were also negative. A follow-up CT scan revealed no fluid collection. The patient recovered well, and was counseled about the high potential for this cancer to recur. He was started on gemcitabine in a 4-week cycle for 6 months.

ANSWERS

1. Approximately 92% of pancreatic cancers are adenocarcinomas, which occur at a mean age of 55 years, and are more common in men. They affect more than 55,000 people annually in the United States, and are usually fatal.
2. Long-term diabetes is a risk factor for pancreatic cancer, increasing the likelihood of it developing by 1.5–2 times. The duration of the diabetes is also important. Those with diabetes for 5 years or longer are more likely to develop pancreatic cancer. Those with new-onset diabetes after the age of 50 have almost 1% higher likelihood of being diagnosed with pancreatic cancer within 3 years. Pancreatic cancer may cause cells to resist insulin, meaning that diabetes can be a symptom of the cancer.
3. The prognosis for pancreatic cancer is very poor. For most patients, the 5-year survival is less than 2 years, since so many have advanced disease by the time it is diagnosed.

LIVER CANCER

The majority of liver cancers arise from the parenchyma and ductal epithelium of the biliary tract. Hepatocellular carcinoma is also referred to as **hepatoma**. It is the most common form of primary liver cancer. Type 2 diabetes is considered a risk factor for liver cancer because of its strong link with obesity. Since obesity may lead to excess fat buildup in the liver, it increases risks for cirrhosis as well as heart disease. Therefore, type 2 diabetes may be associated with increased risks for hepatocellular carcinoma.

Epidemiology

Primary liver cancer is rare in the United States. However, the incidence of hepatocellular carcinoma has been more than tripled in the United States since 1980. Today, the incidence is increasing due to the rising of cases of hepatitis C virus (HCV). Most patients are over 50 years of age. Hepatomas are three times more common in men. They affect people of lower socioeconomic status. Patients with higher rates of cirrhosis and hepatitis generally have higher rates of hepatocellular carcinoma. African American men have the highest mortality rates from hepatoma. In relation to type 2 diabetes mellitus and primary liver cancer, Figure 14.1 shows the percentage of patients in various racial or ethnic groups.

However, hepatomas are more common outside the United States – especially in East Asia and sub-Saharan Africa. There are approximately 1 million people diagnosed with hepatocellular carcinoma annually throughout the world. Primary liver cancer is the sixth most common cancer worldwide. The incidence of liver cancers is similar to the incidence of chronic hepatitis B virus (HBV) infection in East Asia and sub-Saharan Africa. The countries with the highest rates of hepatocellular carcinoma include Mongolia, Egypt, Gambia, Vietnam, Cambodia, Thailand, China, South Korea, North Korea, and Ghana.

Etiology and Risk Factors

The cause of hepatocellular carcinoma is primarily cirrhosis of the liver. However, the presence of the hepatitis B virus increases risks by 100 times in people who carry HBV. The risk factors include alcoholic cirrhosis, hemochromatosis, and chronic HCV infection. In some areas of the world, hepatocellular carcinoma is of higher incidence because of ingesting foods that are contaminated with fungal aflatoxins.

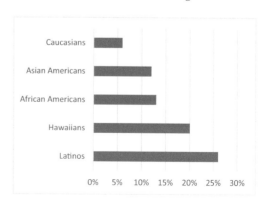

Figure 14.1 Percentage of liver cancer cases in various racial or ethnic groups.

Liver cancer in diabetic patients may be related to medications being taken to control blood glucose. People with type 2 diabetes may develop **fatty liver**, which is a trigger for cirrhosis, fibrosis, and cancer. Fatty liver disease is the most common cause of hepatocellular carcinoma. However, people with type 1 diabetes do not have an increased risk of liver cancer.

Clinical Manifestations

The signs and symptoms may include weight loss, abdominal pain, a right upper quadrant mass, and sometimes, fever. Some patients develop peritonitis, bloody ascites, or shock. Clinical findings may also include hyperlipidemia, hypercalcemia, hypoglycemia, and erythrocytosis. Other potential outcomes include splenomegaly, portal hypertension, **asterixis**, GI bleeding, jaundice, fatigue, cachexia, and encephalopathy.

Pathology

The pathology of hepatocellular carcinoma comprises multiple nodules, with irregular borders. The gross pathology shows a pale mass in the liver that can be unifocal, multifocal, with diffuse infiltration. Larger tumors have macroscopic venous invasion, with or without a fibrous capsule. Smaller tumors lack venous invasion, hemorrhage, or necrosis. The HBV and HCV genomes have genetic material that can predispose cells to accumulate mutations, or to experience disrupted growth. The microscopic appearance ranges from well differentiated to undifferentiated.

Diagnosis

Diagnosis of primary carcinoma may be made by palpating the liver and imaging tests that show an upper right quadrant mass. Along with imaging, alpha fetoprotein (AFP) testing is also performed, which is an indicator of hepatocellular carcinoma. Lower AFP values are not as specific, and may occur along with hepatocellular regeneration, such as in hepatitis. Imaging tests include ultrasound, contrast-enhanced CT, and MRI. Diagnosis is clear when the AFP is elevated and there are characteristic features. Ultrasound may be performed every 6–12 months. Screening is usually advised for patients with chronic hepatitis B, even without cirrhosis.

Treatment

Ablative treatments include hepatic arterial chemoembolization, selective internal radiation therapy, and radiofrequency ablation. All of these provide for palliation and cause tumor growth to become slower. They are done for patients awaiting liver transplantation. The radiofrequency ablation technique can be curative for tumors smaller than 2 cm. For tumors larger than 5 cm that are multifocal, have invaded the portal vein, or are metastatic, radiation therapy is usually ineffective. Sorafenib may slightly improve the patient's condition. Newer agents can prolong survival for a longer time and/or cause fewer side effects. They include regorafenib, lenvatinib, and the immunotherapy agent called nivolumab. Levatinib is an alternative first-line therapy, providing progression-free survival that is better than with sorafenib.

Prevention and Early Detection

Vaccination against HBV can prevent the incidence of hepatocellular carcinoma. Preventing cirrhosis of the liver is important by treating alcoholism, detecting hemochromatosis early, or treating chronic hepatitis C. Hepatocellular carcinoma is usually not detected early in its development. For a person with long-term cirrhosis, various tests for liver cancer are recommended. Physicians also recommend screening with AFP blood tests and ultrasonography every 6 months for high-risk patients.

Prognosis

Unfortunately, prognosis for primary hepatocellular carcinoma is poor, with a 5-year relative survival rate of 18%. For localized disease, this rate is 33%. For regional metastasis, it is 11%, and for distant metastasis, it is only 2.4%. Patients with diabetes, poor glycemic control, or obesity have a poorer prognosis than those without.

CLINICAL CASE

1. Why is type 2 diabetes a risk factor for liver cancer?
2. Which medications may be used for the treatment of liver cancer?
3. What are the prognoses for liver cancer, with and without diabetes?

A 56-year-old man with type 2 diabetes was unexpectedly diagnosed with liver cancer. It shocked him and his wife because they had always thought that tobacco and alcohol were the common causes. The patient had never drank alcohol or smoked cigarettes or any other type of tobacco products. Because there were several tumors in different places throughout the liver, including some near large blood vessels, the patient was considered inoperable, so chemotherapy and radiation therapy were started. The radiation therapy was given in a high dose directly to the tumor. A drug that stops the growth of tumor cells called afatinib dimaleate was also administered since it has shown better results when used along with chemotherapy and radiation. After completion of treatment, the patient was discharged and was doing well after 6 months of follow-up.

ANSWERS

1. Type 2 diabetes is a risk factor for liver cancer because of its strong link with obesity. Since obesity may lead to excess fat buildup in the liver, it increases risks for cirrhosis as well as heart disease. Therefore, type 2 diabetes may be associated with increased risks for hepatocellular carcinoma.
2. Medications used to treat liver cancer include sorafenib, regorafenib, lenvatinib, and nivolumab.
3. The prognosis for primary hepatocellular carcinoma is poor, with a 5-year relative survival rate of 18%. For localized disease, this rate is 33%. For regional metastasis, it is 11%, and for distant metastasis, it is only 2.4%. Patients with diabetes, poor glycemic control, or obesity have a poorer prognosis than those without.

BREAST CANCER

Breast cancer is a malignant neoplastic disease of breast tissue. It is a very common malignancy in women. Breast cancers are usually found as asymptomatic masses during self-examination. Metastasis occurs through the lymphatic system to the axillary lymph nodes and to the bones, lungs, brain, and liver. There is evidence that primary carcinomas of the breast may exist in multiple sites and that tumor cells may enter the bloodstream directly without passing through the lymph nodes. Women with type 2 diabetes have an increased risk for breast cancer – especially after menopause. High insulin levels double the risk of breast cancer in women. Overweight, insulin-resistant women have an 84% higher risk of breast cancer than overweight women that are not insulin-resistant. Since fatty tissue accumulates in the breasts, they become a prime target for unregulated cell growth, which can lead to tumors.

Epidemiology

In the United States, breast cancer is the second most common cause of cancer deaths in women. Approximately 276,500 cases of invasive breast cancer were diagnosed in 2020. Incidence rates are highest in non-Hispanic white women, followed by African American women. Women after age 70 have the highest rates of breast cancer diagnoses. The lowest rates of breast cancer diagnoses are in women before age 30. Breast cancer is rare in men, but it may occur often in older people.

According to the World Health Organization in 2021, breast cancer has now overtaken lung cancer as the most commonly diagnosed cancer throughout the world. Approximately 66% of invasive breast cancer occurs in women aged 55 or older. Caucasian women are diagnosed most often, followed by African women. According to the World Cancer Research Fund in 2020, the countries with the highest rates of breast cancer in women included the Netherlands, Belgium, France, Lebanon, Australia, New Zealand, the United Kingdom, Ireland, Hungary, Germany, Italy, the United States, and Canada (see Figure 14.2).

Etiology and Risk Factors

Breast cancer may develop from cells by inherited susceptibility genes, and hormonal exposures. The most important risk factors are aging and heredity. Women with a first-degree relative with breast cancer have double or triple the risk. The risks are increased by early menarche, late menopause, or a late first pregnancy. Women with a first pregnancy after age 30 have a higher risk for breast cancer than women that have never given birth. Risks are slightly increased if a woman has had a breast lesion that required a biopsy. The use of oral contraceptives increases breast cancer risks. The risk mostly increases when contraceptives are being taken, and reduces within 10 years after stopping them. Risks for breast cancer are also increased by exposure to radiation therapy before the age of 30. Obese postmenopausal women have a higher

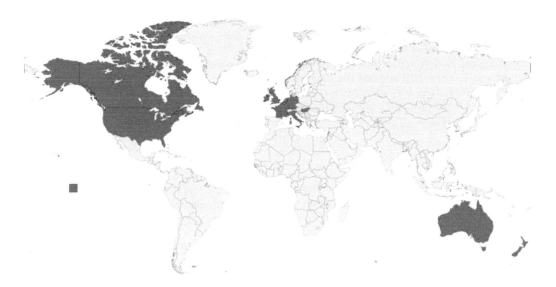

Figure 14.2 Countries with the highest rates of breast cancer in women. (Created by Jahangir Moini.)

risk for breast cancer. If obese women menstruate later than average, risks may be reduced. Smoking and drinking alcohol excessively are other factors.

Diabetes is a definite risk factor for breast cancer, since 10%–20% of patients with breast cancer are diabetic. In studies of 38,000 women, 15% of diabetic women were more likely to develop an advanced stage of breast cancer than for women without diabetes. In other studies, it was shown that risks for breast cancer with diabetes is 20% higher than without diabetes. The links between diabetes and breast cancer are activation of the insulin pathway and insulin-like growth factor pathway, plus the regulation of endogenous sex hormones. Chronic hyperglycemia, via the **Warburg effect**, may also increase risks of breast cancer. An association between diabetes and breast cancer supports the effect of insulin and insulin-like growth factor-1 as a mitogen, plus its influences upon estrogen hormone levels.

Clinical Manifestations

Breast cancers may be suspected by self-examinations or via mammography. The patient may complain of pain or enlargement of the breast. There may be a palpable mass during clinical examination and asymmetry of the breasts. Skin ulcers, edema, and a mass attached to the chest wall may be present. Metastases to the axillary lymph nodes, supraclavicular lymphadenopathy, or infraclavicular lymphadenopathy are common. In some cases, nipple discharge may be observed.

Pathology

Breast cancers most commonly develop from epithelial tumors. Carcinoma in situ is diagnosed when there is cancer cell proliferation in the ducts or lobules. The majority of breast cancers are ductal carcinomas. A small or wide breast area may be affected. If the area is wide, microscopic invasive foci may eventually develop. Metastatic carcinoma is usually adenocarcinoma. The mucinous subtype usually develops in older women, and grows slowly with a much better prognosis. *Inflammatory breast cancer* grows quickly and is often fatal. Breast cancer may spread via the regional lymph nodes, bloodstream, or both. Metastatic breast cancer may spread to the lungs, bones, brain, liver, or skin. The pathophysiological link between diabetes and breast cancer is a bit complicated. When there is increased abdominal fat, there is decreased production of **adiponectin** and increased production of estrogen – all of which lead to increased insulin levels. Increased insulin also increases estrogen and increases the blood supply to cancer cells. Increased estrogen decreases sex hormone binding globulin, further increasing estrogen, and the increased estrogen contributes to breast cancer cell growth.

Diagnosis

Clinical examination and mammography often detects breast cancer. However, the diagnosis can be confirmed by biopsy. Ultrasound is usually performed first to differentiate cancer from a benign tumor. Percutaneous core needle biopsy is preferred. Stereotactic biopsy and ultrasound-guided biopsy are also common. In some cases, a surgical biopsy must be done when a deep lesion is located. Inherited gene mutations can be detected in the saliva or blood. Biomarkers have greatly affected the diagnosis of breast cancer. They help determine risks for developing the disease and guide screening as well as monitoring.

Treatment

Treatments include surgery and radiation therapy. In some cases, mastectomy is required, with *breast-conserving surgery* preserving as much breast tissue as possible. This depends on a determination of tumor size. To describe the extent of breast tissue that must be removed, the terms *lumpectomy, quadrantectomy*, and *wide excision* are used. The patient's preference is important and breast-conserving surgery with radiation therapy has the advantage of less extensive surgery. Therefore, the breast can be kept as intact as possible. Preoperative chemotherapy is often used to shrink the tumor. After the axillary nodes are removed, radiation therapy is required. The patient should exercise every day as instructed. After lymphedema reduces over 1–4 weeks, the patient continues daily exercise and overnight bandaging for as long as the lymphedema is present.

After breast surgery, reconstruction may be *prosthetic* or *autologous*. In prosthetic reconstruction, a silicone or saline implant is placed. In autologous reconstruction, there can be a muscle flap transfer or a muscle-free flap transfer. A primary advantage of breast reconstruction after surgery is improved mental health. Disadvantages include complications from surgery and possible effects of implants over time. Invasive cancer is just as likely to develop in either breast when a woman has a lobular carcinoma in situ in one breast. Therefore, the only way to stop breast cancer in this case is bilateral mastectomy. Women that are of high risk for invasive breast cancer often choose this option.

For patients with lobular carcinoma in situ, daily oral tamoxifen can be administered. Raloxifene is sometimes substituted for tamoxifen in postmenopausal women. With invasive breast cancer, chemotherapy is usually started quickly after surgery. If systemic chemotherapy is not needed, hormone therapy is usually started quickly after surgery. In postmenopausal patients, aromatase inhibitors such as exemestane, letrozole, and anastrozole block peripheral estrogen production. These drugs are more effective than tamoxifen.

Prevention and Early Detection

Prevention of breast cancer primarily includes lifestyle modification, chemoprevention, and surgical prevention. Lifestyle modification involves changes in behavior such as smoking cessation, a healthy diet, alcohol reduction, and regular exercise. Screening for the early detection of breast cancer is important. Monthly self-breast examination is required. Screening with clinical breast examination, mammography, and MRI must be done. Mammography is most accurate for older women. For women with an average risk of breast cancer, screening mammography generally begins at age 40, 45, or 50 and then annually or every 2 years. The patient must be educated about the risks for breast cancer.

Prognosis

The prognosis for breast cancer depends on staging of the tumor and the number and location of affected lymph nodes. Prognosis is worse among younger patients in their 20s or 30s than during middle age. Larger tumors have a worsened prognosis. Patients with poorly differentiated tumors also have a worsened prognosis.

CLINICAL CASE

1. To which other sites does breast cancer commonly metastasize?
2. What is the relationship between diabetes and breast cancer?
3. What is the prognosis for breast cancer in women?

A 37-year-old diabetic woman discovered a mass in her right breast during a self-examination. It was movable and not tender. There was skin dimpling present. Family history revealed that her aunt had died of breast cancer and her father has diabetes mellitus and hypertension. An excision biopsy was done, revealing a grade III invasive ductal carcinoma. A right modified radical mastectomy was performed. Resection margins were negative. Adjuvant radiation therapy and chemotherapy were given. Unfortunately, the breast cancer recurred 2 years later, but this time in the regional lymph nodes. Further evaluation showed that it had also metastasized to the patient's lungs. Aggressive treatments were undertaken, but the patient was unable to be saved, at only age 39.

ANSWERS

1. Metastasis of breast cancer occurs via the lymphatic system to the axillary lymph nodes and to the bones, lungs, brain, and liver.
2. Women with type 2 diabetes have an increased risk for breast cancer – especially after menopause. High insulin levels double the risk of breast cancer in women. Overweight, insulin-resistant women have an 84% higher risk of breast cancer than overweight women that are not insulin-resistant. Since fatty tissue accumulates in the breasts, they become a prime target for unregulated cell growth, which can lead to tumors.
3. The prognosis for breast cancer depends on staging and the number and location of affected lymph nodes. Prognosis is worse among younger patients in their 20s or 30s than during middle age. Larger tumors have a worsened prognosis. Patients with poorly differentiated tumors also have a worsened prognosis.

UTERINE CANCER

Uterine cancer is also known as *endometrial cancer.* It originates from the glandular epithelium of the uterus. It is the most common gynecological cancer, and occurs in the fifth or sixth decade of life. Uterine cancer is diagnosed via biopsy and occurs most often in developed countries that have high-fat diets. In a variety of studies, diabetes has been linked to higher risk for uterine cancer, but there has been some controversy over this relationship.

Epidemiology

According to the American Association for Cancer Research, more than 65,620 new cases are diagnosed, and nearly 12,600 deaths occur annually in the United States. Uterine cancer is the fourth most common cancer in women. Incidence and deaths are increasing continually. Postmenopausal women are mostly affected by uterine cancer. About 92% of cases occur in women aged 50 or older. Caucasian women are affected the most, followed by African American women. However, mortality rates are highest in African American women, possibly because of less access to adequate treatment.

Globally, uterine cancer is the sixth most common female cancer, and is more common in developed countries, affecting 1.6% of the population. The incidence in developed countries is 13 of every 100,000 women. In developing countries, it only affects 0.6% of the population. Africa and Western Asia have the lowest rates, while Northern and Eastern Europe, plus North America, have the highest rates. Unfortunately, global cases of uterine cancer are increasing. More than 75% of cases occur after menopause. The worldwide median age is 63. The countries with the highest rates of uterine cancer are Macedonia, Belarus, Samoa, Ukraine, Lithuania, Greece, Czech Republic, Poland, Canada, the United States, Slovakia, Croatia, Serbia, Jamaica, and Singapore.

Etiology and Risk Factors

The actual cause of uterine cancer is unknown. Inherited gene mutations may be linked. The risk factors include obesity, diabetes mellitus, age over 50, family history of hereditary non-polyposis colorectal cancer, previous pelvic radiation therapy, gallbladder disease, and hypertension. There are possible risk factors of having early *menarche*, estrogen therapy without progesterone, late menopause, and never having given birth. Uterine cancer can be a complication of long-term diabetes mellitus. Increased levels of estrogen heighten the risks of uterine cancer. Women that are overweight or obese are more likely to have high levels of estrogen, increasing risks for uterine cancer. The link between type 2 diabetes and uterine cancer may be regulated through elevated estrogen levels, hyperinsulinemia, or insulin-like growth factor-1.

Clinical Manifestations

The most common clinical manifestation in patients with uterine cancer is abnormal vaginal bleeding. This may include premenopausal or postmenopausal bleeding, or **metrorrhagia** that recurs. Approximately one-third of patients with postmenopausal bleeding are diagnosed with uterine cancer. Lower back pain and lower abdominal pain are also reported. A large, boggy uterus with painful intercourse is usually a sign of advanced uterine cancer.

197

Pathology

Endometrial hyperplasia usually occurs before uterine cancer. Type I tumors are more common than Type II tumors, and are usually responsive to estrogen. They develop usually in young, obese, or perimenopausal women after endometrial hyperplasia. These tumors are usually low grade. The most common histology is endometrioid adenocarcinoma of grade 1 or 2. There may be microsatellite instability, and mutations of the genes. The Type II tumors are higher grade, including grade 3 endometrioid carcinomas and tumors that have nonendometrioid histology that may be clear cell, serous, carcinosarcoma, mixed cell, or undifferentiated. They are more common in older women, with 10%–30% having gene mutations.

Uterine papillary serous carcinomas make up about 10% of uterine cancers. Along with the clear cell carcinomas, they are more aggressive, of higher risk, and linked to more extrauterine disease when discovered. Mucinous carcinomas are usually low grade, with gene mutations. The pathology of uterine tumors involves spreading from the uterine cavity surface to the cervical canal, through the myometrium, to the serosa, into the peritoneal cavity via the lumen of the fallopian tube to the ovary, broad ligament, and peritoneal surfaces. Spreading is also via the bloodstream, which leads to distant metastases, and through the lymphatic system. The higher, more undifferentiated that the tumor grade is, the more chance for deep myometrial invasion, metastases to the pelvic or para-aortic lymph nodes, or extrauterine spread.

Diagnosis

Biopsy can confirm the diagnosis of uterine cancer. A routine Pap test in postmenopausal women, or atypical endometrial cells in any woman, indicates uterine cancer. Transvaginal ultrasound is another alternative, but histologic diagnosis is required. Pelvis and abdominal CT may detect metastatic cancer. The CT scan is indicated for patients that have an abdominal mass.

Treatment

Total hysterectomy or bilateral salpingo-oophorectomy is the preferred treatment. Surgery may be done by the laparoscopic, open, robotic, or vaginal routes. If the tumor is located in the uterus, minimally invasive surgery is preferred. For young women with stage I endometrioid adenocarcinoma, the ovaries must be preserved. For stage II or III tumors, treatments include pelvic radiation therapy, with or without chemotherapy. Patients with combined surgery and radiation therapy have a better prognosis. Total hysterectomy and bilateral salpingo-oophorectomy are avoided if the patient has bulky parametrial disease. Stage IV cancer usually involves surgery combined with radiation and chemotherapy. Hormone therapy is sometimes used.

Prevention and Early Detection

Unfortunately, there is no known method to prevent uterine cancer. However, to decrease the risks, patients should stop smoking, increase physical activity, lose weight, and take hormonal contraceptives. Screening methods to detect uterine cancer early are extremely effective, although Pap tests are not helpful in early stages. Early detection contributes to an excellent treatment outcome in many cases.

Prognosis

The prognosis for uterine cancer is generally good. The average 5-year survival rate is approximately 81%. Early detection improves outlook. Survival rates have been as high as 90%, but these lower as cancer staging increases. Women with stage IV uterine cancer have a low survival rate of about 15%.

CLINICAL CASE

1. What are the risk factors for uterine cancer?
2. Which type of uterine tumors are more common in older women?
3. What factors may decrease the risks of developing uterine cancer?

A 65-year-old woman went to the emergency department because of continued, abnormal uterine bleeding. She told the medical team that she had never gone through menopause. Recently, she had lost weight unintentionally, and started having night-time fever plus severe fatigue. Physical examination revealed uterine inflammation, abdominal tenderness, extruded uterine tissue, and a bloody-white purulent discharge. Pelvic ultrasound showed uterine enlargement and thickening of the endometrium. The patient was hospitalized for further assessment and treatment. The patient's uterus, ovaries, and fallopian tubes were surgically resected. Final microscopic pathological diagnosis was of a stage IIIA invasive uterine tumor. The patient was started on chemotherapy and radiation therapy.

ANSWERS

1. The risk factors for uterine cancer include obesity, diabetes mellitus, age over 50, family history of hereditary nonpolyposis colorectal cancer, previous pelvic radiation therapy, gallbladder disease, and hypertension. Uterine cancer can be a complication of long-term diabetes mellitus. Women that are overweight or obese are more likely to have high levels of estrogen, increasing risks for uterine cancer. The link between type 2 diabetes and uterine cancer may be regulated through elevated estrogen levels, hyper-insulinemia, or insulin-like growth factor-1.

2. The type II uterine tumors with higher grade are the most common. They are more common in older women, with 10%–30% having gene mutations.

3. To decrease risks of uterine cancer, patients should stop smoking, increase physical activity, lose weight, and take hormonal contraceptives. There is no known method to prevent uterine cancer. Screening methods to detect uterine cancer early are extremely effective, although Pap tests are not helpful in early stages. Early detection contributes to an excellent treatment outcome in many cases.

BLADDER CANCER

Cancer of the urinary bladder is also called **transitional cell carcinoma**. It is the most common malignancy of the urinary tract, characterized by multiple growth that tends to recur in a more aggressive form. The majority of bladder malignancies are transitional cell carcinomas and a small percentage are squamous cell carcinomas or adenocarcinomas. The adenocarcinomas may occur as primary tumors, or in rare cases as metastatic tumors from an intestinal carcinoma. They may develop from intestinal metaplasia of the urothelium. Increased incidence of bladder cancer has been linked to type 2 diabetes.

Epidemiology

In the United States, there are about 80,000 new cases of bladder cancer annually, with nearly 18,000 deaths. Bladder cancer occurs more often in men than women. It is more prevalent in urban than in rural areas. Incidence increases with age, and the disease most often affects Caucasians. Worldwide, bladder cancer affects almost 275,000 people annually, and about 108,000 cases are fatal. In developed countries, the majority of cases are transitional cell carcinomas. Only about 1% of all bladder cancers are adenocarcinomas. These tumors also occur most commonly in males. There is no distinct racial or ethnic predilection for adenocarcinomas. Globally, bladder adenocarcinomas appear to make up only 0.5%–2% of all bladder cancers.

Etiology and Risk Factors

The exact cause of bladder cancer is unknown. The risk factors of bladder cancer increase with cigarette smoking. They are also higher with exposure to aniline dyes, beta naphthylamine, mixtures of aromatic hydrocarbons, or benzidine, as used in chemical, paint, plastics, textile, petroleum, and wood industries. Other predisposing factors are chronic urinary tract infections, calculous disease, and schistosomiasis. Adenocarcinomas are caused by extensive intestinal metaplasia known as **cystitis glandularis**, usually occurring at the trigone. Etiology may be related to **exstrophy** of bladder. The diverticula sometimes develop adenocarcinomas. Other causes are endometriosis, pelvic lipomatosis, and infection with *Schistosoma haematobium*. The link between diabetes and bladder cancer mostly concerns use of the diabetes drug pioglitazone (Actos) for 2 years or more. The drug is used to control high blood glucose levels in type 2 diabetes. It is also sold in combination with metformin (as Actoplus Met or Actoplus Met XR) and with glimepiride (Duetact). In the United States, the Food and Drug Administration recommends that pioglitazone not be used in patients with active bladder cancer. It should be used with caution in patients with a previous history of bladder cancer.

Clinical Manifestations

Symptoms of bladder cancer include painless hematuria, frequent urination, burning, dysuria and sometimes, pyuria. Irritation from the tumor may mimic cystitis. The patient may also have anemia. With advanced carcinoma, pelvic pain develops after a pelvic mass becomes palpable.

Pathology

The transitional cell carcinomas of the bladder are superficial and well differentiated, growing outward. They are subclassified as *papillary carcinomas*. They invade early and then metastasize. Approximately 40% of transitional cell carcinomas recur at the same site in the bladder, or in another site – especially if they are large. Bladder cancer often metastasizes to the lungs, liver, intestines, bones, and lymph nodes. Some of these tumors may be linked to faster progression and resistance to chemo-therapeutic agents. Squamous cell carcinoma has cells that similar to the flat cells of the skin. The squamous cells have intracellular bridges, **keratohyalin granules**, and pearls. They must be distinguished from urothelial cancer that has squamous differentiation.

Diagnosis

For diagnosis of bladder cancers, urinalysis, urine cytology, cystoscopy, and excretory urog-raphy are done to detect malignant cells. Biopsy and clinical staging are required. Low-stage tumors make up 75% of bladder cancers. When a biopsy reveals the tumor to be more invasive, another biopsy is required that includes muscle tissue. A stage T2 or higher tumor that invades the muscle requires abdominal and pelvic CT as well as chest X-ray.

Treatment

Complete removal is done via transurethral resection. Risk of recurrence can be reduced by giving repeated instillations of chemotherapies. Immunotherapies may be used for carcinoma in situ and other high-grade superficial tran-sitional cell carcinomas. These include post-transurethral resection instillation of *bacilli Calmette-Guérin* (*BCG*), which is more effective than chemotherapy. The instillation can be done in weekly or monthly intervals over 1–3 years. Before cystectomy, chemotherapy is ordered.

Prevention and Early Detection

The only method of preventing transitional cell carcinoma is to avoid the known risk factors. If detected early, most patients can be cured. Early diagnosis can prevent unexplained weight loss, fatigue, hematuria, back pain, and painful or frequent urination.

Prognosis

Prognosis of bladder cancer depends on the progressive and the staging of tumor. The early stage of superficial bladder cancer is rarely fatal. If the bladder musculature has been invaded, about half of patients survive for 5 years. However, the prognosis of adenocarcinoma of the bladder is poor due to the highly infiltrative nature of the tumor. The 5-year survival rate is only 35%. Staging is the most important factor for prognosis.

CLINICAL CASE

1. What are the classifications of bladder cancers?
2. What does the link between diabetes and bladder cancer mostly concern?
3. Is bladder cancer usually found to be low stage or high stage?

An 83-year-old diabetic man with stage II bladder cancer was evaluated for treatment. Previous diagnoses included hypertension, chronic obstructive pulmonary disease, obe-sity, and obstructive sleep apnea. His symptoms included malaise, weakness, shortness of breath, and a recurring fever. The patient also had pancytopenia. The medical team dis-cussed the patient's medications and found that he had been taking pioglitazone to control his type 2 diabetes. The drug was then stopped. The cancer was found to be in only one part of the patient's bladder. A partial cystectomy was successfully performed to remove the cancerous area of the bladder. There was no cancer in the nearby lymph nodes. The patient eventually was able to go home and was cancer-free with his diabetes well controlled at 1 year of follow-up.

ANSWERS

1. Most bladder cancers are transitional cell carcinomas. A small percentage are squamous cell carcinomas or adenocarcinomas.
2. The link between diabetes and bladder cancer mostly concerns use of the diabetes drug pioglitazone (Actos) for 2 years or more. It is used to control high blood glucose levels in type 2 diabetes, and also sold in combination with metformin and glimepiride.
3. Low-stage tumors make up 75% of bladder cancers. Early stages are rarely fatal, and staging is the most important factor for prognosis.

COLORECTAL CANCER

Colorectal cancer is a malignant neoplastic disease of the large intestine. It is extraordinarily common. Colorectal cancer is the third most commonly *diagnosed* type of cancer in the United States and some other countries. It is almost always an adenocarcinoma, which tends to form bulky exophytic masses or annular constricting lesions. The majority of colorectal cancers are thought to originate from malignant transformation of an adenomatous polyp or a serrated polyp. Being overweight or obese and then developing type 2 diabetes increases risks for colorectal cancer. Type 2 diabetes also means that diagnosed colorectal cancer will have a worsened prognosis.

Epidemiology

Colorectal cancer has more than 140,500 cases and over 50,700 deaths annually in the United States, making it the third most common type of cancer, but the second most common cause of cancer-related deaths. About 5% of men and women will be diagnosed during their lifetimes. Risks average about 1 in every 18–20 people. The disease peaks significantly near the ages of 40 and 50 years, and is slightly more common in men than women. About 55 men of every 100,000 are diagnosed, and also about 40 women of every 100,000. Colorectal cancer disproportionately affects African Americans about 20% more than other racial or ethnic groups, and they are also about 40% more likely to die from the disease. Globally, over 1 million people are diagnosed with colorectal cancer every year, and over 715,000 die. It makes up 10% of cancer diagnoses in men, and 9% in women. Global incidence varies, with the highest rates in Australia, New Zealand, Europe, and the United States. In the United Kingdom, colorectal cancer is the fourth most common type of cancer. The lowest rates are in Africa and South-Central Asia.

Etiology and Risk Factors

The clear cause of colorectal cancer is unknown. Approximately 20% of cases are inherited and 80% cases are sporadic. The risk factors are age, family history, and inflammatory bowel disease such as ulcerative colitis or Crohn colitis. The longer these conditions last, the higher the risks of cancer. Other factors may be genetic, lifestyle, and diet-linked, such as with low fiber but high red meat content, refined carbohydrates, and fat. Though carcinogens may exist in foods, bacterial effects upon substances in the diet more often produce them. The links between diet, weight, exercise, and colorectal cancer strongly relate to the presence of type 2 diabetes.

In part, this is due to the fact that type 2 diabetes and colorectal cancer share risk factors such as excessive weight and lack of physical exercise.

Clinical Manifestations

Colorectal adenocarcinomas grow slowly and may be present for several years before symptoms appear. Symptoms are based on the tumor's site, size, and complications. The first clinical manifestation may be colicky abdominal pain with partial obstruction, or complete obstruction. Bleeding often occurs on an occult basis, and constipation as well as distention are common. Severe anemia may cause fatigue and weakness. Obstruction occurs late if the tumor is within the right colon because of its size, thin walls, and liquid contents. There may be blood mixed or streaked through the stool. In some cases perforation may occur. For some patients, the first clinical manifestations may indicate metastasis and cause hepatomegaly, ascites, or lymph node enlargement.

Pathology

The majority (96%) of colorectal cancers are adenocarcinomas. They develop from columnar glandular epithelium in the mucosa. Colorectal cancer metastasis is via the blood and regional lymph nodes. Most adenocarcinomas are nonmucinous, with the mucinous phenotype making up 20% of all colorectal cancers. Epidermoid carcinomas make up 25% of all colorectal cancers, mostly located in the rectum. Primary colorectal lymphomas make up only 15% of all GI lymphomas, yet less than 1% of colorectal cancers.

Diagnosis

A complete blood count is done to look for anemia. Increased liver biochemical tests, particularly the serum alkaline phosphatase test, are used for metastatic disease. Serum carcinoembryonic antigen (CEA) levels should be measured in all patients with proven colorectal cancer, but these are not sensitive or specific. When the CEA level is high before an operation and low after a colon tumor is removed, it should be monitored so that any recurrence can be found sooner rather than later. Fecal immunochemical tests to find blood in the stool are better than the older guaiac-based tests since many different substances in the diet affect them. Even so, a positive test for blood in the stool can occur because of nonmalignancies such as diverticulosis and ulcers.

Colonoscopy is the diagnostic procedure of choice in patients with a clinical history suggestive of colon cancer. This procedure permits biopsy for pathologist confirmation of malignancy. Virtual colonoscopy uses CT to generate 2D and 3D images of the colon. This test may be good for people who cannot tolerate or are unwilling to have an endoscopic colonoscopy. A colonoscopy should be done every 10 years. However, if a patient has a family history, with a first-degree relative having had colon cancer before the age of 60, a colonoscopy should be done every 5 years starting at age 40 – or every 10 years. When a fecal occult blood test is positive, a colonoscopy is required. A colonoscopy is also required after a lesion is seen in an imaging study or during sigmoidoscopy. All lesions are completely removed and examined.

Treatment

For 70% of patients without metastatic disease, surgery can be curative. There is wide tumor resection, regional lymphatic drainage, and reanastomosis of colon segments. When there is 5 cm or less of normal colon tissue between the lesion and the anal verge, an abdominoperineal resection is usually performed, with a permanent colostomy. For some patients that are not debilitated, subsequent resection of 1–3 liver metastases is recommended. After primary tumor resection, criteria for this include those with liver metastases in one hepatic lobe, without any extrahepatic metastases. A small amount of patients with liver metastases qualify, but 5-year survival after surgery is 25%. Surgical procedures may involve laparotomy with hemicolectomy, lymph node dissection, and for some patients, appendectomy.

For rectal cancer with 1–4 positive lymph nodes, combined radiation and chemotherapy are used. When there are more than four positive lymph nodes, this combination is not as effective. Presurgical radiation therapy and chemotherapy improve resectability rates of rectal cancer, or can decrease incidence of lymph node metastasis. Following curative surgery for colorectal cancer, there must be a surveillance colonoscopy 1 year later. This can also be done 1 year after the preoperative colonoscopy. Another surveillance colonscopy is done 3 years after the 1-year surveillance colonoscopy when no tumors or polyps are found. After that, surveillance colonscopy is done every 5 years. When a presurgical colonoscopy was not complete due to an obstructing cancer, a "completion colonscopy" is done 3–6 months after surgery, to find synchronous cancers, and to find and remove any precancerous polyps. Further screening for recurrence must include patient history, physical examination, and measurement of CEA levels every 3 months, for 3 years. After that, it is done every 6 months, for 2 years. A CT or MRI is recommended once per year, though these are of unproven benefit for regular follow-up when there are no abnormalities during examinations or blood tests.

When surgery will not be curative or there are extreme surgical risks, limited palliative surgery may be performed, such as to resect an area of perforation or relieve an obstruction. The median survival time is only 7 months, however. Electrocoagulation can debulk some obstructive tumors, or the colon can be held open by stents. Chemotherapy has the ability to reduce tumor size and extend life for several months. Newer medications can be used alone or combined with others, and include capecitabine, irinotecan, and oxaliplatin. The monoclonal antibodies are sometimes effective, and include bevacizumab, cetuximab, and panitumumab. There is no "best" regimen for metastatic colorectal cancer, though some chemotherapy can delay progression. If colon cancer is advanced, a highly experienced person manages the chemotherapy, with access to drugs that are under investigation.

Prevention and Early Detection

There is no proven method of preventing colorectal cancer. However, some of the risk factors can be controlled by regular colorectal cancer screening, maintaining a normal body weight via physical activity and a good diet, limiting red and processed meats, and increasing intake of fruits, vegetables, and whole grains. Avoiding or limiting alcohol intake is also suggested, and smoking should be avoided. Some studies indicate that daily multivitamins that contain folic acid, plus calcium and magnesium supplements, may be helpful. Studies have also shown that people who regularly take aspirin and other nonsteroidal anti-inflammatory drugs (NSAIDs) have lower risks of colorectal polyps and cancer. Estrogen and progesterone replacement therapy after menopause may be helpful for women in reducing risks for colorectal cancer. Early detection of colorectal polyps or cancer can occur via regular screening methods. If found earlier, this can improve treatment and prognosis, and regular screening may even prevent the disease, since a polyp may take 10–15 years to become cancerous.

Prognosis

The prognosis for colorectal cancer is greatly dependent upon the staging. If the cancer is limited only to the mucosa, the 10-year survival rate is close to 90%. If there is extension through the colon wall, this rate is 70%–80%. However, if there are positive lymph nodes the rate is 30%–50%, and for metastasis, the rate is less than 20% for 10-year survival.

CLINICAL CASE

1. How is diabetes related to colorectal cancer?
2. Which dietary factors are linked to colorectal cancer?
3. What is the overall prognosis for colorectal cancer?

A 58-year-old diabetic woman received a diagnosis of stage II colorectal cancer. She also had been diagnosed earlier with gout and hyperlipidemia. Colonoscopy had revealed a descending colon mass that was biopsied and found to be an adenocarcinoma. The patient was started on chemotherapy, which stabilized the cancer after 2 months. However, she developed severe hypertension that also had to be treated. The patient did very well with her various treatments, and at 5 years of follow-up is doing well without cancer recurrence.

ANSWERS

1. Being overweight or obese and then developing type 2 diabetes increases the risk for colorectal cancer. Type 2 diabetes also means that diagnosed colorectal cancer will have a worsened prognosis.
2. Diets with low fiber but high red meat content, refined carbohydrates, and fats are linked to colorectal cancer.
3. The prognosis for colorectal cancer is greatly dependent upon the staging. If limited only to the mucosa, the 10-year survival rate is close to 90%. With extension through the colon wall, the rate is 70%–80%. If there are positive lymph nodes, the rate is 30%–50%. With metastasis, the rate is less than 20% for 10-year survival.

KEY TERMS

- Adiponectin
- Asterixis
- Carney complex
- Cowden's syndrome
- Cystitis glandularis
- Desmoplastic stroma
- Exstrophy
- Fatty liver
- Hepatoma
- Keratohyalin granules
- Metrorrhagia
- Transitional cell carcinoma
- Warburg effect
- Werner's syndrome

REFERENCES

Abbas, G., and Choudhary, M.I. (2014). *The Management of Diabetes Mellitus and Late Diabetic Complications: Anti-diabetic Therapy*. Lap Lambert Academic Publishing.

Adeghate, E., Saadi, H., Adem, A., and Obineche, E. (2006). *Diabetes Mellitus and Its Complications: Molecular Mechanisms, Epidemiology, and Clinical Medicine* (Annals of the New York Academy of Sciences, Volume 1084). Wiley-Blackwell.

Agbanashi, L. (2020). *Liver Cancer: Comprehensive and Perfect Guide on Liver Cancer*. Agbanashi.

American Cancer Society. (2021). *Colorectal Cancer Causes, Risk Factors, and Prevention*. American Cancer Society. https://www.cancer.org/content/dam/CRC/PDF/Public/8605.00.pdf

Aydiner, A., Igci, A., and Soran, A. (2019). *Breast Disease – Management and Therapies*, Volume 2 (2nd Edition). Springer.

Behl, T., Kaur, I., and Kotwani, A. (2016). *Insights into Pathways Leading to Diabetes Mellitus and Complications*. Lap Lambert Academic Publishing.

BMC – Springer Nature – Cancer. (2019). *The Effect of Diabetes on the Risk of Endometrial Cancer: An Updated Systematic Review and Meta-Analysis*. BioMed Central Ltd. https://bmccancer.biomedcentral.com/articles/10.1186/s12885-019-5748-4

Chadha, M. (2020). *Complications in Diabetes Mellitus: Bench to Bedside*. Jaypee Brothers Medical Publishers Ltd.

Christiakov, D.A. (2006). *New Advances in the Genetics and Treatment of Type 1 Diabetes Mellitus and Late Diabetic Complications*. Nova Biomedical.

Diabetes.co.uk – The Global Diabetes Community – Diabetes Complications. (2019a). *Bladder Cancer*. Diabetes Digital Media Ltd. https://www.diabetes.co.uk/diabetes-complications/bladder-cancer.html

Diabetes.co.uk – The Global Diabetes Community – Diabetes Complications. (2019b). *Liver Cancer*. Diabetes Digital Media Ltd. https://www.diabetes.co.uk/diabetes-complications/liver-cancer.html

Diabetes.co.uk – The Global Diabetes Community – Diabetes Complications. (2019c). *Uterine Cancer*. Diabetes Digital Media Ltd. https://www.diabetes.co.uk/diabetes-complications/uterine-cancer.html

Engin, O. (2021). *Colon Polyps and Colorectal Cancer*, 2nd Edition. Springer.

Food and Drug Administration (FDA). (2010). *FDA Drug Safety Communication: Update to Ongoing Safety Review of Actos (Pioglitazone) and Increased Risk of Bladder Cancer*. Food and Drug Administration. https://www.fda.gov/drugs/drug-safety-and-availability/fda-drug-safety-communication-update-ongoing-safety-review-actos-pioglitazone-and-increased-risk

Fried, R., and Carlton, R.M. (2018). *Type 2 Diabetes: Cardiovascular and Related Complications and Evidence-Based Complementary Treatments*. CRC Press.

Goonewardene, S.S., Persad, R., Motiwala, H., and Albala, D. (2020). *Management of Non-Muscle Invasive Bladder Cancer*. Springer.

Grani, G., Cooper, D.S., and Durante, C. (2020). *Thyroid Cancer: A Case-Based Approach*, 2nd Edition. Springer.

Hameed, A., Qureshi, J.A., and Malik, S.A. (2012). *Diabetes Mellitus: Epidemiology, Late Diabetic Complications and Association with Hepatitis C Virus (HCV) Infection*. Lap Lambert Academic Publishing.

Jordan, P. (2018). *Targeted Therapy of Colorectal Cancer Subtypes*. Springer.

Lindsey Elmore. (2021). *The Link between Diabetes and Breast Cancer*. Lindsey Elmore. https://lindseyelmore.com/the-link-between-diabetes-and-breast-cancer/?q=/the-link-between-diabetes-and-breast-cancer/&

Luster, M., Duntas, L.H., and Wartofsky, L. (2019). *The Thyroid and Its Diseases: A Comprehensive Guide for the Clinician*. Springer.

Mbayo, F.I. (2021). *Acute Metabolic Complications of Diabetes Mellitus*. Our Knowledge Publishing.

Michalski, C.W., Rosendahl, J., Michl, P., and Kleeff, J. (2020). *Translational Pancreatic Cancer Research: From Understanding of Mechanisms to Novel Clinical Trials (Molecular and Translational Medicine)*. Humana Press.

Mir, S.H. (2017). *Experimental Diabetology-Biochemistry, Histopathology and Therapeutics: Diabetes Mellitus – Complications and Treatment*. Lap Lambert Academic Publishing.

Mirza, M.R. (2020). *Management of Endometrial Cancer*. Springer.

Mohamed, A.S. (2015). *Diabetes Mellitus: Types – Mechanisms – Complications*. CreateSpace Independent Publishing Platform.

Mohan Bose, S., Chander Sharma, S., Mazumdar, A., and Kaushik, R. (2021). *Breast Cancer – Comprehensive Management*. Springer.

Moschini, M. (2020). *Outcomes and Therapeutic Management of Bladder Cancer*. Mdpi AG.

NCBI – PMC – U.S. National Library of Medicine – National Institutes of Health – Cureus. (2020). *Diabetes as a Risk Factor for Breast Cancer*. National Center for Biotechnology Information – U.S. National Library of Medicine. https://www.ncbi.nlm.nih.gov/pmc/articles/PMC7279688/

NIH – National Library of Medicine – National Center for Biotechnology Information. (2019). *Exploring the Link between Diabetes and Pancreatic Cancer*. National Library of Medicine.

Pancreatic Cancer Action Network. (2021). *6 Things You Need to Know about Diabetes and Pancreatic Cancer*. Pancreatic Cancer Action Network. https://www.pancan.org/news/6-things-need-know-diabetes-pancreatic-cancer/

Rymore, R. (2014). *Diabetes Mellitus Explained. Types of Diabetes, Symptoms, Treatments, Diet, Complications and Self-Management All Included*. IMB Publishing.

Wartofsky, L., and Van Nostrand, D. (2016). *Thyroid Cancer: A Comprehensive Guide to Clinical Management*, 3rd Edition. Springer.

WebMD – Diabetes – News. (2013). *Type 2 Diabetes Might Raise Risk of Liver Cancer*. WebMD LLC. https://www.webmd.com/diabetes/news/20131208/type-2-diabetes-might-raise-risk-of-liver-cancer

Winter, W.E., and Signorino, M.R. (2002). *Diabetes Mellitus: Pathophysiology, Etiologies, Complications, Management, and Laboratory Evaluation: Special Topics in Diagnostic Testing*. AACC Press.

Glossary

Acanthosis nigricans: A skin pigmentation disorder involving dark patches of skin, with a thick but soft texture, in various areas of the body; it may be a sign of pre-diabetes.

Acromegaly: Excessive enlargement of the limbs due to thickening of bones and soft tissues, caused by hypersecretion of growth hormone, usually from a tumor of the pituitary gland.

Addison's disease: A disorder involving disrupted functioning of the part of the adrenal cortex. This results in decreased production of two hormones by the adrenal cortex: cortisol and aldosterone.

Adipokines: A protein hormone produced and secreted by adipocytes into the systemic circulation; it causes sensitivity of peripheral tissues to insulin.

Adiponectin: A protein hormone produced and secreted by adipocytes into the systemic circulation; it causes sensitivity of peripheral tissues to insulin.

Afterload: The tension developed by the heart during contraction.

Agnosia: Inability to recognize incoming sensations.

Aldosterone: A steroid hormone that is produced by the adrenal cortex and regulates salt balance, blood volume, and blood pressure in the body.

Alport syndrome: A hereditary kidney disease that causes hematuria, hearing loss, and eye problems.

Amaurosis fugax: Loss of sight without an obvious eye lesion, from a neurological condition.

Amygdala: One of the four basal ganglia, part of the limbic system, consisting of gray matter in the anterior portion of the temporal lobe.

Amyloidosis: A progressive metabolic disease involving abnormal protein deposits.

Angiotensinogen: An inactive precursor of angiotensin; it is a large protein synthesized by the liver, secreted into the bloodstream, and converted into angiotensin by renin.

Anhedonia: Inability to enjoy what is usually pleasurable.

Anticipatory anxiety: Expectation of anxiety or panic in a particular situation.

Antiphospholipid syndrome: An autoimmune, hypercoagulable state caused by antibodies that provokes blood clots and pregnancy-related complications.

Antroduodenal manometry: The measurement of pressure in the gastric antrum and proximal small intestine.

Aortic regurgitation: Backflow of blood from the aorta into the left ventricle because of insufficiency of the aortic valve.

Apolipoproteins: Non-lipid protein portions in plasma lipoproteins.

Arcus corneae: A white or gray opaque ring in the margin of the cornea.

Arterial tone: The resistance to elongation or stretch in an artery.

Arteriosclerosis: Thickening and loss of elasticity of the arterial walls.

Ascites: An abnormal accumulation of fluid in the abdomen.

Asterixis: A motor disturbance, with lapses of assumed postures of muscle groups; commonly called a "liver flap."

Ataxia: A neurological sign, with lack of voluntary coordination of muscle movements; it may include gait abnormality, speech changes, and eye movement abnormalities.

Atheromas: Abnormal masses of fatty or lipid materials with a fibrous covering, forming raised plaques in the intima of an artery.

Atherosclerosis: The buildup of a waxy plaque on the inside of blood vessels.

Athlete's foot: A common fungus infection between the toes, also known as tinea pedis or foot ringworm.

Atypical angina: A type of chest pain that is not typical in its presentation, and is usually caused by respiratory, musculoskeletal, gastrointestinal, or psychological conditions.

Autoantigens: Antigens that are targets of a humoral or cell-mediated immune response.

Azotemia: An excess of nitrogenous waste products in the blood.

Bariatric surgery: A technique that changes the anatomy of the digestive system to limit the amount of food that can be eaten and digested, promoting weight loss.

Baroreflex: A reflex triggered by stimulation of a baroreceptor, responding to distension of the great vessels of the head and neck.

Basal ganglia: Also called the basal nuclei; subcortical nuclei in the forebrain involved in voluntary motor movements, learning, eye movements, cognition, and emotions.

Beriberi: A disease caused by deficiency of vitamin B1, usually caused by chronic alcoholism, and affecting multiple body systems.

Berry aneurysm: A sac formed by local dilatation of the wall of an artery, vein, or the heart.

Beta-hydroxybutyrate: An acid involved in fatty acid metabolism that is increased in diabetic ketoacidosis.

Blood-brain barrier: The semipermeable capillary border that allows selective passage of blood constituents into the brain.

Bradykinin: A powerful vasodilator that increases capillary permeability, constricts smooth muscle, and stimulates pain receptors.

Brittle diabetes: A form of diabetes that involves unexplained oscillation between hypoglycemia and diabetic ketoacidosis.

Bruit: A harsh or intermittent auscultatory sound that is usually abnormal.

Cachexia: A profound state of constitutional disorder involving general ill health and malnutrition.

Cajal cells: Interstitial cells of the gastrointestinal tract implicated in muscle contraction and neurotransmission.

Candida albicans: A fungal species that causes cutaneous, mucocutaneous, or severe systemic infections.

Candidate population: A group of people being considered as likely candidates to develop a certain disease, or to not develop it.

Carbohydrate tolerance: The amount of a carbohydrate (commonly glucose) that can be tolerated without adverse reactions as part of a test.

Cardiac biomarker: Enzymes, hormones, and proteins that are linked to heart conditions, such as troponin, creatinine kinase, and myoglobin.

Cardiomyopathy: A chronic disease of the myocardium, in which it becomes enlarged, thickened, and/or stiffened.

Carney complex: An autosomal dominant condition, with myxomas, skin hyperpigmentation, and endocrine overactivity.

Catecholamine: Sympathomimetic amines, including dopamine, epinephrine, and norepinephrine, which are important for physiological responses to stress.

Cavernous sinus: An irregular venous channel between the layers of dura mater through which several cranial nerves penetrate.

Celiac disease: A disease that damages the small intestine and interferes with absorption of nutrients from food; it occurs when the body reacts abnormally to gluten.

Ceramide: The basic unit of sphingolipids, consisting of sphingosine or a related base, attached via its amino group to a long-chain fatty acid anion.

Ceruloplasmin: An alpha$_2$-globulin of the plasma in which most plasma copper is transported.

Chagas disease: A bloodborne disease caused by *Trypanosoma cruzi*, transmitted by insects, causing fever, lymphadenopathy, hepatosplenomegaly, and facial edema.

Charcot's joint: A joint with reduced sensation of pain or position caused by tabes dorsalis, diabetic neuropathy, amyloidosis, or leprosy.

Cheyne-Stokes respirations: Breathing with rhythmic waxing and waning depth of respirations, repeated every 45 seconds to 3 minutes.

Cholelithiasis: Presence or formation of gallstones in the gallbladder or common bile duct.

Chylomicrons: Microscopic globules of various materials that are 80–1,000 nanometers in diameter.

Cingulate cortices: Parts of the brain in the medial aspect of the cerebral cortex, including the cingulate gyrus, and the cingulate sulcus.

Circle of Willis: A circulatory anastomosis that supplies blood to the brain and surrounding structures.

Circumduction gait: Also called a hemiplegic gait; the leg is stiff without flexion at the knee and ankle, and each step is rotated away from the body, and then towards it.

Claw hand deformity: Atrophy of the interosseous muscles with hypertension of the metacarpophalangeal joints and flexion of the interphalangeal joints.

Coarctation of the aorta: Stenosis of the arch aorta, a congenital heart defect, with localized deformity of the tunica media that causes narrowing of the vessel's lumen.

Cognition: The mental action or process of acquiring knowledge and understanding, via thoughts, experiences, and the senses.

Corona: An eminence or encircling structure that resembles a crown.

Corpectomy: Removal of a vertebral body during spinal surgery.

Corpus callosum: A thick, wide nerve tract of commissural fibers, beneath the cerebral cortex, which allows communication between the cerebral hemispheres.

Cowden's syndrome: A condition of benign hamartomas and increased risk of breast, thyroid, uterine, and other cancers.

Crenation: The process of forming a notch in a body structure.

Cultural sensitivity: Being aware of and accepting cultural differences between people.

Cumulative incidence: A measure of disease frequency during a period of time.

Curvilinear: Having a formation of curved lines.

Cushing syndrome: A disorder due to secretion of cortisol from a tumor or excessive corticosteroids; there is fat accumulation in the torso, bruising, and a moon-shaped face.

Cystitis glandularis: Chronic cystitis with gland-like metaplasia of urothelium.

Cystoid fluid: Liquid that resembles the fluid contained within a cyst.

Cytokines: Small proteins important in cell signaling; involved in autocrine, paracrine, and endocrine signaling as immunomodulating agents.

DASH diet: A diet high in fruits, vegetables, low-fat dairy products, and fiber; low in saturated and total fats; and low in cholesterol.

Delusions: Fixed belief that cannot be changed even when conflicting evidence is presented, often a component of psychotic disorders.

Dermatome: The skin area supplied with afferent nerve fibers by one posterior spinal root; also, the lateral part of an embryonic somite.

Desmoplastic stroma: In a neoplasm, fibrosis in the vascular tissues that form the ground substance, framework, or matrix of a body organ.

Diabetic amyotrophy: Diabetes-related painful wasting and weakness of muscle – most commonly, the deltoid muscle.

Diapedesis: Outward passage of blood cells though intact vessel walls.

Dilated cardiomyopathy: Decreased function of the left ventricle with dilation that usually causes global hypokinesia and overall cardiac failure.

Down syndrome: The most common cause of mental retardation and malformation in a newborn, due to the presence of an extra chromosome.

Dyslipidemia: An abnormal amount of lipids and lipoproteins in the blood.

Dyspareunia: Painful sexual intercourse due to medical or psychological causes.

Ebstein anomaly: Congenital downward displacement of the tricuspid valve into the right ventricle.

Eclampsia: A life-threatening disorder during pregnancy, with hypertension, general edema, proteinuria, and seizure.

Ecology: The study of the distribution and abundance of organisms and their interactions with the environment.

Eisenmenger syndrome: A condition that results from abnormal blood circulation caused by a defect in the heart.

Electrogastrography: The recording of electrical activity of the stomach, as measured between its lumen and the body surface.

Eosinophil-derived neurotoxin: An enzyme with cytotoxic properties that can reduce activity of single-strand RNA viruses, and is also an attractant to immune cells.

Ergonomic: Maximizing productivity by reducing fatigue and discomfort.

Ergonomics: The applied science of designing equipment to maximize productivity by reducing fatigue and discomfort.

Eructation: The release of air or gas from the stomach or esophagus through the mouth.

Eruptive xanthomatosis: A metabolic disorder characterized by excessive accumulation of lipids in the body and a resulting spread of xanthomas by skin eruptions.

Erythropoietin: A glycoprotein hormone that acts on stem cells of the bone marrow to stimulate red blood cell production.

Euglycemia: A normal level of glucose in the blood.

Exstrophy: Congenital absence of a portion of the abdominal wall and bladder wall, the bladder appearing to be turned inside out, with the internal surface of its posterior wall showing through the opening in the anterior wall.

Exudation: The escape of fluid, cells, or cellular debris from blood vessels and deposition in or on the tissue.

Fabry disease: An X-linked lysosomal storage disease marked by progressive symptoms including burning pain in the hands and feet, sweating, and purple skin lesions, with death resulting from renal, cardiac, or cerebrovascular complications.

Facet syndrome: A low back pain syndrome attributed to osteoarthritis of the interarticular vertebrae.

Fatty acid: Monoprotic acids, especially those found in animal and vegetable fats and oils, made up of saturated or unsaturated compounds having an even number of carbon atoms; examples include palmitic, stearic, and oleic acids.

Fatty liver: Also called steatosis, fatty liver can be a temporary or long-term condition, which is not harmful itself, but may indicate some other type of problem. Left untreated, it can contribute to other illnesses.

Fatty streak: Early evidence of atherosclerosis, in which cholesterol, macrophages, and smooth muscle cells accumulate in the intima of arteries.

Floaters: Translucent specks that float across the visual field, due to small objects floating in the vitreous humor.

Fluorescein angiography: Fluorescein angiography (FA) involves the color radiographic examination of the retinal vasculature following rapid IV injection of a sodium fluorescein contrast medium.

Foam cells: Cells with abundant, pale-staining, finely vacuolated cytoplasm, usually histiocytes that have ingested or accumulated material that dissolves during tissue preparation, especially lipids.

Frank-Starling principle: A mathematical expression stating that stroke volume increases with diastolic volume.

Free fatty acids: Any acid derived from fats by hydrolysis.

Friction rub: The sound heard on auscultation made by the rubbing of two opposed serous surfaces roughened by an inflammatory exudate, or, if chronic, by nonadhesive fibrosis.

Frontotemporal dementia: A form of dementia that affects speech and personality, while stimulating visual perception.

Funduscopy: Ophthalmoscopy; a test that allows visualization of the fundus of the eye and other structures using a funduscope (ophthalmoscope).

Genome: A complete set of chromosomes derived from one parent, the haploid number of a gamete.

Gestational diabetes mellitus: A condition during pregnancy, involves a defect in how the body processes and uses glucose in the diet; the pancreas is not involved, while the placenta is implicated.

Glomerular sclerosis: Hyaline deposits or scarring within the renal glomeruli, a degenerative process occurring in association with renal arteriosclerosis or diabetes.

Glomerulus: A network of vascular tufts encased in the capsule of the kidney.

Gluconeogenesis: The metabolic pathway resulting in generation of glucose from non-carbohydrate carbon substrates; it aids in maintaining blood glucose levels.

Glycemic index: A number associated with carbohydrates in a food source indicating their effect upon the blood glucose level; a value of 100 represents the standard, an equivalent amount of pure glucose.

Glycemic load: A number estimating how much a food source will raise the blood glucose level after it is eaten; one unit of glycemic load approximates the effect of consuming one gram of glucose.

Glycerol: Also called glycerine; a simple polyol compound that is the "backbone" of all triglycerides; it is widely used as a food sweetener.

Glycogenesis: The process of glycogen synthesis, in which glucose molecules are added to chains of glycogen for storage.

Glycogenolysis: The breakdown of glycogen to glucose-1-phospahte and glycogen.

Glycolytic pathway: The principal series of phosphorylates reactions involved in pyruvic acid production in phosphorylates fermentations.

Glycosylation: A chemical reaction in which glycosyl groups are added to a protein to produce a glycoprotein.

Goodpasture syndrome: A rare autoimmune disease in which antibodies attack the basement membrane in the lungs and kidneys, leading to bleeding from the lungs.

Graves' disease: A disease characterized by an enlarged thyroid and increased basal metabolism due to excessive thyroid secretion.

Guillain-Barre syndrome: A temporary inflammation of the nerves, causing pain, weakness, and paralysis in the extremities and often progressing to the chest and face. It typically occurs after recovery from a viral infection or, in rare cases, following immunization for influenza or COVID-19.

Haptoglobin: A plasma protein that is a normal constituent of blood serum and functions in the binding of free hemoglobin in the bloodstream.

Hemiparesis: Muscle weakness on one side of the body.

Hemiplegia: Unilateral paralysis of the body.

Hemochromatosis: A disorder of iron metabolism characterized by excessive accumulation of iron in the liver and other tissues and by development of severe cirrhosis.

Hemodynamics: The study of the forces involved in the circulation of blood.

Hemoptysis: The expectoration of blood or of blood-streaked sputum from the larynx, trachea, bronchi, or lungs.

Hepatoma: A usually malignant tumor occurring in the liver.

Heterogeneous: A trait that can be produced by different genes or combinations of genes.

Hippocampus: A part of the limbic system that is important for consolidation of information from short-term to long-term memory, and in spatial memory.

Holter monitoring: Continuous monitoring of the electrical activity of a patient's heart muscle for 24 hours, using a special portable device called a Holter monitor. Patients wear the Holter monitor while carrying out their usual daily activities.

Homocysteine: A naturally occurring amino acid found in blood plasma. High levels of homocysteine in the blood are believed to increase the chance of heart disease, stroke, Alzheimer's disease, and osteoporosis.

Huntington's disease: A rare hereditary condition that causes progressive chorea (jerky muscle movements) and mental deterioration that ends in dementia.

Hyperaldosteronism: The body's overproduction of aldosterone, a hormone that controls sodium and potassium levels in the blood. Its overproduction leads to retention of salt and loss of potassium, which leads to high blood pressure.

Hyperglycemia: An abnormally high concentration of glucose in the circulating blood, seen especially in patients with diabetes mellitus.

Hyperhomocysteinemia: Elevated levels of homocysteine in the bloodstream. High levels of homocysteine are found in the blood of patients with homocystinuria.

Hyperinsulinism: Higher than normal levels of insulin in the blood; associated with reduced insulin sensitivity, hyperglycemia, excessive insulin secretion, and hypoglycemia.

Hyperpneic: Increase in depth of breathing, which may or may not be accompanied by an increase in the respiratory rate. Maximal hyperpnea occurs during strenuous exercise.

Hypertrophic cardiomyopathy: An ongoing disease process that damages the muscle wall of the lower chambers of the heart and thickens abnormally.

Hyperviscosity: Increased blood viscosity, which means "thickness."

Hypoglycemia: Low blood sugar; it occurs when blood glucose concentration falls below the level necessary to support the body's need for energy and stability throughout its cells.

Hypokinetic: Relating to or characterized by slow movement.

Iatrogenic: Pertaining to disease or disorder caused by doctors. The disorders may be unforeseeable and accidental, may be the result of unpredictable or unusual reactions, may be an inescapable consequence of necessary treatment, or may be due to medical incompetence or carelessness.

Immunoassay: Detection and assay of substances by serologic (immunologic) methods; in most applications, the substance in question serves as antigen, both in antibody production and in measurement of antibody by the test substance.

Immunoscintigraphy: The imaging of specific tissues by means of their binding to radioactively labeled monoclonal antibodies; used to detect metastatic cancer. The release of radiation from the antibodies is detected and quantified.

Incentives: Any stimuli that encourages a desired response. Incentives may be provided to patients, or to practitioners.

Incidence: The rate at which a certain event occurs, as the number of new cases of a specific disease occurring during a certain period in a population at risk.

Incidence rate: A measure of the frequency with which a disease or other incident occurs over a specified time period.

Indurative: Pertaining to causing an area of hardened tissue.

Insula: An oval region found in each hemisphere of the cerebral cortex, lateral to the lentiform nucleus and situated within the sylvian fissure, involved in sensation, emotion, and autonomic function.

Insulin resistance: A pathological condition in which the cells fail to normally respond to insulin; it is linked to poor diet.

Insulinoma: A tumor of the beta cells of the islets of Langerhans; it is usually benign and causes hypoglycemia.

Internal capsule: A white matter structure in the inferomedial part of each cerebral hemisphere that provides passage to ascending and descending fibers that run to and from the cerebral cortex.

Intestinal micelles: Tiny aggregates of fatty acids and monoglycerides formed by the detergent action of the bile acids on digested fats so that these materials can be made soluble and absorbed into the intestinal villi.

Iontophoresis: The introduction of ions of soluble salts into the body by an electric current.

Ipsilaterally: Located on or affecting the same side of the body.

Isodisomy: A trait caused by both copies of a chromosomal set being inherited from the biological mother or the father;

it may result in the expression of recessive traits in the offspring.

Kawasaki disease: An acute disease of young children characterized by a rash and swollen lymph nodes and fever with unknown cause.

Keratohyalin granules: Irregularly shaped basophilic granules in the cells of the stratum granulosum of the epidermis.

Ketone bodies: Water-soluble molecules (acetoacetate, beta-hydroxybutyrate, and their breakdown product, acetone) that contain the ketone group produced by the liver from fatty acids during fasting, starvation, carbohydrate restrictive diets, prolong intense exercise, alcoholism, or in poorly treated type 2 diabetes mellitus.

Kussmaul sign: Deep, labored breathing patterns often associated with severe metabolic acidosis – especially diabetic ketoacidosis, but also with kidney failure; the respirations are described as "gasping for air."

Lacunar infarction: A small stroke deep within the brain (as in the internal capsule, basal ganglia, thalamus, or pons) caused by damage to or a blockage of a tiny penetrating artery.

Laser photocoagulation: Surgical coagulation of tissue by means of intense light energy, such as a laser beam, performed to destroy abnormal tissues or to form adhesive scars, especially in ophthalmology.

Lenticulostriate arteries: Any of the anterolateral central arteries of the sphenoidal part of middle cerebral artery.

Leprosy: Leprosy is a slowly progressing bacterial infection that affects the skin, peripheral nerves in the hands and feet, and mucous membranes of the nose, throat, and eyes. Destruction of the nerve endings causes the affected areas to lose sensation.

Leptin: A hormone mostly made by adipose cells; it helps regulate energy balance by inhibiting hunger; it is opposed by the hormone ghrelin; in obesity, a decreased sensitivity to leptin occurs.

Lewy bodies: Abnormal aggregations of protein that develop inside nerve cells and contribute to Parkinson's disease and Lewy body dementia.

Ligamentous laxity: A chronic body pain characterized by loose ligaments.

Lipemia retinalis: A white appearance of the retina that can occur from lipid deposition in lipoprotein lipase deficiency.

Lipodystrophy: A group of genetic or acquired disorders in which the body is unable to produce and maintain healthy fat tissue.

Lipoproteins: Substances made of protein and fat that carry cholesterol through your bloodstream. There are two main types of cholesterol: high-density lipoprotein and low-density lipoprotein.

Locus ceruleus: A nucleus in the pons that is involved in physiological responses to stress and panic, and is part of the reticular activating system.

Löffler syndrome: A disease in which eosinophils accumulate in the lung in response to a parasitic infection. The symptoms include irritable bowel syndrome, abdominal pain, cramping, skin rashes, and fatigue.

Lyme disease: An inflammatory disease caused by a spirochete (*Borrelia burgdorferi*) that is transmitted by ticks and usually characterized by an initial rash followed by flulike symptoms including fever, joint pain, and headache. If left untreated, the disease can result in chronic arthritis, and nerve and heart dysfunction.

Macrosomia: "Long body"; when an infant's body is longer than normal while the weight may be varied; sometimes confused with "large for gestational age," which describes infant birth weight greater than the 97th percentile of most infants.

Macular edema: An eye disease caused by a swelling of the macula resulting from leakage and accumulation of fluid.

Mallory hyaline bodies: An inclusion body found in liver cells, especially in diseases caused by the excessive consumption of alcohol. Mallory bodies are composed of collections of intermediate filaments.

Maltese cross pattern: A term of art referring to a light microscopic appearance of a crystal or crystalloid structure which is likened to a Maltese cross, which may correspond to granules of talc or cholesterol or bacteria.

Marantic endocarditis: Nonbacterial thrombotic endocarditis associated with cancer and other debilitating diseases.

Membranous nephropathy: A glomerular disease of unknown cause that produces nephrotic syndrome. It may be distinguished from lipoid nephrosis by immunofluorescence and electron microscopy.

Mesangial cell: A specialized cell, or cells, in the kidney making up the mesangium of the glomerulus; they help form the vascular pole of the renal corpuscle and account for 30%–40% of the total cells of the glomerulus.

Metrorrhagia: Any irregular, acyclic bleeding from the uterus between periods.

Minimal change disease: The form of nephrotic syndrome most often found in children, in which renal biopsies reveal little if any pathological change under the light microscope.

Mitral regurgitation: Backflow of blood from the left ventricle into the left atrium, owing to insufficiency of the mitral valve and usually due to mitral valve prolapse, or rheumatic heart disease.

Mood swings: Periods of variation in how one feels, changing from a sense of well-being to one of depression. This occurs normally, but may become abnormally intense in persons with manic-depressive states.

Muehrcke lines: Parallel white lines in the fingernails and toenails associated with hypoalbuminemia.

Müller cells: Supporting cells that extend through the retina to form its inner and outer limiting membranes.

Mycosis: Any disease caused by a fungus (filamentous or yeast).

Natriuretic peptides: Peptides present in the blood and found in elevated levels in people with chronic heart failure. They arise in the upper chambers of the heart, probably as a result of stretching, and cause blood vessels to widen, and the output of urine to increase.

Neonatal diabetes: A disease that affects infants and their ability to produce or use insulin; it is a monogenic form that occurs in the first 6 months of life, and only occurs rarely; its two forms are permanent and transient.

Nephrotic syndrome: A collection of symptoms that occur because the glomeruli in the kidney become leaky. This allows protein to leave the body in large quantities.

Neurofibromatosis: A group of three conditions in which tumors grow in the nervous system: NF1, NF2, and schwannomatosis.

Neuroglycopenia: Hypoglycemia of sufficient duration and degree to interfere with normal brain metabolism. Patients with an insulinoma or hypoglycemia due to an insulin overdose may have this condition, which produces confusion, agitation, coma, or brain damage.

Neurotrophins: Growth factors of the nervous system, such as brain-derived neurotrophic factor, nerve growth factor, and glia-derived neurotrophic factor.

Nocturnal angina: A type of unstable angina that occurs while resting at night.

Omental: Referring to an omentum, which is a layer of peritoneum that surrounds abdominal organs.

Optical coherence tomography: A radiographical method used to obtain high-resolution cross-sectional image of the structures of the eye.

Orthopnea: Difficulty in breathing that occurs while the patient is lying down.

Osteophyte: A bony outgrowth occurring usually adjacent to an area of articular cartilage damage in a joint affected by osteoarthritis. Osteophytes are also common around the intervertebral discs of the spine.

Oxidated: A state in which oxidation has occurred; a loss of electrons, or an increase in the oxidation state by a molecule, atom, or ion.

Oximetry: Measurement of oxygen saturation of the blood using an oximeter.

Paranoia: An unfounded or exaggerated distrust of others, sometimes reaching delusional proportions.

Parenchyma: The essential or functional elements of an organ, as distinguished from its framework, which is called the stroma.

Paresthesia: An abnormal dermal sensation with no apparent physical causes; it is most common in the extremities and often related to metabolic disorders such as diabetes mellitus.

Parotid glands: The largest of the three main pairs of salivary glands, located on either side of the face, just below and in front of the ears.

Paroxysmal nocturnal dyspnea: Sudden attacks of dyspnea that usually occur when patients are asleep in bed. The affected patient awakens gasping for air and tries to sit up to relieve the symptom.

Penumbras: The regions of partial illumination or radiation caused by light or X-rays not originating from a point source.

Pericytes: Elongated, contractile cells wrapped around precapillary arterioles outside the basement membrane.

Period prevalence: The number of people with a specific disease at one point in time, divided by the total number of people in the population.

Periodontium: A band of fibrous tissue connecting bones or cartilages, serving to support and strengthen joints.

Pheochromocytoma: A tumor of the chromaffin cells, most often found in the medulla of the adrenal gland.

Plasmin: The active principle of the fibrinolytic or clot-lysing system, a proteolytic enzyme with a high specificity for fibrin and the ability to dissolve formed fibrin clots.

Point prevalence: The measure of the proportion of people within a population who have a disease or condition at a certain time or date.

Polycystic ovary syndrome: A condition in which a female has little or no menstruation, is infertile, has excessive body hair, and is obese; the ovaries may contain several cysts.

Polycythemia: An increase in the total red blood cell mass of the blood.

Polyol pathway: The polyol pathway is a two-step process that converts glucose to fructose. In this pathway, glucose is reduced to sorbitol, which is subsequently oxidized to fructose.

Polypol: An organic compound containing multiple hydroxyl groups.

Polysomnography: A type of sleep study that is used in the study of sleep and as a diagnostic tool in sleep medicine.

Porphyria: A group of liver disorders in which substances called porphyrins build up in the body, negatively affecting the skin or nervous system.

Pott's disease: A disease of the spine, usually caused by tubercular infection and characterized by weakening and gradual disintegration of the vertebrae and the intervertebral discs.

Pragmatics: The study of how language context contributes to meaning, involving speech act theory, conversational implications, and interactive talk.

Preeclampsia: A disorder of pregnancy characterized by high blood pressure, and often, a significant amount of protein in the urine; it begins after 20 weeks of pregnancy and influences the risk of poor outcomes for both mother and baby; risk factors include obesity, prior hypertension, older age, and diabetes mellitus.

Preload: Maximum stretch of the heart at the end of diastole.

Prevalence: In epidemiology, the proportion of a particular population found to be affected by a medical condition; usually expressed as a fraction, percentage, or as the number of cases per 10,000 or 100,000 people.

Proprioception: The sense of the relative position of the parts of one's own body and strength of effort being employed in movement.

Proteobacteria: A major phylum of Gram-negative bacteria. They include a wide variety of pathogenic genera, such as *Escherichia*, *Salmonella*, *Vibrio*, *Helicobacter*, and *Yersinia*.

Pylorospasm: A disturbance of the motor function of the stomach accompanied by spasmodic intensification of the tonus of its sphincter.

Radiculopathy: A set of conditions in which one or more nerves are affected and do not work properly.

Resistant hypertension: Hypertension that does not normalize with the use of a diuretic medication plus optimal doses of two additional antihypertensive drugs.

Resistin: Cytokine secreted by adipocytes into the circulation; causes resistance of peripheral tissues to insulin; possible link between obesity and type 2 diabetes mellitus.

Restrictive cardiomyopathy: A form of cardiomyopathy in which the walls of the heart become rigid.

Rhabdomyolysis: A condition in which damaged skeletal muscle breaks down rapidly; it may damage the kidneys and lead to kidney failure.

Saccades: Rapid intermittent eye movements made as the attention switches from one point to another.

Saccular aneurysm: A sac formed by the localized dilatation of the wall of an artery, a vein, or the heart.

Sarcoidosis: A disease that can affect many organs within the body. It causes the development of granulomas. They are made up of clumps of cells from the immune system.

Sciatica: Pain or discomfort associated with the sciatic nerve. This nerve runs from the lower part of the spinal cord, down to the back of the leg.

Shingles: Also called herpes zoster or zona. Any person who has had chickenpox can develop shingles. This condition erupts along the course of the affected nerve, producing lesions anywhere on the body and may cause severe nerve pain.

Silhouette: A drawing consisting of the outline of something, especially a human profile, filled in with a solid color.

Sjögren's syndrome: A chronic autoimmune disease of the lacrimal and salivary glands, and often of the lungs, kidneys, and nervous system.

Stable angina: Chest pain of cardiac origin that has not changed in character, frequency, intensity, or duration for 60 days.

Steatohepatitis: Liver disease characterized by fatty change of hepatocytes, accompanied by intralobular inflammation and fibrosis. Most often caused by alcohol abuse, diabetes, or obesity.

Steatorrhea: Excess fat in the feces due to a malabsorption syndrome caused by disease of the intestinal mucosa (e.g., sprue) or pancreatic enzyme deficiency.

Sterol: Any of a group of predominantly unsaturated solid alcohols of the steroid group, such as cholesterol and ergosterol, found in animals, plants, and fungi, especially as components of cell membranes.

Stroke volume: The volume of blood pumped from the left ventricle per beat.

Stromal cells: Differentiating cells found in abundance within bone marrow, but can also be seen all around the body. Stromal cells can become connective tissue cells of any organ.

Subclavian steal syndrome: A constellation of signs and symptoms that arise from reversed blood flow in the vertebral artery or the internal thoracic artery, due to a proximal stenosis or occlusion of the subclavian artery.

Summation gallop: An extra "galloping" heart sound caused by tachycardia, best heard over the apex of the heart.

Supernatant: The liquid lying above a layer of precipitated insoluble material.

Susceptibility gene: A gene that increases a person's likelihood of contracting a heritable illness.

Syndrome X: A group of metabolic risk factors linked to insulin resistance and associated with increased risk of cardiovascular disease. It consists of increased waist circumference, elevated triglycerides, low HDL cholesterol, hypertension, and impaired fasting glucose.

Syringomyelia: The presence of longitudinal cavities lined by dense, gliogenous tissue in the spinal cord, which is not caused by vascular insufficiency. Syringomyelia is marked clinically by pain and paresthesia, followed by muscular atrophy of the hands and analgesia with thermoanesthesia of the hands and arms.

Systemic lupus erythematosus: A disease where a person's immune system attacks and injures the body's own organs and tissues. Almost every system of the body can be affected by SLE.

Tabes dorsalis: A slowly progressive nervous disorder, from degeneration of the dorsal columns of the spinal cord and sensory nerve trunks, resulting in disturbances of sensation and interference with reflexes and consequently with movements.

Tangier disease: High-density lipoprotein deficiency; an inheritable disorder of lipid metabolism characterized by almost complete absence from plasma of high-density lipoproteins and by storage of cholesterol esters in the tonsil.

Thenar atrophy: Decrease in size of the fleshy part of the hand at the base of the thumb.

Thrombolysis in situ: Dissolution of a thrombus in the original position and not having been moved.

Thrush: Infection of the oral mucous membrane by the fungus called *Candida albicans.*

Thyrotoxicosis: A condition resulting from excessive concentrations of thyroid hormones in the body, as in hyperthyroidism.

Tissue plasminogen activator: A protein involved in the breakdown of blood clots.

Toxic megacolon: An acute form of colonic distension. It is characterized by a very dilated colon, accompanied by abdominal distension, and sometimes fever, abdominal pain, or shock.

Toxoplasmosis: An infectious disease caused by the one-celled protozoan parasite *Toxoplasma gondii.* Although most individuals do not experience any symptoms, the disease can be very serious, and even fatal, in individuals with weakened immune systems.

Transitional cell carcinoma: Bladder cancer in which the cells lining the urinary bladder lose the ability to regulate their growth and start dividing uncontrollably.

Transudation: Passage of a body fluid through a membrane or tissue surface.

Troponin: A complex of muscle proteins which, when combined with Ca^{++}, influence tropomyosin to initiate contraction.

Tuberous xanthomas: A nodular, papule, or plaque in the skin due to lipid deposits; it is usually yellow, but may be brown, reddish, or cream colored.

Ulnar claw: A sharp, curved, horny structure at the end of ulna bone.

Unilateral foot drop: Affecting only one side, loss of the ability to bend the ankle so that the foot rises. This may be due to disorders of the lower spinal cord or of the nerves to the muscles that flex the ankle.

Unstable angina: Chest pain of cardiac origin that is variable, usually increasing in frequency and intensity and with irregular timing.

Vagus nerve (X): The cranial nerves that interface with parasympathetic control of the heart, lungs, and digestive tract; they are implicated in heart rate, gastrointestinal peristalsis, sweating, mouth muscle movements, speech, the gag reflex, vomiting, satiety, bladder control, and glucose production.

Valsalva maneuver: Inappropriate cardiac slowing and arteriolar dilatation, which reflect autonomic neural changes.

Variant angina: The attacks occur during rest, exercise capacity is well preserved, and attacks are associated electrocardiographically with elevation of the ST segment. It is cyclic in nature and is believed to be caused by coronary artery spasm.

Vasa nervorum: The blood vessels supplying nerves.

Visuospatial deficits: A lack or deficiency of denoting the ability to comprehend and conceptualize visual representations and spatial relationships in learning and performing a task.

Vitrectomy: The surgical removal of the vitreous (transparent gel that fills the eye from the iris to the retina).

Warburg effect: The reliance of most cancer cells on glycolysis rather than oxidation to meet their metabolic needs.

Werner's syndrome: Premature aging in the adult, transmitted as an autosomal recessive trait, and characterized principally by scleroderma like skin changes, involving especially the extremities, cataracts, subcutaneous calcification, muscular atrophy, a tendency to diabetes mellitus, aged appearance of the face, white hair and/or baldness, and a high incidence of neoplasms.

Wernicke-Korsakoff syndrome: The combined presence of Wernicke encephalopathy and alcoholic Korsakoff syndrome.

White coat syndrome: A transient increase in blood pressure that occurs in apprehensive patients on seeing a "white coat," especially if the patient is female and the doctor male. This may result in mislabeling the patient as having hypertension.

Wilson's disease: A genetic disorder in which excess copper builds up in the body, causing vomiting, weakness, ascites, leg swelling, yellow skin, itching, tremors, muscle stiffness, speech difficulties, personality changes, anxiety, and psychosis.

Wolff-Parkinson-White syndrome: A disorder due to a problem with the heart's electrical system; symptoms may include tachycardia, palpitations, shortness of breath, lightheadedness, syncope, and, in rare cases, cardiac arrest.

Xanthelasma: Soft, yellow-orange plaques on the eyelids or medial canthus, the most common form of xanthoma; may be associated with low-density lipoproteins, especially in younger adults.

Xanthochromia: Yellowish discoloration of the skin or spinal fluid.

Xanthoma: A papule, nodule, or plaque in the skin due to lipid deposits; it is usually yellow, but may be brown, reddish, or cream colored.

Xerostomia: Dryness of the mouth from salivary gland dysfunction.

Zygomycosis: A fungal infection associated with genera of the class Zygomycetes.

Index

Note: **Bold** page numbers refer to tables and *italic* page numbers refer to figures.